Study Guide to Accompany

Introductory Clinical Pharmacology

EIGHTH EDITION

SALLY S. ROACH, MSN, RN, AHN-BC
Associate Professor
University of Texas at Brownsville and Texas Southmost College
Brownsville, Texas

SUSAN M. FORD, MN, RN, OCN
Associate Dean for Nursing
Tacoma Community College
Tacoma, Washington

 Wolters Kluwer | Lippincott Williams & Wilkins
Health

Philadelphia · Baltimore · New York · London
Buenos Aires · Hong Kong · Sydney · Tokyo

Ancillary Editor: Audrey Lickwar
Production Editor: Mary Kinsella
Director of Nursing Production: Helen Ewan
Managing Editor / Production: Erika Kors
Design Coordinator: Holly Reid McLaughlin
Senior Manufacturing Manager: William Alberti
Manufacturing Coordinator: Karin Duffield
Compositor: Aptara
Printer: R. R. Donnelley, Willard

9 8 7 6 5 4 3

ISBN13: 978-0-7817-8184-8
ISBN: 0-7817-8184-1

Contents

Preface

This study guide has been designed to help you get the most benefit from the eighth edition of *Introductory Clinical Pharmacology*. Completely updated, this study guide provides current and comprehensive coverage of the newest pharmacological aspects along with basic nursing skills needed in administering medications and caring for patients.

As you read your textbook, this guide will be an important tool in helping you discover whether your reading and study habits are allowing you to identify the most important ideas in each chapter. To help you accomplish this goal, the following types of exercises are provided in this study guide:

ASSESSING YOUR UNDERSTANDING

This section includes fill-in-the-blank questions as well as matching exercises. The types of questions included will follow the same format in most study guide chapters.

- **Matching Exercises**
  Matching exercises help you to distinguish among several key terms, drugs, or adverse reactions.
- **Fill-in-the-Blanks**
  These questions correlate very closely with the textbook and focus on important information in each chapter.

APPLYING YOUR KNOWLEDGE

These questions challenge you to reflect on the critical thinking and blended skills developed in the classroom and apply them to your own practice.

- **Dosage Calculations**
  These problems give you practice in solving common medication dosage problems related to the specific medications in each chapter. Doing these calculations reinforces your ability to solve dosage problems and allows you to gain practice as well as confidence in preparation for the clinical setting.
- **Short Answer Questions**
  Requiring more critical thinking than the exercises in the Assessing Your Understanding section, these short answer questions offer an exciting and practical means to challenge you and "stretch" your application of the concepts.

PRACTICING FOR NCLEX

Each chapter contains a section of multiple choice questions presented in NCLEX exam format.

Enjoy your studies, and know that this study guide is a tool that will help you better understand the sometimes complicated world of pharmacology.

CHAPTER 1

General Principles of Pharmacology

SECTION I: ASSESSING YOUR UNDERSTANDING

Activity A MATCHING

1. Match the drug reaction in Column A with its action in Column B.

Column A	Column B
____ 1. Additive	**A.** One drug interferes with the action of the other, causing neutralization or decrease in effect
____ 2. Synergistic	**B.** Combined effect of two drugs equal to sum of each drug given alone
____ 3. Antagonistic	**C.** Drugs interact with each other and produce an effect greater than the sum of their separate actions

2. Match each term in Column A with its process in Column B.

Column A	Column B
____ 1. Absorption	**A.** Changes a drug to a more or less active form
____ 2. Distribution	**B.** Eliminates drugs from the body
____ 3. Metabolism	**C.** Moves drug particles within the gastrointestinal tract
____ 4. Excretion	**D.** Dispenses drugs to body tissues or target sites

Activity B FILL IN THE BLANKS

1. When a drug is given orally, food may impair or enhance its _____.

2. _____ administration of a drug produces the most rapid drug action.

3. A/An _____ drug reaction occurs when one drug interferes with the action of another.

4. Drug _____ occurs when drugs interact with each other and produce an effect that is greater than the sum of their separate actions.

5. A/An _____ disorder is a genetically determined abnormal response to normal doses of a drug.

SECTION II: APPLYING YOUR KNOWLEDGE

Activity C SHORT ANSWERS

The role of a nurse is to educate patients about a prescribed drug, its adverse reactions, signs and symptoms of those adverse reactions, and any related implications. Answer the following questions that involve the nurse's role managing such situations.

1. A nurse is educating a patient about how drugs act on the body by altering the cellular environment. What are the changes that occur because of alteration of cellular environment?

_____

_____

_____

2. Which organization is responsible for approving new drugs? How long does the process of drug development take?

_____

_____

_____

Activity D

1. A patient with digestion problems visits the health care center to obtain information about certain herbs and dietary supplements. The patient is already taking prescription drugs for indigestion.

   a. What are some of the adverse reactions that the nurse will have to convey to the patient concerning consumption of botanicals?

   _____

   _____

   _____

   b. How can a nurse ensure that the patient does not misuse herbs and natural supplements?

   _____

   _____

   _____

2. List the processes that take place before the U.S. Food and Drug Administration (FDA) phase of drug development?

   _____

   _____

   _____

3. A teaching plan for a pregnant patient includes information about harmful effects to a fetus caused by smoking and alcohol

consumption. What should the nurse tell the patient?

_____

_____

_____

SECTION III: PRACTICING FOR NCLEX

Activity E

Answer the following questions.

1. At times it is confusing for the nurse to recognize a drug by its name because there are different categories of drug names. To which of the following categories of drug names should the nurse refer to avoid confusion?
   a. Official name
   b. Scientific name
   c. Trade name
   d. Generic name

2. What is the purpose of the *Controlled Substances Act* of 1970? Select all that apply.
   a. Report adverse effects of drugs
   b. Regulate manufacture of drugs
   c. Organize distribution of drugs
   d. Control dispensing of drugs
   e. Encourage drug development

3. A patient wants to know what happens physiologically to the liquid medications that he has been taking for an illness. How should the nurse explain the process to the patient?
   a. Disintegrates in the gastrointestinal tract
   b. Is quickly absorbed by the body system
   c. Disintegrates in the small intestine
   d. Disintegrates into small pieces

4. A patient is admitted to a local health care center with severe dehydration. Which route of drug administration would the nurse apply to counter the dehydration quickly?
   a. Oral
   b. Subcutaneous
   c. Intravenous
   d. Intramuscular

5. A nurse explains to a patient (who is not allergic to drugs) that drugs alter the functions of the body's cells. Which of the following symptoms will the nurse monitor for altered cellular function in the patient? Select all that apply.
   a. Blood pressure
   b. Impaired vision
   c. Urine output
   d. Slurred speech
   e. Heart rate

6. A cancer patient requests information from the nurse on the activity of drugs that are prescribed to him. Which of the following should the nurse use to describe the method of action of cancer drugs? Select all that apply.
   a. Acts on the cell membrane
   b. Causes change in the cells' pH levels
   c. Acts on cellular processes
   d. Creates chemical change in body fluids
   e. Causes cell starvation and death

7. A primary health care provider prescribes reduced doses of a drug and lengthened durations between doses for a patient with kidney disease. Which of the following are reasons for such a prescription? Select all that apply.
   a. Patient could exhibit drug toxicity
   b. Provides longer duration of drug action
   c. Patient could exhibit drug tolerance
   d. Prevents accumulation of the drug
   e. Prevents drug dependency

8. When assessing a patient for an illness, the nurse takes note of certain factors that influence drug response. Which of the following factors should the nurse note? Select all that apply.
   a. Patient's age
   b. Existing disease
   c. Patient's weight
   d. Patient's appetite
   e. Patient's height

9. A patient is to undergo frequent diagnostic tests during the course of treatment at a health care facility. In which of the following conditions should the nurse perform frequent diagnostic tests?
   a. Impaired vision
   b. Impaired speech
   c. Impaired liver function
   d. Impaired hearing

Administration of Drugs

SECTION I: ASSESSING YOUR UNDERSTANDING

Activity A MATCHING

1. Match the administration routes in Column A with their commonly used administration sites in Column B.

Column A

____ 1. Transdermal

____ 2. Intradermal

____ 3. Intramuscular

____ 4. Subcutaneous

Column B

A. Upper arm, hip, and thigh

B. Upper arms, upper abdomen, and upper back

C. Chest, flank, and upper arm

D. Inner part of forearm and upper back

2. Match the drugs in Column A with their usual administration routes in Column B.

Column A

____ 1. Lozenges

____ 2. Heparin

____ 3. Scopolamine

____ 4. Mucolytics

Column B

A. Inhalation

B. Transdermal

C. Buccal

D. Subcutaneous

Activity B FILL IN THE BLANKS

1. Electronic infusion devices are classified as either infusion _____ or infusion pumps.

2. The Z-track method of intramuscular injection is used when a drug is highly irritating to _____ tissues.

3. In the _____ dose system of dispensing medications, the pharmacist dispenses each dose in a package that is labeled with the drug name and dosage.

4. Nitroglycerin is commonly given by the _____ route.

5. The nurse should instruct the patient to place _____ drugs against mucous membranes of the cheek.

6. Escape of fluid from a blood vessel into surrounding tissues while the needle or catheter is in the vein is known as _____.

SECTION II: APPLYING YOUR KNOWLEDGE

Activity C SHORT ANSWERS

The administration of a drug is a fundamental responsibility of the nurse. An understanding of the basic concepts of administering drugs is critical if the nurse is to perform this task safely and accurately. Answer the following questions, which involve the nurse's role in the administration of drugs.

1. The physician has asked a nurse to administer a drug to a patient. How can the nurse iden-

tify the patient prior to administering the medication?

_____

_____

_____

2. After administering a drug to the patient, the nurse realizes that she has given an incorrect dosage of the drug. Why should the nurse report drug errors?

_____

_____

_____

Activity D CASE STUDY

1. A nurse is caring for a group of patients. The physician has asked him to administer different drugs to the different patients. The nurse becomes confused when he finds some drug names that sound similar and a few that are spelled similarly. How can the nurse ensure that he is administering the right drug to the right patient?

_____

_____

_____

2. After administering a drug to a patient, the nurse records the process immediately. Why is it important to document administration of drugs immediately?

_____

_____

_____

3. A nurse is required to administer a drug to a patient through the transdermal route. What are the nurse's responsibilities when administering a drug through this route?

_____

_____

_____

SECTION III: PRACTICING FOR NCLEX

Activity E

Answer the following questions.

1. A nurse administers a drug on an as-needed (PRN) basis. Which of the following interventions should the nurse perform immediately after administering the drug to the patient? Select all that apply.
   a. Record administration of the drug
   b. Evaluate patient's response to the drug
   c. Record the site used for parenteral administration
   d. Inform physician about the drugs administered

2. What nursing intervention should be performed to minimize risk of skin irritation when administering drugs by the transdermal route?
   a. Shave the area before applying the patch
   b. Always apply patches on the same site
   c. Moisten skin before applying patches
   d. Remove the old patch for the next dose

3. A nurse is caring for a patient with a superficial skin infection. What information should the nurse obtain from the primary health care provider before administering the prescribed topical drug to the patient?
   a. Cause of the skin infection
   b. Instructions for drug application
   c. Reasons for selecting the drug
   d. Composition of the drug

4. While assessing a patient, a nurse is required to perform the tuberculin test. The drug is to be administered by an intradermal injection. Which of the following sites is ideal for administering the intradermal injection to the patient?
   a. Thigh
   b. Hairy areas
   c. Inner forearm
   d. Upper arm

5. A nurse has been assigned to perform venipuncture for a patient. Three attempts to perform venipuncture have been unsuccessful. Which of the following steps should the nurse perform in this situation?

    a. Keep trying until venipuncture is successful

    b. Ask for assistance from a skilled nurse

    c. Inject the drug intramuscularly

    d. Shift the patient into a more conducive position

6. A nurse is required to administer 5 mL of a drug intramuscularly to an adult patient. Which of the following interventions should the nurse perform while administering the drug to the patient?

    a. Divide the drug and give it as two separate injections

    b. Use a needle with a ½-inch length for the injection

    c. Administer the drug at the upper back

    d. Insert the needle at an angle of 45°

7. The physician has asked a nurse to administer a subcutaneous injection to a patient. The nurse observes that the patient is very thin. Which of the following sites should the nurse select to administer the injection to this patient?

    a. Upper arm

    b. Lower back

    c. Upper abdomen

    d. Thigh muscle

8. A nurse is caring for a patient with a nasogastric feeding tube. The nurse is required to administer drug tablets to the patient. Which of the following interventions should the nurse perform during the administration of the drug? Select all that apply.

    a. Ensure that the tablets are completely dissolved

    b. Put the tablets in water without crushing them

    c. Flush the tube with water to clear the tubing

    d. Mix the drug after the tube is fixed

    e. Check the tube for placement

Review of Arithmetic and Calculation of Drug Dosages

SECTION I: ASSESSING YOUR UNDERSTANDING

Activity A MATCHING

1. Match the terms in Column A with the descriptions in Column B.

Column A

___ **1.** Proper fraction

___ **2.** Improper fraction

___ **3.** Mixed number

___ **4.** Lowest common denominator

Column B

A. A whole number and a proper fraction

B. Part of a whole or any number less than a whole number

C. The lowest number divisible by all the denominators

D. Fraction having a numerator the same as or larger than the denominator

2. Match the computations in Column A with the procedures in Column B.

Column A

___ **1.** To change a mixed number to an improper fraction

___ **2.** To add fractions with like denominators

___ **3.** To add mixed numbers or fractions with mixed numbers

___ **4.** To divide a whole number by a fraction

Column B

A. Add the numerators and place the sum of the numerators over the denominator

B. First change the mixed number to an improper fraction

C. Change the whole number to an improper fraction by placing the whole number over 1

D. Multiply the denominator of the fraction by the whole number, add the numerator, and place the sum over the denominator

Activity B FILL IN THE BLANKS

1. When fractions with like _____ are compared, the fraction with the largest numerator is the largest fraction.

2. To compare fractions with unlike denominators, the _____ common denominator must first be determined.

3. When _____ are multiplied, the numerators are multiplied, and the denominators are multiplied.

4. When whole numbers are multiplied with fractions, the _____ is multiplied by the whole number, and the product is placed over the denominator.

5. A fraction having a numerator the same as or _____ than the denominator is an improper fraction.

6. _____ numbers are changed to improper fractions and then multiplied.

7. To multiply a whole number and a mixed number, both numbers must be changed to _____ fractions.

8. Part of a whole or any number less than a whole number is a _____ fraction.

9. A/An ____ is a way of expressing a part of a whole or the relation of one number to another.

10. A proportion is a method of expressing _____ between two ratios.

CHAPTER 4

The Nursing Process

SECTION I: ASSESSING YOUR UNDERSTANDING

Activity A MATCHING

1. Match the phases of the nursing process in Column A with their functions in Column B.

Column A

_____ 1. Assessment

_____ 2. Nursing diagnosis (analysis)

_____ 3. Planning

_____ 4. Implementation

_____ 5. Evaluation

Column B

A. Describing steps for carrying out nursing activities or interventions that are specific and will meet the expected outcomes

B. Carrying out a plan of action

C. Collecting objective and subjective data

D. Determining the effectiveness of the nursing interventions in meeting the expected outcomes

E. Identifying problems that can be solved or prevented by independent nursing actions

2. Match the nursing diagnoses related to drug administration in Column A with their meanings in Column B.

Column A

_____ 1. Effective Therapeutic Regimen Management

_____ 2. Ineffective Therapeutic Regimen Management

_____ 3. Deficient Knowledge

_____ 4. Noncompliance

_____ 5. Anxiety

Column B

A. Patient may not take the medication correctly or follow the medication regimen prescribed by the health care provider

B. Behavior of the patient fails to coincide with the therapeutic plan agreed on by the patient and the health care provider

C. Patient lacks sufficient knowledge to administer the drug regimen correctly, lacks interest in learning, has a cognitive limitation, or has an inability to remember

D. Patient experiences reduced ability to focus on details

E. Patient is willing to regulate and integrate the treatment regimen into daily living

Activity B FILL IN THE BLANKS

1. _____ data are facts obtained by means of a physical assessment or examination.

2. An _____ assessment is one that is made at the time of each patient contact and may include the collection of objective data, subjective data, or both.

3. A nursing _____ is a description of the patient's problems and their probable or actual related causes based on the subjective and objective data in the database.

4. Planning anticipates the _____ phase or the carrying out of nursing actions that are specific for the drug being administered.

5. The nursing care must be planned on an _____ basis after a careful collection and analysis of the subjective and objective data.

SECTION II: APPLYING YOUR KNOWLEDGE

Activity C SHORT ANSWERS

A nurse's role in performing various nursing processes involves assisting patients in their treatment therapy. The nurse also helps patients to understand and effectively manage the therapeutic regime. Using the nursing process requires practice, experience, and a constant updating of knowledge. Answer the following questions related to the nursing process.

1. a. What is the nursing process?

   _____

   _____

   _____

   b. What are the five phases of the nursing process?

   _____

   _____

   _____

2. What are initial and ongoing assessments?

   _____

   _____

   _____

SECTION III: PRACTICING FOR NCLEX

Activity D

Answer the following questions.

1. A nurse is assigned to care for a patient with a respiratory problem. During assessment, what intervention should the nurse perform to obtain subjective data from the patient?

   a. Inquire about the number of cigarettes smoked per day

   b. Monitor the patient's pulse rate and rhythm

   c. Monitor the patient's blood pressure

   d. Assess the patient's body temperature

2. A nurse is caring for a patient of childbearing age. Which of the following is the most relevant assessment that the nurse should perform before administering a drug to this patient?

   a. Family history

   b. Relationship with spouse

   c. Pregnancy status

   d. Menstruation history

3. What should a nurse focus on when developing expected outcomes for a patient?

   a. The type of drug administered

   b. The patient's condition or illness

   c. Dosage pattern administered to the patient

   d. The patient's ability to recuperate

4. A nurse is assigned to care for a patient in a health care facility. Which of the following should the nurse include in her nursing diagnosis?

   a. Problems that can be solved by independent nursing actions

   b. Problems that have a treatment marking a definite cure

   c. Identification of the patient's condition and criticality

   d. Problems that cannot be prevented by nursing actions

5. A nurse is assigned to care for a patient who has just been admitted to a health care facility. What is the significance of planning for nursing actions specific to the drug to be administered? Select all that apply.

  a. It allows greater accuracy in drug administration

  b. It allows absolute prevention of relapse

  c. It allows patient understanding of the drug regimen

  d. It promotes an optimal response to therapy in minimal time

  e. It promotes patient compliance with prescribed drug therapy

6. A nurse is caring for a patient who has to continue with the drug regimen on an outpatient basis. Routine assessments of the patient reveal that the patient is not complying with the medication regimen. What intervention should the nurse perform to combat the patient's noncompliant attitude?

  a. Prepare a fixed schedule for the patient to take the drug

  b. Find out the reason for noncompliance if possible

  c. Teach the patient the importance of following a drug regimen

  d. Frequently monitor the patient's condition to identify a relapse

7. Prioritize the following nursing interventions of the nursing process, which are given in random order.

  a. Analyze the data collected during assessment

  b. Formulate one or more nursing diagnoses

  c. Collect the objective and subjective data

  d. Identify the patient's needs or problems

  e. Develop expected outcomes for the patient

CHAPTER 5

Patient and Family Teaching

SECTION I: ASSESSING YOUR UNDERSTANDING

Activity A MATCHING

1. Match the learning domains in Column A with the corresponding patient activities in Column B.

Column A	Column B
___ 1. Psychomotor	A. Making decisions and drawing conclusions
___ 2. Affective	B. Learning physical skills
___ 3. Cognitive	C. Attitudes, feelings, and beliefs

2. Match the nursing diagnoses in Column A with their corresponding characteristics in Column B.

Column A	Column B
___ 1. Effective Individual Therapeutic Regimen Management	A. Teaches patients with deficient cognitive knowledge and psychomotor skills
___ 2. Deficient Knowledge	B. Involves discharge teaching
___ 3. Ineffective Therapeutic Regimen Management	C. Teaches adverse drug reactions and effects as well as their management

Activity B FILL IN THE BLANKS

1. The psychomotor domain involves learning _____ skills or tasks.

2. The _____ domain includes the patient's and the caregiver's attitudes, feelings, beliefs, and opinions.

3. It is important not to _____ capsules before swallowing.

4. Exposing a drug to excessive _____, heat, cold, or moisture may cause the drug to deteriorate.

5. A daily calendar is an inexpensive, yet effective means for _____ drug administration.

SECTION II: APPLYING YOUR KNOWLEDGE

Activity C SHORT ANSWERS

A nurse's role in determining the effectiveness of patient teaching involves evaluating the patients' knowledge of materials presented. The nurse also helps the patients answer their queries and difficulties by conducting interactive sessions with them. Answer the following questions, which involve the nurse's role in evaluating the effectiveness of patient teaching.

1. A patient has been taught exercises for strengthening eye muscles. How should the nurse

ensure that the patient perfectly remembers all the exercises that were taught to him or her?

_____

_____

_____

2. A patient's relative has been instructed on how to measure the patient's temperature by using an electronic thermometer. How does the nurse ensure that the patient's relative has understood the procedure?

_____

_____

_____

Activity D

In using the nursing process as a framework for patient teaching, the nursing diagnosis stage comes immediately after the assessment stage. The systematic method of the nursing process differs from the teaching plan. The systematic method encompasses all the patient health care needs; whereas, the teaching plan focuses on the patient's learning needs and the learning domains. Answer the following questions, which involve the nurse's role in the preparation of a framework for patient teaching.

1. A patient admitted to a health care facility for malaria is to be trained in the administration of antimalarial drugs. The patient is deficient in cognitive knowledge and psychomotor skills.

   a. What nursing diagnosis should the nurse use for this patient?

   _____

   _____

   _____

2. An asthma patient in a local health care facility is due to be discharged. The patient is to be taught how to perform breathing exercises at home.

   a. What patient skills are involved in this case?

   _____

   _____

   _____

b. Which nursing diagnosis should be used to teach breathing exercises to the patient?

_____

_____

_____

3. An obese patient visits a local health care center for a weight-loss program. The weight-loss program recommends strict dietary control and regular physical exercise. However, the patient claims to be a dietitian herself and expects her opinions to be respected as well.

   a. What learning domain is accessed when the patient implements the weight-loss program?

   _____

   _____

   _____

SECTION III: PRACTICING FOR NCLEX

Activity E

Answer the following questions.

1. A patient admitted to a health care facility for diabetes receives insulin injections. The patient is improving and is expected to be discharged in a couple of days. The nurse assigned to the patient needs to teach him how to administer the postdischarge doses of insulin. The patient feels that administering insulin at home could be a bit too complicated for him. For which of the following reasons should the nurse adopt the nursing diagnosis Ineffective Therapeutic Regimen Management for this patient? Select all that apply.

   a. Is useful in discharge teaching
   b. Manages complicated medication regimen
   c. Helps patients in achieving positive results
   d. Informs the patient about drug reactions
   e. Teaches management of adverse effects of the drug

2. A patient is admitted to a local health care center for jaundice and is prescribed a number of drugs. The nurse in charge of the patient wants to teach him how to administer the prescribed drugs and has formulated a

teaching plan. When and how should the teaching plan be implemented? Select all that apply.

a. A day or two before the patient's discharge

b. When the patient is alone, alert, and not sedated

c. As soon as the patient is admitted

d. By dividing the material in sessions

e. By teaching everything all at once

3. A nurse caring for a patient with typhoid needs to formulate a teaching plan to instruct the patient on drug administration. Which of the following reasons are most important for a nurse to perform a patient assessment before formulating a teaching plan? Select all that apply.

a. To determine barriers in the learning process

b. To improve patient motivation

c. To improve patient participation

d. To choose the best teaching methods

e. To develop an effective teaching plan

4. A nurse is assigned to care for a patient with gangrene on his toes. The nurse needs to teach the patient how to bandage the wound at home. What learning domain should the nurse employ to teach the patient?

a. Cognitive

b. Psychomotor

c. Affective

d. Intellectual

5. A patient admitted to a local health care facility for chronic acidity and heartburn is administered certain drugs. The assigned nurse formulates a teaching plan listing all the interventions to be conducted for the patient. What should the nurse do during the implementation of the teaching plan?

a. Perform the interventions identified in teaching plan

b. Determine the effectiveness of patient teaching

c. Begin with expected outcomes

d. Use the patient's past experiences

6. A nurse preparing a teaching plan for a patient needs to identify the suitable learning domain. Which of the following are learning domains that patients, at any given time, might be using? Select all that apply.

a. Intellectual

b. Intuitive

c. Psychomotor

d. Cognitive

e. Affective

7. A patient admitted to a health care facility for bronchial asthma is prescribed drugs in the form of spray inhalers. The patient needs to be taught about the administration of the drugs. Which of the following would be the main obstacle in the learning process?

a. Patient has low grasping power

b. Patient is nervous about using inhalers

c. Patient has a different literacy level

d. Patient is not aware of the drug's action

8. A gastroenteritis patient is admitted to a health care facility. The nurse in charge prepares a teaching plan to help the patient follow a restricted diet at home. The patient is moody and irritable at times and wants his opinions to be respected. What learning domain should the nurse involve when teaching the patient?

a. Affective

b. Cognitive

c. Intellectual

d. Psychomotor

CHAPTER 6

Sulfonamides

SECTION I: ASSESSING YOUR UNDERSTANDING

Activity A MATCHING

1. Match the conditions caused by sulfonamides in Column A with their related symptoms in Column B.

Column A

_C_ 1. Stomatitis

_D_ 2. Adverse reaction of sulfasalazine

_A_ 3. Crystalluria

_B_ 4. Pruritus

Column B

A. Crystals in the urine

B. Itching

C. Inflammation of the mouth

D. Orange-yellow urine and skin

2. Match the conditions in Column A with their related symptoms in Column B.

Column A

_D_ 1. Thrombocytopenia

_A_ 2. Aplastic anemia

_B_ 3. Leukopenia

_C_ 4. Calculi

Column B

A. Decrease in red blood cells in the bone marrow

B. Decrease in number of white blood cells

C. Formation of stone in genitourinary tract

D. Decrease in platelet count

Activity B FILL IN THE BLANKS

1. Sulfonamides are contraindicated in patients with hypersensitivity to sulfonamides, during lactation, and in children less than ___2___ years old.

2. Sulfonamides are primarily _Bacteriostatic_ because of their ability to inhibit the activity of folic acid in bacterial cell metabolism.

3. To avoid the adverse effects of _Photosensetivity_ during sulfonamide therapy, patients should be cautioned to wear protective clothing or sunscreen when outside.

4. _Cranberry_ juice is a commonly used remedy for preventing and relieving symptoms of urinary tract infections (UTIs).

5. _Thrombocytopenia_ is manifested by easy bruising and unusual bleeding after moderate to slight trauma to the skin or mucous membranes.

SECTION II: APPLYING YOUR KNOWLEDGE

Activity C SHORT ANSWERS

A nurse's role in managing patients involves assisting the patients in answering any queries regarding the treatment that is being provided. The nurse also helps the patients by educating them about precautions to be taken. Answer the following questions, which involve the nurse's role in management of such situations.

1. A patient has been admitted to a health care facility and the primary health care provider has prescribed sulfonamide therapy. What are the activities that the nurse is required to perform as part of the preadministration assessment?

_____

_____

_____

2. A patient has been admitted to a health care facility and is on sulfonamide therapy. What should the nurse include in the teaching plan for the patient and his family?

_____

_____

_____

Activity D DOSAGE CALCULATION

1. The primary health care provider has prescribed oral sulfadiazine, 3 g per day, as a maintenance dose to be given in equal doses. The drug is available in the form of a 500-mg tablet. How many tablets will the nurse administer to the patient for each day? _____

2. A patient has been prescribed 2 g of Azulfidine per day in four equal doses. The drug is available in a 500-mg tablet. How many tablets will the nurse administer to the patient for each dosage? _____

3. The primary health care provider has prescribed 4 g of erythromycin/sulfisoxazole per day, to be given orally 4 times a day in equal dosages. After reconstitution, the concentration of the drug in the solution is 250 mg per 5 mL. How many milliliters of the solution should the nurse administer to the patient for each dosage? _____

4. The primary health care provider has prescribed 1500 mg sulfasalazine per day. The drug is available in 500-mg tablets. How many tablets should be administered to the patient in a day? _____

5. The primary health care provider has prescribed sulfamethoxazole/trimethoprim tablets, 2 g initially for a day. The drug is available in 400-mg tablets. How many tablets should the nurse administer to the patient in a day? _____

SECTION III: PRACTICING FOR NCLEX

Activity E

Answer the following questions.

1. A patient with second-degree burns is admitted to a health care facility. Which of the following interventions should the nurse perform to improve the patient's treatment?
   a. Clean the surface of the skin
   b. Apply a ½-inch layer of cream
   c. Apply the drug with naked hands
   d. Apply cream over debris on skin surface

2. A patient on sulfonamide therapy develops thrombocytopenia. Which of the following interventions should the nurse perform to alleviate the patient's condition?
   a. Prevent patient from being moved until therapy is over
   b. Instruct patient to avoid brushing teeth
   c. Palpate the patient's skin to assess for trauma
   d. Inspect the patient's skin daily

3. A nurse is educating a patient, who is being discharged, about the measures to combat the effects of photosensitivity. Which of the following precautions should the nurse instruct the patient to follow regarding the effects of photosensitivity while on sulfadiazine therapy?
   a. Stop using contact lenses during the treatment
   b. Apply sunscreen to exposed areas when outdoors
   c. Avoid lights while indoors
   d. Wear protective clothing while outdoors

4. A patient is admitted to a health care facility, and the primary health care provider has prescribed sulfonamide therapy. The patient has also been instructed to increase fluid intake by 2000 mL per day. Which of the following reasons should the nurse give to the patient for increasing fluid intake? Select all that apply.
   a. Removes microorganisms from urinary tract
   b. Allows for easy absorption of drug by gastrointestinal (GI) system
   c. Prevents formation of crystals in urine
   d. Allows for easy excretion by kidneys
   e. Prevents stone formation in genitourinary tract

5. Which of the following adverse reactions should the nurse assess for in a patient during or after the application of mafenide?

   a. Orange-yellow urine

   b. Crystals in urine

   c. Edema

   d. Burning sensation in skin

6. A patient has been admitted to a health care facility and the primary health care provider has prescribed sulfasalazine. The patient is using soft contact lenses. Which of the following information should the nurse provide to the patient about the use of contact lenses during the treatment?

   a. Burning sensation in eyes

   b. Headache and dizziness

   c. Permanent yellow stain in lenses

   d. Impaired vision

7. A patient has been diagnosed with ulcerative colitis and is being administered sulfasalazine. Which of the following interventions should the nurse perform while caring for the patient? Select all that apply.

   a. Check the number and appearance of stool samples

   b. Administer drug during meals or immediately afterwards

   c. Check appearance of urine and measure output

   d. Assess for a loss of appetite or anorexia

   e. Monitor patient for relief or intensification of the symptoms

8. Sulfonamide therapy has been prescribed for a 30-year-old patient with a urinary tract infection. Which of the following information should the nurse give to the patient about the use of cranberries during the treatment?

   a. Prevents bacteria from attaching to walls of the urinary tract

   b. Prevents crystals from forming in the urine

   c. Prevents effect of photosensitivity

   d. Prevents formation of clots

9. A patient with a urinary tract infection is admitted to a health care facility. The physician has prescribed sulfonamide therapy. Which of the following is an advantage of sulfonamide therapy?

   a. Is easily absorbed by the GI system

   b. Kills bacterial cells to fight infection

   c. Decreases the number of white blood cells

   d. Does not have life-threatening adverse reactions

10. A 40-year-old patient is on sulfonamide therapy. Which of the following symptoms should the nurse assess for in the patient to detect Stevens-Johnson syndrome?

    a. Inflammation of the mouth

    b. Lesions on mucous membranes

    c. Crystals in urine

    d. Diarrhea

Penicillins

SECTION I: ASSESSING YOUR UNDERSTANDING

Activity A MATCHING

1. Match the conditions caused by penicillins in Column A with their symptoms in Column B.

Column A

C **1.** Pseudomem-
      branous colitis

D **2.** Anaphylactic
      shock

A **3.** Candidiasis

B **4.** Fungal superin-
      fection (oral
      cavity)

Column B

A. Lesions of the
      mouth or tongue,
      vaginal discharge,
      and anal or vaginal
      itching

B. Inflamed oral
      mucous mem-
      branes, swollen and
      red tongue, swollen
      gums, and pain in
      the mouth and
      throat

C. Diarrhea or bloody
      diarrhea, rectal
      bleeding, fever, and
      abdominal cramp-
      ing

D. Severe hypoten-
      sion, loss of conscious-
      ness, and acute res-
      piratory distress

2. Match the groups of penicillins in Column A with their features in Column B.

Column A

C **1.** Natural peni-
      cillins

D **2.** Penicillinase-
      resistant peni-
      cillins

B **3.** Aminopeni-
      cillins

A **4.** Extended-spec-
      trum peni-
      cillins

Column B

A. Penicillin effective
      against a wide
      range of bacteria,
      including
      pseudomonads

B. Combinations of
      penicillins with
      beta-lactamase
      inhibitors

C. First large-scale
      antibiotics used to
      combat infection

D. Antibiotic devel-
      oped to combat
      pencillinase

Activity B FILL IN THE BLANKS

1. A patient may develop phlebitis, an administration route reaction, when penicillin is
administered via the _IV_ route.

2. _Extended_ -spectrum penicillins are a
group of penicillins used to destroy bacteria
such as pseudomonads.

3. Adverse reactions associated with penicillin
include _hematopoietic_ changes, such as anemia,
leukopenia, and thrombocytopenia.

4. Treatment of minor hypersensitivity reactions
caused by penicillins may include administration of _antihistamine_ such as diphenhydramine (Benadryl) for a rash or itching.

5. An example of bacterial resistance is the ability of certain bacteria to produce _penicillinase_, an enzyme that inactivates penicillin.

SECTION II: APPLYING YOUR KNOWLEDGE

Activity C   SHORT ANSWERS

A nurse's role in managing patients who are being administered penicillin involves monitoring them and implementing interventions that aid in their recovery. Answer the following questions, which involve the nurse's role in management of such situations.

1. A patient with pneumonia has been prescribed penicillin. What should a nurse assess for in the patient before administering the first dose of penicillin?

   _____

   _____

   _____

2. A patient receiving penicillin is showing signs of impaired oral mucous membranes. What are the appropriate interventions a nurse should take to ensure the patient's well-being?

   _____

   _____

   _____

Activity D   DOSAGE CALCULATION

1. A doctor prescribes 375 mg of ampicillin for a patient. The available solution contains 125 mg/5cc. How many cc of the available solution will the nurse administer? _____

2. 1.5 million units of penicillin G (aqueous) have been prescribed for a patient. The available solution contains 500,000 units per cc. How many cc of the available solution is needed to meet the prescribed drug level?

   _____

3. A patient has been prescribed 500 mg of oxacillin sodium intramuscularly. After reconstitution, the vial contains 250 mg of active drug per 1.5 mL solution. How much of the reconstituted solution will be administered to the patient? _____

4. A doctor prescribes 500 mg of Nafcillin every 4 hours for a patient. After reconstitution, the concentration of the drug is 250 mg/mL. How many milliliters of the reconstituted solution should be administered to the patient?

   _____

5. A patient has been prescribed 1g of penicillin V. The available penicillin V tablet is 500 mg. How many tablets will the nurse administer to the patient? _____

6. A doctor prescribes 1.5 g of Unasyn (ampicillin/sulbactam) for a patient. After reconstitution, the concentration of Unasyn in the vial is 600 mg/mL. How many milliliters of the reconstituted solution will be administered to the patient? _____

SECTION III: PRACTICING FOR NCLEX

Activity E

Answer the following questions.

1. A patient has developed a rash after the administration of penicillin. The primary health care provider has diagnosed it as a mild hypersensitivity reaction. Which of the following interventions should the nurse perform to alleviate the patient's skin condition?

   a. Reduce the dosage to provide relief to the patient

   b. Instruct the patient to avoid taking baths

   c. Tell the patient to avoid clothing contact with the affected areas

   d. Administer frequent skin care to the patient

2. A 27-year-old married woman is prescribed penicillin intramuscularly for an infection. Which of the following points should a nurse inform this patient when educating her about penicillin therapy?

   a. Take the drug at the prescribed times of the day

   b. Discontinue dosage as soon as symptoms of the condition disappear

   c. Stop taking birth control pills during the medical regimen

   d. Take the drug on an empty stomach, an hour before or 2 hours after meals

3. A nurse is caring for a patient who is receiving penicillin. Which of the following drug reactions is a cause for concern and should be reported immediately to the primary health care provider?

   a. Pain at injection site

   b. Redness or soreness at previous penicillin injection site

   c. Mild nausea

   d. Decrease in body temperature

4. Given below, in random order, are important interventions when caring for a patient receiving antibiotics for an infection. Arrange the interventions in the order they would occur in most situations.

   3 1. Identify the appropriate penicillin

   2 2. Order a culture and sensitivity test

   5 3. Record improvement on patient's chart

   4 4. Administer penicillin to patient

   1 5. Obtain general history of patient

5. A nurse is caring for a patient who is receiving penicillin. Which of the following assessments will a nurse perform as part of the ongoing assessment process? Select all that apply.

   a. Obtain patient's general health history

   b. Save sample of stool for tests

   c. Evaluate patient daily for response to therapy

   d. Record improvement on patient's chart

   e. Perform additional culture and sensitivity tests

6. A patient who is receiving penicillin complains of diarrhea. Arrange the interventions a nurse will perform in the most likely sequence.

   4 1. If the stool tests positive for blood, save sample

   2 2. Notify primary health care provider if diarrhea confirmed

   1 3. Inspect all stools for signs of diarrhea

   3 4. Save a sample of the stool to test for occult blood

7. A nurse has just administered penicillin intramuscularly to a patient as prescribed. The nurse suspects that the patient is developing signs of anaphylactic shock. Which of the following reactions should a nurse monitor for in this patient? Select all that apply.

   a. Severe hypotension

   b. Nausea and vomiting

   c. Loss of consciousness

   d. Acute respiratory distress

   e. Pain at injection site

8. Which of the following interventions should a nurse perform in the event of impaired comfort or increased fever in a patient after he or she has been administered penicillin? Select all that apply.

   a. Discontinue administering the drug immediately

   b. Take vital signs every 4 hours or more

   c. Report any rise in temperature to the primary health care provider

   d. Change the patient's diet to a soft, nonirritating diet

   e. Administer antipyretic drug according to primary health provider's instructions

9. When caring for a patient who is receiving penicillin, a nurse is required to monitor for symptoms of a bacterial superinfection of the bowel. Which of the following symptoms should a nurse monitor for in the patient? Select all that apply.

   a. Diarrhea/bloody diarrhea

   b. Vomiting

   c. Abdominal cramping

   d. Lesions

   e. Rectal bleeding

10. Given below, in random order, are the steps for administering a crystalline drug intramuscularly. Arrange the steps in the correct order.

   4 1. Extract the penicillin from the vial

   1 2. Read manufacturer's directions on label

   5 3. Administer the drug to the patient

   3 4. Reconstitute the drug to a liquid form

   2 5. Obtain the appropriate diluent

CHAPTER 8

Cephalosporins

SECTION I: ASSESSING YOUR UNDERSTANDING

Activity A MATCHING

1. Match the cephalosporin group in Column A with its appropriate drug in Column B.

Column A	Column B
_D_ 1. First generation	A. Cefepime (Maxipime)
_C_ 2. Second generation	B. Cefoperazone (Cefobid)
_B_ 3. Third generation	C. Cefoxitin (Mefoxin)
_A_ 4. Fourth generation	D. Cefazolin (Ancef)

2. Match the nursing diagnoses in Column A with their appropriate causes in Column B.

Column A	Column B
_C_ 1. Risk for Impaired Skin Integrity	A. Related to ineffectiveness of cephalosporin to treat the infection
_A_ 2. Risk for Impaired Comfort	B. Related to superinfection
_D_ 3. Impaired Urinary Elimination	C. Related to hypersensitivity to cephalosporin therapy
_B_ 4. Diarrhea	D. Related to nephrotoxic effects on kidneys

Activity B FILL IN THE BLANKS

1. Administration route reactions to cephalosporins include pain, tenderness, and _inflammation_ at the injection site when given intramuscularly.

2. A _disulfiram_ -like reaction may occur if alcohol is consumed within 72 hours after certain cephalosporin administration.

3. The needle insertion site and the area above the site are inspected several times a day for signs of redness, which may indicate _Thrombophlebitis_

4. The nurse should not administer cephalosporins if the patient has a history of allergies to cephalosporins or _penicillins_

5. When cephalosporins are given intravenously (IV), the nurse inspects the needle insertion site for signs of _extravasation_ or infiltration.

SECTION II: APPLYING YOUR KNOWLEDGE

Activity C SHORT ANSWERS

A nurse's role in managing patients who have received cephalosporins involves monitoring them and implementing interventions that lead to their recovery. Answer the following questions, which involve the nurse's role in management of patients receiving cephalosporin therapy.

1. A patient diagnosed with a lung infection has been prescribed cephalosporins. What are the factors the nurse should consider before the first dose of the drug is administered?

   _____

   _____

   _____

2. An elderly patient has been prescribed cephalosporin.

   a. What nursing interventions are important when the patient is to be administered cephalosporin by IV?

      _____

      _____

      _____

   b. What nursing interventions are important when the patient is to be administered cephalosporin intramuscularly (IM)?

      _____

      _____

      _____

Activity D   DOSAGE CALCULATION

1. A middle-aged patient has been prescribed 500 mg of Cefzil every 24 hours. The available form of drug is 250-mg tablets. To meet the recommended dose, how many tablets should the nurse administer each time? _____

2. A patient undergoing treatment of infection has been prescribed 400 mg of loracarbef orally every 12 hours. For the first dosage, the nurse administers the patient four 100-mg capsules at 8 AM. For the next dosage, the drug is available only in 200-mg capsules. To meet the recommended dose, how many capsules should the nurse administer at the next dosage and at what time? _____

3. A patient has been prescribed 250 mg of cefuroxime drug orally b.i.d. every day. The available drug is in 250-mg tablets. To meet the recommended dose, how many tablets should the nurse administer and how many times a day? _____

4. A patient undergoing hemodialysis has been prescribed a single 400-mg dose of ceftibuten orally two times weekly. After reconstitution, the vial contains 90 mg/5mL of the drug. Approximately how many milliliters of the reconstituted solution should be administered to the patient for each dosage? _____

5. A patient has been prescribed 250 mg of Velosef every 12 hours for infections caused by susceptible microorganisms. The available drug is in a 500-mg capsule. How many capsules should the nurse administer to the patient each time? _____

6. A patient is being administered 300 mg of cefdinir orally q12h. However, the physician has prescribed a change in the dosage amount for each administration, in which the amount of drug the patient receives per day is the same but is administered with an interval of 24 hours between each administration. How many milligrams of the drug should the nurse administer after every 24 hours? _____

7. A patient has been prescribed 200 mg of cefditoren orally t.i.d. The available drug is in 100-mg tablets. To meet the recommended dose, the nurse will require how many tablets each day? _____

SECTION III: PRACTICING FOR NCLEX

Activity E

Answer the following questions.

1. A patient with renal impairment is currently being administered cephalosporins. What are the nursing interventions the nurse should perform when caring for this patient?

   a. Inspect each bowel movement

   b. Administer antipyretic drugs

   c. Record the fluid intake and output

   d. Monitor for excessive perspiration

2. The nurse has administered IV cephalosporin to a 32-year-old patient. What specific condition should the nurse monitor for when this drug is given intravenously?

   a. Phlebitis

   b. Angina

   c. Fever

   d. Tenderness

3. A patient has been administered oral anticoagulants while on cephalosporin therapy. What should the nurse identify as a maximized risk in this patient?

   a. Increased risk for bleeding
   b. Increased risk for nephrotoxicity
   c. Increased risk of hypertension
   d. Increase in the number of white blood cells (WBCs)

4. A physician has prescribed loracarbef to a 45-year-old patient. Which of the following instructions should the nurse give this patient?

   a. Avoid direct sunlight for 1 hour after taking the drug
   b. Take the drug with milk or fruit juice
   c. Minimize consumption of alcohol while on therapy
   d. Take the drug 1 hour before or 2 hours after meals

5. A 72-year-old patient with paralysis has been prescribed cephalosporin intramuscularly for an infection. Why should the nurse monitor this patient carefully?

   a. The patient may experience a stinging or burning sensation
   b. There is an increased risk for hypersensitivity reaction
   c. The large muscle may be atrophied
   d. There is an increased risk for thrombophlebitis

6. Which of the following are expected outcomes in a patient receiving cephalosporin? Choose all that apply.

   a. Complete recovery
   b. Optimal response to therapy
   c. Understanding the treatment
   d. Improved dietary patterns
   e. Compliance with treatment

7. The test reports of a patient on cephalosporin therapy show a deficient production of red blood cells (RBCs). Which of the following adverse effects has the patient developed?

   a. Nephrotoxicity
   b. Anorexia
   c. Aplastic anemia
   d. Toxic epidermal necrolysis

8. A patient on cephalosporin therapy has developed diarrhea. Which of the following is an ideal nursing intervention in this case? Select all that apply.

   a. Save samples of the stool
   b. Administer an antipyretic drug
   c. Discontinue the drug
   d. Immediately report to the physician
   e. Institute treatment for diarrhea

CHAPTER 9

Tetracyclines, Macrolides, and Lincosamides

SECTION I: ASSESSING YOUR UNDERSTANDING

Activity A MATCHING

1. Match the drugs in Column A with the effect of their interaction with macrolides in Column B.

Column A

C 1. Antacids

A 2. Digoxin

D 3. Anticoagulants

B 4. Lincomycin

Column B

A. Increased serum levels of digoxin

B. Decreased therapeutic activity of macrolides

C. Decreased absorption and effectiveness of macrolides

D. Increased risk of bleeding

2. Match the drugs in Column A with their adverse reactions in Column B.

Column A

B 1. Tetracyclines

C 2. Macrolides

A 3. Lincosamides

Column B

A. Blood dyscrasias

B. Epigastric distress

C. Abdominal pain or cramping

Activity B FILL IN THE BLANKS

1. **Macrolides** antibiotics are used for upper respiratory infections caused by *Haemophilus influenzae*.

2. Myasthenia gravis is a disease that affects the **Myoneural** junction in nerves and is manifested by extreme weakness and exhaustion of the muscles.

3. **Lincosamides** act by inhibiting protein synthesis in susceptible bacteria, causing cell death.

4. **Telithromycin** should not be ordered if a patient is taking cisapride or pimozide.

5. Food or drugs containing calcium, magnesium, aluminum, or iron prevent the absorption of the **tetracyclines** if ingested concurrently.

SECTION II: APPLYING YOUR KNOWLEDGE

Activity C SHORT ANSWERS

A nurse's role in managing patients involves assisting the patients in answering inquiries regarding the treatment being provided. The nurse also helps patients by educating them about the precautions to be taken. Answer the following questions, which involve the nurse's role in managing such situations.

1. A patient with upper respiratory infections caused by *Haemophilus influenzae* is prescribed azithromycin. What is the role of the nurse in monitoring and managing the patient's needs?

_____

_____

_____

2. A patient is to be discharged from a health care facility. His physician prescribed demeclocycline to take for 4 days. What should the nurse include in her teaching plan to educate the patient regarding the medication?

_____

_____

_____

Activity D DOSAGE CALCULATION

1. A physician has prescribed 600 mg of demeclocycline per day for an adult patient. The physician has suggested four separate doses of 150 mg. Only 300-mg tablets are available. How many doses should the nurse administer per day? _____

2. A physician prescribes doxycycline for a 7-year-old patient who weighs 75 lb. Two types of capsules are available. One capsule contains 50 mg of doxycycline. How many capsules should the nurse administer per day if the child should be given 2 mg/lb per day for severe infection? _____

3. A patient has been prescribed 500 mg of clarithromycin, twice a day. The tablets contain 250 mg of clarithromycin. How many tablets should the nurse administer to the patient each time? _____

4. The physician has prescribed 500 mg of erythromycin to be given every 12 hours for a patient. How many tablets should the nurse administer every 12 hours if they are available in tablets of 250 mg? _____

5. The physician has prescribed 2250 mg of clindamycin for a patient with severe infection. Each milliliter of Cleocin Phosphate Sterile Solution contains clindamycin phosphate equivalent to 150 mg of clindamycin. What amount of Cleocin Phosphate Sterile Solution should the nurse give to the patient?

_____

6. The physician has prescribed 600 mg of lincomycin for a patient, which is to be administered intramuscularly every 24 hours. Lincocin Sterile Solution is available, which contains 300 mg of lincomycin per milliliter. What amount of the Lincocin Sterile Solution should the nurse give to the patient? _____

SECTION III: PRACTICING FOR NCLEX

Activity E

Answer the following questions.

1. Which of the following categories of patients are contraindicated for lincosamides?
   a. Patients with viral infections
   b. Patients younger than 9 years old
   c. Patients who are lactating
   d. Patients with liver disease

2. A patient being treated with lincosamides is to undergo an operation under anesthesia. If a neuromuscular blocking drug is to be administered for anesthesia, what are the possible complications?
   a. Increased risk for bleeding
   b. Severe and profound respiratory depression
   c. Decreased absorption of the lincosamide
   d. Increased risk for digitalis toxicity

3. A nurse is assigned to take care of a patient with an infection. The nurse is required to identify and record signs and symptoms of the infection. The nurse should closely monitor the patient for which of the following symptoms? Select all that apply.
   a. General malaise
   b. Diabetes
   c. Blood dyscrasias
   d. Chills and fever
   e. Redness

4. A patient with high fever has been prescribed doxycycline. Which of the following tests should be performed before the first dose of drug is given? Select all that apply.
   a. Stress test
   b. Sensitivity test
   c. Glucose tolerance test
   d. Renal function test
   e. Urinalysis

5. A patient has been given a tetracycline drug. Which of the following should the nurse immediately report to the primary health care provider during the ongoing assessment of the patient? Select all that apply.
   a. Drop in blood pressure
   b. Regular urine output

(c) Increase in pulse rate

d. Normal blood sugar level

(e) Increase in temperature

6. A patient has been administered Ketak as part of a dental treatment. The nurse should inform the patient of which adverse effects?

a. Esophagitis

(b) Difficulty focusing

c. Photosensitivity

d. Development of skin rashes

7. A patient has been prescribed oral preparations of tetracycline. Which of the following must the nurse include in the patient education plan?

(a) Take the drug on an empty stomach

b. Take the drug just before a meal

c. Take the drug along with milk

d. Take the drug only at bedtime

8. A nurse is caring for a 12-year-old patient who has been prescribed dirithromycin. The patient's father inquires about the risks associated with the drug before it is administered. Which of these risks should the nurse include in her reply?

(a) Anorexia, constipation, dry mouth, or electrolyte imbalance

b. Visual disturbance, headache, or dizziness

c. Abdominal pain, esophagitis, skin rash, or blood dyscrasias

d. Photosensitivity reactions, hematologic changes, or discoloration of teeth

9. A patient is admitted to a health care facility for diarrhea. The patient's stool tested positive for blood and mucus. What immediate nursing intervention should follow this observation?

a. Save urine sample for tests

b. Measure and record vital signs

c. Check patient's blood pressure

(d) Save stool sample for occult blood test

10. A physician has prescribed lincomycin to a patient. How should the nurse administer this drug to the patient?

a. Administer the drug on empty stomach

(b) Administer the drug 1 to 2 hours before and after giving food

c. Administer the drug 4 hours after food (between meals)

d. Administer the drug with some fruit juice

CHAPTER 10

Fluoroquinolones and Aminoglycosides

SECTION I: ASSESSING YOUR UNDERSTANDING

Activity A MATCHING

1. Match the interacting drugs used with fluoroquinolones in Column A with their common uses in Column B.

Column A	Column B
C 1. Theophylline	A. Blood thinners
D 2. Cimetidine (Tagamet)	B. Relief of pain and inflammation
A 3. Oral anticoagulants	C. Management of respiratory problems
B 4. Nonsteroidal anti-inflammatory drugs (NSAIDs)	D. Management of gastrointestinal (GI) upset

2. Match each adverse reaction of aminoglycosides in Column A with its signs and symptoms in Column B.

Column A	Column B
B 1. Nephrotoxicity	A. Numbness, skin tingling, circumoral paresthesia
C 2. Ototoxicity	B. Proteinuria, hematuria, increase in blood urea nitrogen (BUN) level
A 3. Neurotoxicity	C. Tinnitus, dizziness, roaring in the ears

Activity B FILL IN THE BLANKS

1. **Enteric-coated** tablets have a special coating that prevents the drug from being absorbed in the stomach.

2. **Theophylline** is a fluoroquinolone that is used in the management of respiratory problems, such as asthma.

3. Fluoroquinolones exert their **bactericidal** effect by interfering with the synthesis of bacterial DNA.

4. Kanamycin, neomycin, and paromomycin are used orally in the management of **hepatic** coma.

5. **Respiratory** paralysis is a serious adverse effect caused by administration of aminoglycosides.

SECTION II: APPLYING YOUR KNOWLEDGE

Activity C SHORT ANSWERS

A nurse's role in managing patients who are using fluoroquinolones and aminoglycosides involves monitoring and managing interventions that aid in their recovery. Answer the following questions that involve the nurse's role in the management of such situations.

1. A patient with acute pain caused by tissue injury is prescribed intravenous fluoroquinolones. What interventions should the

nurse perform when caring for the patient taking fluoroquinolones?

_____

_____

_____

2. A nurse is assigned to care for a patient with a high fever. What interventions should the nurse perform when caring for this patient?

_____

_____

_____

Activity D DOSAGE CALCULATION

1. A patient has been diagnosed with infections caused by susceptible microorganisms. The physician has prescribed 500 mg of ciprofloxacin every 12 hours. The available drug is in the form of a 250-mg tablet. To meet the recommended dose, how many tablets should the nurse administer each time? _____

2. The physician has prescribed 200 mg of gati-floxacin every 24 hours. The available drug is in the form of a 50-mg tablet. To meet the recommended dose, how many tablets should the nurse administer each time? _____

3. The physician has prescribed 960 mg of gemi-floxacin mesylate. The available drug is in the form of a 320-mg tablet. To meet the recommended dose, how many tablets should the nurse administer each time? _____

4. The physician has prescribed 20 mg/mL of gentamicin. The available drug is in the form of 10 mg/mL. To meet the recommended dose, how many injections should the nurse administer each time? _____

5. The physician has prescribed a 400-mg total dose to a patient. The available drug is in the form of a 20-mg tablet. The drug regimen has to continue over a period of 10 days. How many tablets should the patient have each day? _____

6. The physician has prescribed 750 mg of amikacin to be administered through the intravenous (IV) route. The available drug is in the form of 1 g/4 mL. How much amikacin dosage should the nurse prepare to be administered IV? _____

SECTION III: PRACTICING FOR NCLEX

Activity E

Answer the following questions.

1. A nurse is required to care for a patient who is to receive fluoroquinolones. Under which of the following conditions should the nurse administer fluoroquinolones cautiously?
   a. Patients with a history of seizures
   b. Patients with renal failure
   c. Patients with neuromuscular disorders
   d. Patients who are elderly

2. A patient is being administered cephalosporins with aminoglycosides. The nurse should be aware that the interaction of cephalosporins with aminoglycosides can create this effect:
   a. Increased risk of ototoxicity
   b. Increased risk of nephrotoxicity
   c. Increased risk of neuromuscular blockage
   d. Increased serum theophylline levels

3. A nurse is caring for a patient who is taking aminoglycosides for a gram-negative bacter-ial infection. Which of the following inter-ventions should the nurse perform as part of the preadministration assessment for the patient?
   a. Obtain patient's blood count
   b. Monitor vital signs every 4 hours
   c. Record findings in patient's chart
   d. Ensure that urinalysis is conducted
   e. Ensure that hepatic function tests are con-ducted

4. A nurse is caring for a patient with a low res-piratory rate. The patient is administered flu-oroquinolones. The nurse is required to assess the client for which of the following adverse effects caused by administration of fluoroquinolones?
   a. Urticaria
   b. Anorexia
   c. Rash
   d. Dizziness

5. A nurse is assigned to care for a patient with hepatic coma who has been prescribed kanamycin. Which of the following

observations is the nurse most likely to make when monitoring the client's condition?

a. Lethargy

b. Abdominal pain

c. Numbness

d. Muscle twitching

6. A nurse is caring for a patient who is being administered aminoglycosides. When assessing the patient, the nurse understands that the patient has developed apnea. The nurse knows that the patient has developed a risk for which of the following conditions?

a. Neuromuscular blockade

b. Nephrotoxicity

c. Pseudomembranous colitis

d. Ototoxicity

7. A nurse is caring for a patient who is receiving fluoroquinolones through the intravenous route. Which of the following nursing interventions should the nurse perform to avoid the occurrence of phlebitis or thrombophlebitis?

a. Check the rate of infusion every 2 hours

b. Frequently inspect the vein used for infusion

c. Alternate the vein used for infusion

d. Share observations with physicians

e. Frequently perform assessments

8. A nurse is caring for a patient with a sexually transmitted disease who will be administered fluoroquinolones. Which of the following should the nurse confirm to establish that fluoroquinolone is not contraindicated in the patient?

a. Patient is not younger than 18 years of age

b. Patient does not have preexisting hearing loss

c. Patient does not have myasthenia gravis

d. Patient does not have parkinsonism

9. A nurse is caring for a patient who is receiving fluoroquinolones. Which of the following instructions should the nurse offer to help the patient protect herself against photosensitive reactions?

a. Wear brimmed hats

b. Wear cover-up clothing

c. Limit sun exposure to hazy days

d. Wear sunscreen

e. Wear light makeup

10. A nurse is caring for a patient with a severe fracture to his hand and wrist. The physician has prescribed Pavulon. The nurse knows that Pavulon is most commonly used for which of these reasons?

a. Management of edema

b. As an anti-infective agent

c. Anesthesia

d. Blood thinner

CHAPTER 11

Miscellaneous Anti-Infectives

SECTION I: ASSESSING YOUR UNDERSTANDING

Activity A MATCHING

1. Match the anti-infective drugs given in Column A with their uses in Column B.

Column A	Column B
A 1. Spectinomycin	A. Treats gonorrhea in patients who are allergic to penicillins, cephalosporins, or probenecid
C 2. Fosfomycin tromethamine	
D 3. Aztreonam	B. Treats vancomycin-resistant *Enterococcus faecium*
B 4. Quinupristin	C. Treats urinary tract infections
	D. Treats gram-negative microorganisms

2. Match the anti-infective drugs in Column A with their most adverse reactions in Column B.

Column A	Column B
D 1. Linezolid	A. Nephrotoxicity
C 2. Daptomycin	B. Urticaria
B 3. Spectinomycin	C. Vein irritation
A 4. Vancomycin	D. Pseudomembranous colitis and thrombocytopenia

Activity B FILL IN THE BLANKS

1. Linezolid is a ___oxazolidinone___ that acts by binding to a site on a specific ribosomal RNA.

2. Linezolid is contraindicated in patients with ___Phenylketonuria___

3. ___Ertapenem___ is used to treat serious infections and community-acquired pneumonia caused by bacteria.

4. ___Carbapenems___ are used cautiously in patients with central nervous system (CNS) disorders, seizure disorders, and renal or hepatic failure.

5. Nephrotoxicity and ototoxicity may be seen with the administration of ___Vancomycin___

SECTION II: APPLYING YOUR KNOWLEDGE

Activity C SHORT ANSWERS

A nurse's role in managing patients who are receiving anti-infective drugs involves monitoring the patients and implementing interventions that aid their recovery. Answer the following questions that involve the nurse's role in management of such situations.

1. A nurse has been caring for a client with gonorrhea. After treatment, the nurse has to evaluate the effectiveness of the treatment plan. What factors should the nurse consider

to determine the success of the treatment plan?

_____

_____

_____

2. A nurse has been caring for a patient with a bacterial infection. The nurse has to ensure that the patient complies with his medicine regimen on an outpatient basis. What instructions should the nurse provide to the patient and patient's family to decrease the chance of noncompliance by the patient?

_____

_____

_____

3. A nurse is assigned to care for a patient admitted in a health care facility because of a gram-negative bacterial infection. The nurse must assess the client and prepare the nursing diagnosis. What are the drug-specific diagnoses that the nurse should focus on for a patient taking miscellaneous anti-infectives?

_____

_____

_____

Activity D DOSAGE CALCULATION

1. A patient is prescribed 500 mg of aztreonam every 12 hours. The drug is available in 125-mg tablets. How many tablets should the nurse administer per day to meet the recommended dose? _____

2. A patient is prescribed 400 mg of vancomycin per day. The drug is available in 80-mg tablets. How many tablets should the nurse administer per day?_____

3. A patient with a bacterial infection is prescribed daptomycin to be administered intravenously (IV). The normal dosage for daptomycin is 4 mg/kg. The patient weighs 65 kg. The normal dose of daptomycin available is 500 mg/10mL. How much drug solution should the nurse prepare? _____

4. A patient with a rash on the hand is prescribed 500 mg of Trobicin every 12 hours. The drug is available in 100-mg tablets. How

many tablets should the nurse administer in 2 days?

5. A patient with pneumonia is prescribed 300 mg of ertapenem every 8 hours. The drug is available in 150-mg tablets. How many tablets should the nurse administer per day to meet the recommended dose? _____

6. A patient with bacterial infection is prescribed 700 mg of aztreonam to be taken intramuscularly (IM). The drug is available in 50 mL/g. How much of drug in solution should the nurse prepare for the IM administration? _____

SECTION III: PRACTICING FOR NCLEX

Activity E

Answer the following questions.

1. A nurse is assigned to care for a patient who has developed a serious bacterial infection. The patient has been prescribed linezolid, which has to be administered orally. Which of the following most serious adverse reactions of linezolid should the nurse monitor for in the patient?
   a. Thrombocytopenia
   b. Nephrotoxicity
   c. Ototoxicity
   d. Phlebitis

2. A nurse has been caring for a patient who was treated for bacterial infection. The patient is now scheduled to receive treatment on an outpatient basis. Which of the following instructions should the nurse offer to the patient and patient's family under continuing care?
   a. Complete the full course of treatment
   b. Always take the drug with food
   c. Avoid drinking alcoholic beverages
   d. Understand potential adverse reactions
   e. Monitor for adverse symptoms for 3 days

3. A nurse is caring for a 35-year-old patient with gonorrhea. The physician has prescribed a dosage of 4 g of spectinomycin to be given intravenously to the patient. The available dosage of this drug is 5 mL/2 g.

How much of the drug solution should the nurse prepare?

a. 2 mL

b. 10 mL

c. 15 mL

d. 4 mL

4. A nurse is caring for a patient with gonorrhea who is being prescribed spectinomycin. The nurse should monitor for which of the following adverse effects when caring for this patient?

a. Sudden decrease in blood pressure

b. Headache

c. Urticaria

d. Throbbing neck pain

5. A nurse is assigned to care for a patient whose physician prescribed quinupristin/dalfopristin. Which of the following precautions should the nurse take when administering quinupristin/dalfopristin?

a. Monitor for cross-sensitivity if administering the drug with a cephalosporin

b. Monitor for secondary bacterial or fungal infections

c. Monitor for bone marrow depression

d. Monitor for hearing or kidney problems

6. A nurse is caring for a patient with a bacterial infection. The nurse has to administer vancomycin to the patient through the parenteral route. The nurse ensures that every dose of vancomycin is administered over 60 minutes. She should remain alert for which of the following conditions when caring for this patient?

a. Shock

b. Severe hypotension

c. Sudden decrease in blood pressure

d. Ringing in the ears

7. A patient with a urinary tract infection is administered fosfomycin tromethamine. The nurse is required to conduct an ongoing patient assessment. What are the required elements of this ongoing assessment? Select all that apply.

a. Monitor for sudden decrease in pulse and respiratory rate

b. Monitor vital signs every 4 hours

c. Observe for sudden increase in temperature

d. Observe patient frequently during first 48 hours of therapy

e. Determine signs of any infection

8. A nurse is caring for a patient with a gram-negative bacterial infection. The patient has to be administered aztreonam. The nurse has to assess the patient's medical history to determine the medications that the patient uses. He knows aztreonam has to be administered cautiously in case the patient is taking which of the following drugs?

a. Antiplatelet drugs

b. Nephrotoxic drugs

c. Warfarin

d. Penicillin

9. A nurse is assigned to care for a patient who has to receive an anti-infective drug intramuscularly (IM). Which of the following nursing interventions should the nurse perform when caring for this patient?

a. Check the infusion site every 12 hours

b. Rotate injection sites

c. Inspect previous injection sites

d. Assess for vein irritation

e. Adjust rate of infusion every 30 minutes

10. A patient with a bacterial infection has been admitted to a health care facility. The patient has an infection caused by *Enterococcus faecium*, which is resistant to the effect of vancomycin. The nurse knows that which of the following drugs will help reduce the infection in the patient?

a. Daptomycin

b. Quinupristin/dalfopristin

c. Fosfomycin tromethamine

d. Spectinomycin

CHAPTER 12

Antitubercular Drugs

SECTION I: ASSESSING YOUR UNDERSTANDING

Activity A MATCHING

1. Match the drugs in Column A with the effects of their interaction with isoniazid in Column B.

Column A

_D_ 1. Aluminum salts

_C_ 2. Anticoagulants

_A_ 3. Phenytoin

_B_ 4. Tyramine

Column B

A. Increases serum levels

B. Produces exaggerated sympathetic-type response

C. Increases risk for bleeding

D. Reduces absorption of isoniazid

Activity B FILL IN THE BLANKS

1. Nephrotoxicity and ototoxicity may be seen with the administration of 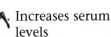 _Vancomycin_

2. People with human 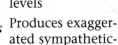 _immunodeficiency_ virus are at risk for tuberculosis (TB) because of their compromised immune systems.

3. 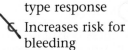 _Extrapulmonary_ tuberculosis is the term used to distinguish TB affecting the lungs from infection with the *M. tuberculosis* bacillus in other organs of the body.

4. When isoniazid is taken with foods containing _tyramine_, an exaggerated sympathetic-type response can occur.

5. The recommended treatment regimen is for the administration of rifampin, isoniazid, pyrazinamide, and ethambutol for a minimum of _2_ months.

SECTION II: APPLYING YOUR KNOWLEDGE

Activity C SHORT ANSWERS

A nurse's role in managing patients who are diagnosed with tuberculosis and administered antitubercular drugs involves instructing the patients about adverse reactions and precautions to be taken during recovery. Answer the following questions regarding the nurse's role in the management of such situations.

1. The nurse is caring for a 24-year-old patient with tuberculosis (TB). What interventions should the nurse perform as part of the preadministration assessment when providing care for this client?

_____

_____

_____

2. A nurse has been caring for a patient with TB. After treatment, the nurse has to care for the patient on an outpatient basis. What instructions should the nurse offer the patient and patient's family to decrease the chances of noncompliance?

_____

_____

_____

3. A nurse has been caring for a patient with TB. After the patient's treatment, the nurse has to evaluate the effectiveness of the treatment plan. What should the nurse keep in mind when evaluating the success of this plan?

_____

_____

_____

Activity D DOSAGE CALCULATION

1. A patient has been prescribed 150 mg of isoniazid per day. Each available tablet of isoniazid contains 100 mg of the drug. How many tablets will need to be administered to the patient in 2 days? _____

2. A physician prescribes 600 mg of rifampin per day for a patient. Rifampin is available as 300-mg tablets. How many tablets will need to be administered to the patient per day?

_____

3. A patient has been prescribed 1 gram of pyrazinamide per day. If this antitubercular drug is available as 500-mg tablets, then how many tablets per day will have to be administered to the patient? _____

SECTION III: PRACTICING FOR NCLEX

Activity E

Answer the following questions.

1. A nurse is required to care for a patient who has been administered rifampin. Which of the following generalized adverse reactions should the nurse monitor for in the patient?

   a. Myalgia

   b. Jaundice

   c. Reddish-orange color of body fluids

   d. Dermatitis and pruritus

2. A nurse is assigned to care for a patient with TB who has to be administered ethambutol. Which of the following conditions should the nurse ensure to confirm that ethambutol is not contraindicated in the patient? Select all that apply.

   a. Patient is not younger than 13 years of age

   b. Patient does not have cataracts

   c. Patient does not have a hypersensitivity to the drug

   d. Patient does not have diabetes mellitus

   e. Patient does not have acute gout

3. A nurse has been caring for a patient with TB in a health care facility. After treatment, the nurse has to ensure that the patient follows his drug regimen regularly without missing a dose. The nurse suggests that the patient follow an alternative-dosing regimen of twice weekly. How can this mode of taking the dosage help the client?

   a. Decreases gastric upset and promotes nutrition

   b. Promotes fluid balance in the patient's body

   c. Prevents the occurrence of neuropathy

   d. Prevents the occurrence of liver dysfunction

4. A nurse is assigned to care for a client with extrapulmonary tuberculosis in a health care facility. The nurse knows that which of the following organs can be affected by extrapulmonary tuberculosis? Select all that apply.

   a. Heart

   b. Liver

   c. Spleen

   d. Brain

   e. Kidneys

5. A nurse is assigned to care for a patient with TB. When conducting the preadministration assessment, the nurse should know that the patient is taking which of the following drugs so that she can closely monitor the patient when he is receiving rifampin? Select all that apply.

   a. Oral anticoagulants

   b. Digoxin

   c. Oral contraceptives

   d. Colchicine

   e. Allopurinol

6. A nurse is caring for a TB patient who has been administered isoniazid. The treatment has lasted for many months, and ongoing assessment reveals that the patient is developing a severe toxic reaction. The nurse should monitor for which of the following manifestations of a severe toxic reaction to isoniazid?

a. Hepatotoxicity

b. Anaphylactoid reactions

c. Severe hepatitis

d. Epigastric distress

7. A patient with tuberculosis is administered pyrazinamide as prescribed. The nurse caring for the patient suspects that the patient is developing signs of hepatotoxicity as an adverse reaction of pyrazinamide. Which of the following manifestations of a hepatotoxic reaction should the nurse look for in the patient?

a. Severe jaundice

b. Epigastric distress

c. Severe hepatitis

d. Hematologic changes

8. A nurse is required to care for a TB patient who has been administered antitubercular drugs. The nurse has to provide care to the patient on an outpatient basis. Which of the following interventions should the nurse perform to prevent the risk of hepatitis in the TB patient?

a. Administer antitubercular drugs in combination

b. Use DOT to administer drugs on outpatient basis

c. Instruct patient to take pyridoxine according to prescription

d. Instruct the patient to minimize alcohol consumption

9. A nurse is assigned to care for a TB patient who has received rifampin. Under which of the following conditions is the use of rifampin contraindicated?

a. Patients who have tested positive for human immunodeficiency virus (HIV)

b. Patients with hepatic or renal impairment

c. Patients with diabetes mellitus

d. Patients with diabetic retinopathy

CHAPTER 13

Leprostatic Drugs

SECTION I: ASSESSING YOUR UNDERSTANDING

Activity A MATCHING

1. Match the generic names of the leprostatic drugs in Column A with their trade names in Column B.

Column A	Column B
___ 1. Dapsone	A. Rifadin
___ 2. Clofazimine	B. Trecator
___ 3. Rifampin	C. Udolic (ICI)
___ 4. Ethionamide	D. Lamprene

2. Match the leprostatic drugs in Column A with their adverse reactions in Column B.

Column A	Column B
___ 1. Dapsone	A. Vertigo (dizziness)
___ 2. Clofazimine	B. Hemolysis
___ 3. Rifampin	C. Abdominal/epigastric pain

Activity B FILL IN THE BLANKS

1. Clofazimine is used for primary combined leprosy therapy and the inflammation of _____ disease.

2. Leprostatic drugs are administered orally with food to minimize _____ upset.

3. Patients with leprosy can experience changes in the _____ of their skin.

4. _____ and jaundice are adverse reactions of administering dapsone.

SECTION II: APPLYING YOUR KNOWLEDGE

Activity C SHORT ANSWERS

A nurse's role in managing leprosy involves helping patients deal with the adverse effects caused by leprostatic drug therapy. The nurse also educates patients and their families about the treatment regimen. Answer the following questions, which involve the nurse's role in management of such situations.

1. The nurse is assessing a patient who is receiving a leprostatic drug. What should the nurse focus on in the following stages:

   a. Preadministration assessment

   _____

   _____

   _____

   b. Ongoing assessment

   _____

   _____

   _____

2. A patient on leprostatic drugs is feeling self-conscious about her appearance. What steps can the nurse take to help this patient?

   _____

   _____

   _____

Activity D DOSAGE CALCULATION

1. A patient has received a prescription for 100 mg of dapsone every day. On hand are 50-mg tablets. To meet the recommended dose, how many tablets of dapsone should the nurse administer every day? _____

2. A patient has been prescribed 600 mg of rifampin every 12 hours. The available drug is a 300-mg capsule. To meet the recommended dose, how many capsules should the nurse administer each time? _____

SECTION III: PRACTICING FOR NCLEX

Activity E

Answer the following questions.

1. Which of the following is most important for the nurse to assess in a patient when initiating clofazimine therapy?
   a. Gastrointestinal disorders
   b. Cardiopulmonary disease
   c. Liver dysfunction
   d. Renal impairment

2. What are the severe adverse reactions a nurse should closely monitor for in a patient on dapsone therapy? Select all that apply.
   a. Jaundice
   b. Hemolysis
   c. Toxic epidermal necrolysis (TEN)
   d. Abdominal/epigastric pain
   e. Conjunctiva

3. What nursing intervention is important when administering leprostatic drugs?
   a. Administer with aluminum salts
   b. Administer with anticoagulants
   c. Administer on an empty stomach
   d. Administer orally with food

4. A female patient who has recently given birth is undergoing treatment for leprosy. She wishes to know the effects of dapsone in case she decides to breast-feed her infant. What should the nurse identify as the effects of dapsone on a newborn dependent on mother's milk?
   a. The drug will have no effect on the neonate
   b. The neonate may experience hemolytic reactions
   c. The neonate may experience skin eruptions
   d. The neonate may reject the breast milk

5. During the treatment of leprosy, a patient experiences changes in the pigmentation of his skin. He is depressed about this physical change in his body. What should a nurse do to help the patient?
   a. Note the patient's compliance with drug regimen
   b. Note the signs of depression or indifference
   c. Allow patient to verbalize his feelings
   d. Instruct the patient to adapt to the changes

6. How can the nurse ensure that a patient on leprostatic drug therapy complies with his or her treatment regimen?
   a. Communicate with the family members for the response of the patient
   b. Explain the prescribed dosage regimen to the patient
   c. Report the adverse drug reactions to the primary health care provider
   d. Listen to the patient about the dosage problems and make necessary changes

CHAPTER 14

Antiviral Drugs

SECTION I: ASSESSING YOUR UNDERSTANDING

Activity A MATCHING

1. Match the interactant drug in Column A with its uses in Column B.

Column A		Column B
C	1. Antifungals	A. Treat bacterial infection
A	2. Clarithromycin	B. Relieve pain
D	3. Sildenafil	C. Eliminate or manage fungal infections
B	4. Opioid analgesics	D. Treat erectile dysfunction

2. Match the interactant drug in Column A with its common uses in Column B.

Column A		Column B
A	1. Probenecid	A. Gout treatment
D	2. Cimetidine	B. Pain relief
B	3. Ibuprofen	C. Anti-infective agent
C	4. Imipenem/cilastatin	D. Gastric upset, heartburn

Activity B FILL IN THE BLANKS

1. **Lemon** balm is a perennial herb with heart-shaped leaves that has been used for hundreds of years. Its scientific name is *Melissa officinalis*.

2. **Cidofivir**, also called Vistide, should not be given to patients who have renal impairment or in combination with medications that are nephrotoxic, such as aminoglycosides.

3. **Ritonavir**, also called Norvir, is contraindicated if the patient is taking bupropion (Wellbutrin), zolpidem (Ambien), or an antiarrhythmic drug.

4. The drug **Indanivir** has been known to cause kidney and/or bladder stones in patients.

5. **Antiretroviral** drugs are used to treat human immunodeficiency virus (HIV) and acquired immunodeficiency syndrome (AIDS).

SECTION II: APPLYING YOUR KNOWLEDGE

Activity C SHORT ANSWERS

A nurse's role in managing patients who are being administered antiviral drugs includes observing and monitoring their progress and performing any necessary interventions as required. Answer the following questions, which involve the nurse's role in managing such situations.

1. A patient is diagnosed with herpes simplex virus (HSV), and the physician has prescribed antiviral drugs for him. What should the nurse assess for before administering the antiviral drug?

_____

_____

_____

2. A patient has hepatitis B, and the physician has prescribed an antiviral drug. What should the nurse assess for while administering the antiviral drug to the patient?

_____

_____

_____

Activity D DOSAGE CALCULATION

1. A primary health care provider has prescribed 120 mg of Foscavir per day to be given intravenously. The strength of the drug in the available solution is 24 mg/mL. How many milliliters of the solution should the nurse administer to the patient in a day?

_____

2. The primary health care provider has prescribed intravenous acyclovir to a patient. The standard dosage of the drug is 5 mg/kg to be given once a day. The patient weighs 50 kg, and the available drug solution is 10 mL/500 mg. How much of the drug dosage should the nurse prepare for the client for a week?

_____

3. The primary health care provider has prescribed 100 mg of amantadine daily for a patient. The drug is available as syrup with a concentration of 50 mg/5 mL. How many milliliters of the syrup should the nurse prepare for the patient to be administered for a week?

_____

4. The primary health care provider has prescribed 500 mg of famciclovir per dose. The drug is available in 125-mg tablets. How many tablets should the nurse administer to the patient per dose? _____

5. The primary health care provider has prescribed 300 mg of cidofovir for a patient. The drug is available as syrup with a concentration of 375 mg/5 mL. How many milliliters of the given syrup should the nurse administer to the patient? _____

6. The primary health care provider has prescribed 1 mg of entecavir per dose. The drug is available in 0.05 mg/mL oral solution. How many milliliters for six such doses should the nurse prepare for the patient?

_____

SECTION III: PRACTICING FOR NCLEX

Activity E

Answer the following questions.

1. A nurse is required to administer ribavirin to a patient. Which of the following points should the nurse keep in mind while administering the drug? Select all that apply.
   a. Discard and replace the solution every 24 hours
   b. The drug can worsen respiratory status
   c. The drug increases risk of nephrotoxicity in patient
   d. Use a small particle aerosol generator
   e. The drug induces anorexia and weight loss

2. A patient on an antiretroviral drug is also taking clarithromycin. Which of the following effects occur when antiretroviral therapy is combined with clarithromycin?
   a. Increased serum level of the antiretroviral
   b. Increased serum level of both drugs
   c. Risk of toxicity
   d. Decreased effectiveness of the antiretroviral

3. A patient with HSV 1 has been prescribed antiretroviral therapy. Before beginning the treatment, what is the most appropriate intervention that the nurse should perform considering the patient's infection?
   a. Save a sample of the patient's urine
   b. Record patient's temperature
   c. Inspect areas with lesions
   d. Check the patient's blood pressure

4. A nurse is caring for a patient who is on antiretroviral therapy for HIV. The patient has developed anorexia and nausea because of the therapy. Which of the following interventions should the nurse perform in the given situation? Select all that apply.
   a. Reduce the frequency but increase the quantity of meals
   b. Ensure that client's diet includes soft, non-irritating foods
   c. Keep the atmosphere clean and free of odors
   d. Eliminate carbonated beverages or hot tea from diet
   e. Provide good oral care before and after meals

5. In which of the following cases should a nurse monitor for phlebitis in a patient?

   a. Patient is given drugs orally

   b. Patient is given drugs intramuscularly

   c. Patient is given drugs intravenously

   d. Patient is given drugs transdermally

6. In which of the following cases should the nurse exercise caution while caring for clients who have been administered indinavir?

   a. Patients with renal impairment

   b. Patients with cardiac disorders

   c. Patients with sulfonamide allergy

   d. Patients with history of bladder stone formation

7. A nurse is required to administer didanosine to an HIV patient. Which of the following points should the nurse keep in mind while administering the drug?

   a. Administer drug with meals

   b. Administer with 2 oz of water

   c. Avoid generating dust

   d. Refrigerate solution

8. A primary health care provider has prescribed 5400 mg of Foscavir per day to be administered intravenously. The strength of the drug in the available solution is 24 mg/mL. How many milliliters of the solution should the nurse administer to the patient in a day?

   a. 250 mL

   b. 225 mL

   c. 275 mL

   d. 200 mL

$$\frac{1mL}{24mg} = \frac{x}{5400mg}$$

$$24x = 5400 \, mg$$

9. The primary health care provider has prescribed 800 mg of acyclovir per dose. The drug is available in 200-mg tablets. How many tablets should the nurse administer to the patient per dose?

   a. 1

   b. 2

   c. 4

   d. 8

10. The primary health care provider has prescribed 200 mg of amantadine daily. The drug is available as syrup with a concentration of 50 mg/5 mL. How many milliliters of the given syrup should the nurse administer to the patient?

   a. 10 mL

   b. 15 mL

   c. 20 mL

   d. 25 mL

Antifungal Drugs

SECTION I: ASSESSING YOUR UNDERSTANDING

Activity A MATCHING

1. Match the antifungal drug in Column A with its uses in Column B.

Column A

B **1.** Flucytosine

D **2.** Ketoconazole

A **3.** Griseofulvin

E **4.** Miconazole

C **5.** Micafungin sodium

Column B

A. Treats infections of the skin, hair, or nails

B. Inhibits DNA and RNA synthesis in fungi

C. Prevents stem cell transplantation

D. Treats systemic fungal infections

E. Treats vaginal infections

Activity B FILL IN THE BLANKS

1. **Systemic** fungal infections are serious infections that occur when fungi gain entrance into the interior of the body.

2. **Superficial** mycotic infections occur on the surface of, or just below, the skin or nails.

3. **Creatnine** clearance tests are done before administering fluconazole to an elderly patient or patient with renal impairment.

4. The use of griseofulvin is contraindicated for patients having severe **Liver** disease.

5. The systemic agent itraconazole should not be used to treat fungal nail infections in patients with a history of **heart** problems.

6. Use of amphotericin B for patients who have **electrolyte** imbalances can cause severe bone marrow suppression.

7. **Lesions** caused by fungal infections may create anxiety for a patient undergoing antifungal treatment.

SECTION II: APPLYING YOUR KNOWLEDGE

Activity C SHORT ANSWERS

A nurse's role in managing a patient who is prescribed an antifungal drug involves preadministration assessment. The nurse also monitors patients who are taking an antifungal drug. Answer the following questions, which involve the nurse's role in management of patients on antifungal therapy.

1. A patient with vaginal fungus is prescribed an antifungal drug. What preadministration assessments should the nurse conduct before administration of this drug?

_____

_____

_____

2. After the preadministration assessment, the patient is administered an antifungal drug for

a vaginal infection. What is the nurse's role when caring for the patient using a topical antifungal infection preparation?

_____

_____

_____

Activity D DOSAGE CALCULATION

1. A patient has been prescribed 400 mg of fluconazole drug every 24 hours. The available drug is in a 200-mg tablet. To meet the prescribed dose, how many tablets should the nurse administer each day?

   _____

2. A patient has been prescribed 200 mg of fluconazole every 12 hours. The available drug is in a 50-mg tablet. To meet the prescribed dose, how many tablets should the nurse administer each time? _____

3. A patient has been prescribed 100 mg of flucytosine every 6 hours. The available drug is a 50-mg tablet. To meet the prescribed dose, how many tablets should the nurse administer each day? _____

4. An athletic patient has been prescribed 500 mg of griseofulvin in four doses every day. The available drug is in the form of a 125-mg/5-mL suspension. To meet the prescribed dose, how many milliliters should the nurse administer for each dose?

   _____

5. A patient with a nail infection has been prescribed 200 mg of itraconazole twice daily. The drug is available in the form of 100-mg capsules at the local pharmacy. The patient would like to know the total number of capsules he should buy for a 3-day course to meet the prescribed dose. What is the total number of capsules required for this patient?

   _____

6. A patient with a fungal infection has been prescribed 400 mg of ketoconazole in two doses every day. The available drug is in 200-mg capsules. To meet the prescribed dose, how many capsules should the nurse administer each time? _____

SECTION III: GETTING READY FOR NCLEX

Activity E

Answer the following questions.

1. A nurse is required to assess a patient for symptoms of deep myotic infection. Which parts of the body should the nurse check for deep mycotic infections?
   a. Liver
   b. Lungs
   c. Mouth
   d. Heart

2. A patient with a fungal infection is admitted to the health care facility. The physician prescribes topical administration of an antifungal drug. What kinds of reactions should the nurse monitor for in the patient?
   a. Dehydration
   b. Nausea
   c. Stinging
   d. Diarrhea

3. The nurse is documenting the history of a patient who will start itraconazole therapy. In which of the conditions is itraconazole contraindicated?
   a. Bone marrow suppression
   b. Severe liver disease
   c. History of heart failure
   d. History of asthma

4. What care should the nurse take when administering an intravenous (IV) solution of amphotericin B?
   a. Ensure that the IV solution is protected from light
   b. Freeze the unused IV solution
   c. Ensure that the IV solution is used within 24 hours
   d. Store the drug in a heated environment

5. A patient has been prescribed intravenous amphotericin B to cure a fungal infection. What adverse reactions should a nurse monitor for in the patient?
   a. Vomiting
   b. Abdominal pain
   c. Muscle pain
   d. Anorexia

6. A patient is undergoing antifungal treatment. The patient has lesions caused by fungal infections, and the reaction to the treatment is slow. As a result, the patient is anxious. What should the nurse do to help reduce the anxiety of the patient undergoing treatment?

   a. Check the patient's blood pressure

   b. Encourage the patient to verbalize his or her feelings

   c. Provide the patient with a warm blanket

   d. Keep the patient away from light

7. A patient who is being treated for a fungal infection is to be discharged. The nurse needs to instruct the patient how to take care of the infection after the discharge. What important instructions should the nurse include in the patient's teaching plan?

   a. Abstain from sexual contact while lesions are present

   b. Avoid sunlight when going outdoors

   c. Avoid physical activities

   d. Keep towels separate from those of other family members

8. A patient undergoing treatment with keto-conazole will soon be discharged. What drug reactions should the nurse instruct the patient to expect?

   a. Unusual fatigue, yellow skin, and darkened urine

   b. Fever, sore throat, or skin rash

   c. Headache, dizziness, and drowsiness

   d. Nausea, vomiting, or diarrhea

CHAPTER 16

Antiparasitic Drugs

SECTION I: ASSESSING YOUR UNDERSTANDING

Activity A MATCHING

1. Match the anthelmintic in Column A with its effect on helminthic infections in Column B.

Column A

_B_ **1.** Albendazole

_C_ **2.** Mebendazole

_D_ **3.** Pyrantel

_A_ **4.** Thiabendazole

Column B

A. Interrupts the life cycle of the helminth

B. Interferes with the synthesis of helminth microtubules

C. Blocks uptake of glucose by the helminth

D. Paralyzes the helminth

2. Match the drug in Column A with its effect when combined with an anthelmintic drug in Column B.

Column A

_C_ **1.** Cimetidine

_A_ **2.** Phenobarbital

_B_ **3.** Warfarin

Column B

A. Increased metabolism of metronidazole

B. Increased risk of bleeding

C. Decreased metabolism of metronidazole

Activity B FILL IN THE BLANKS

1. _Mebendazole_ or Vermox blocks the helminth's uptake of glucose, resulting in a depletion of the helminth's own glycogen.

2. Parenteral injection of the antimalarial drug _Chloroquine_ is avoided because the drug can cause cardiovascular collapse when given intramuscularly (IM) or intravenously (IV).

3. _Paromomycin_ is an aminoglycoside with amebicidal activity and is used to treat intestinal amebiasis.

4. _Iodoquinol_ interferes with the results of thyroid function tests up to 6 months after therapy.

5. Irreversible _Retinal_ damage has occurred in patients on long-term therapy with antimalarial drugs.

SECTION II: APPLYING YOUR KNOWLEDGE

Activity C SHORT ANSWERS

A nurse's role in managing patients who are receiving anthelmintic drugs involves monitoring them and implementing interventions that aid in their recovery. Answer the following questions, which involve the nurse's role in the management of such situations.

1. A patient with a pinworm infection has been prescribed an anthelmintic drug. What should a nurse assess for in the patient before administering the drug?

_____

_____

_____

2. A patient receiving an anthelmintic drug is showing signs of nausea, vomiting, and abdominal pain. What are the appropriate interventions a nurse should take to ensure the patient's well-being?

_____

_____

_____

Activity D   **DOSAGE CALCULATION**

1. A doctor prescribes 500 mg per day of chloroquine. The available chloroquine tablet is 250 mg. How many tablets should the patient consume daily? _____

2. A patient has been prescribed 780 mg of quinine sulfate per day (divided into three equal doses). The available quinine sulfate tablet is 260 mg. How many tablets should the nurse administer to the patient every day?

_____

3. A doctor prescribes 50 mg of intravenous (IV) pyrimethamine per day. After reconstitution, the concentration of the drug is 10 mg/mL. How many milliliters of the reconstituted solution should be administered to the patient? _____

4. A primary health care provider prescribes 1250 mg of mefloquine hydrochloride tablets. The available mefloquine hydrochloride tablet is 250 mg. How many tablets should the nurse administer to the patient? _____

5. A doctor prescribes 750 mg of atovaquone twice daily. Atovaquone is available as syrup, and 1 mL contains 150 mg of the drug. How many milliliters should the nurse administer to the patient daily? _____

SECTION III: PRACTICING FOR NCLEX

Activity E

Answer the following questions.

1. A nurse is required to care for a patient with malaria who is acutely ill. Which of the following interventions should the nurse perform?

   a. Record vital signs of the patient every 12 hours

   b. Observe the patient every 4 hours for malaria symptoms

   c. Collect urine samples of the patient and send them for testing

   d. Carefully measure and record the fluid intake and output

2. For which of the following patients is the antimalarial drug quinine contraindicated?

   a. Patients with myasthenia gravis

   b. Patients with thyroid disease

   c. Patients with blood dyscrasias

   d. Patients with diabetes

3. Which of the following are adverse effects associated with anthelmintic drugs? Select all that apply.

   a. Drowsiness and dizziness

   b. Nausea and vomiting

   c. Visual disturbances

   d. Abdominal pain and cramps

   e. Tinnitus (ringing sound in ears)

4. A nurse is caring for a patient with a helminthic infection. Which of the following interventions should the nurse perform?

   a. Save stool samples only during the first day of treatment

   b. Follow hospital procedure for transporting stool to the laboratory

   c. Visually inspect stools only if patient reports anything unusual

   d. Use any container to save a sample of the stool

5. A nurse is caring for a patient who has been administered chloroquine. Which of the following conditions is a cause for concern that the nurse should report immediately to the primary health care provider?

   a. Unusual muscle weakness

   b. Peripheral neuropathy

   c. Yellow or brown urine color

   d. Ringing in the ears

   e. Visual changes

6. Which of the following information should be given to women of childbearing age regarding possible effects of albendazole?

   a. Albendazole can cause serious harm to a developing fetus

   b. Albendazole increases the risk of miscarriage

c. Albendazole may decrease the chances of conception

d. Albendazole may adversely affect the estrogen hormone

7. A female patient is prescribed pyrantel for roundworms. Which of the following should a nurse inform the patient when educating her about taking an anthelmintic drug?

a. Use birth control pills instead of the barrier method for contraception

b. Discontinue dosage as soon as symptoms of the affected condition disappear

c. Use chlorine bleach to disinfect toilet facilities or shower stalls after bathing

d. Take the drug with milk and not water unless the patient is lactose intolerant

8. Which of the following adverse effects associated with paromomycin should a nurse monitor for in a patient?

a. Vertigo and hypotension

b. Nephrotoxicity and ototoxicity

c. Thrombocytopenia

d. Peripheral neuropathy

9. Which of the following pieces of information should a nurse give to a patient who has been prescribed metronidazole?

a. Take the drug with meals or immediately afterwards

b. Avoid alcohol for the first week of treatment

c. Take cimetidine for gastric upset or other stomach problems

d. Wear protective clothing to guard against photosensitivity

10. A patient has been prescribed doxycycline for malaria. Which of the following should the nurse inform the patient regarding the side effects of the drug?

a. Photosensitivity

b. Skin eruptions

c. Cinchonism

d. Thrombocytopenia

CHAPTER 17

Nonopioid Analgesics: Salicylates and Nonsalicylates

SECTION I: ASSESSING YOUR UNDERSTANDING

Activity A MATCHING

1. Match the interactant drug in Column A with its effect in Column B when taken with a salicylate.

Column A

_B_ **1.** Anticoagulant

_D_ **2.** Activated charcoal

_A_ **3.** Antacid

_C_ **4.** Carbonic anhydrase inhibitor

Column B

A. Decreased effects of the salicylates

B. Increases risk of bleeding

C. Increased risk for salicylism

D. Decreased absorption of the salicylates

2. Match the nursing diagnosis checklist options in Column A with their nursing diagnoses in Column B.

Column A

_C_ **1.** Impaired Comfort

_A_ **2.** Chronic or Acute Pain

_D_ **3.** Impaired Physical Mobility

_B_ **4.** Disturbed Sensory Perception

Column B

A. Peripheral nerve damage and/or tissue inflammation

related to aspirin therapy

B. Auditory: related to adverse drug reactions

C. Related to fever of the disease process (e.g., infection or surgery)

D. Related to muscle and joint stiffness

Activity B FILL IN THE BLANKS

1. The analgesic action of the salicylates is caused by the inhibition of _prostaglandins_ which are fatty acid derivatives found in almost every tissue of the body and body fluids.

2. Aspirin prolongs bleeding time by inhibiting the aggregation (clumping) of _platelets_

3. _Pancytopenia_ is a reduction in all cellular components of the blood.

4. The use of aspirin may be involved in the development of _Reye's_ syndrome in children who have chickenpox or influenza.

5. _Tinnitus_, a ringing sound in the ear, is one of the symptoms of salicylism.

SECTION II: APPLYING YOUR KNOWLEDGE

Activity C SHORT ANSWERS

A nurse's role in managing discomfort of patients involves assisting them with relieving their pain. The nurse also helps administer drugs and provide physical comfort. Answer the following questions, which involve the nurse's role in the management of such situations.

1. What are the different ways in which a nurse can assess patients' pain?

_____

_____

_____

2. A patient has been prescribed salicylates. How can the nurse monitor and manage this patient's discomfort?

_____

_____

_____

Activity D DOSAGE CALCULATION

1. A patient has been prescribed 650 mg of aspirin every 4 hours. The available tablets are 325 mg. How many tablets will the nurse administer to the patient daily? _____

2. The physician prescribes 500 mg of Dolobid, to be taken orally every 8 hours. The available tablets are 250 mg. How many tablets will the nurse administer to the patient daily?

_____

3. Salsalate, 3000 mg daily, has been prescribed for a patient. The available tablet contains 500 mg of salsalate. How many tablets are needed daily to meet the prescribed drug level?

_____

4. A patient has been prescribed 600 mg of acetaminophen every day. The available drug is a 300-mg tablet, which is to be administered every 6 hours. To meet the recommended dose, how many tablets should the nurse administer each time? _____

5. A patient can be given 650 mg of buffered aspirin every 4 hours. The available tablets are 325 mg. How many tablets will the nurse

administer to the patient each time if the tablets are to be administered every 8 hours? _____

6. A patient is prescribed 650 mg of Ecotrin every 4 hours. The nurse has 325-mg tablets. How many tablets should the nurse administer every 4 hours? _____

SECTION III: PRACTICING FOR NCLEX

Activity E

Answer the following questions.

1. A patient has been prescribed salicylates as an analgesic agent. The nurse should monitor for which of the following adverse reactions?

   a. Skin eruptions
   b. Gastrointestinal (GI) bleeding
   c. Jaundice
   d. Bleeding disorders

2. For which of the following patients are salicylates contraindicated? Select all that apply.

   a. Patients with hypersensitivity to the drug
   b. Patients with a history of heart failure
   c. Patients with influenza or viral illness
   d. Patients with bleeding disorders
   e. Patients with hepatic disorders

3. In which of the following patients is acetaminophen preferred over aspirin?

   a. Patients with severe pain
   b. Patients with high fever
   c. Patients with bleeding tendencies
   d. Patients with inflammatory disorders

4. A patient has been administered acetaminophen. Which of the following interventions should the nurse perform as part of the ongoing assessment?

   a. Reassess patient's pain rating 3 hours after administration
   b. Monitor vital signs every 8 hours
   c. If stools are dark, immediately send a sample for testing
   d. Assess for decrease in inflammation and greater mobility

5. Which of the following symptoms can be observed in a patient with salicylate levels between 150 and 250 mcg/mL?

   a. Nausea

   b. Respiratory alkalosis

   c. Hemorrhage

   d. Asterixis

6. Which of the following is an effect of combining loop diuretics with acetaminophen?

   a. Increased possibility of toxicity

   b. Decreased effect of acetaminophen

   c. Increased risk for bleeding

   d. Decreased effectiveness of the diuretic

7. Which of the following information should a nurse provide to a patient who has been prescribed salicylates regarding their purchase and storage?

   a. Do not use over-the-counter drugs containing aspirin

   b. Include paprika, licorice, prunes, and raisins in diet

   c. Store the drug in a cool, ventilated area

   d. Purchase salicylates in small amounts

   e. Notify the physician before surgery or a dental procedure

8. Which of the following adverse reactions should a nurse monitor for in a patient who has received salsalate?

   a. GI bleeding

   b. Hypoglycemia

   c. Pancytopenia

   d. Hemolytic anemia

9. In patients with which of the following conditions can aspirin be used?

   a. Hemophilia

   b. Rheumatoid arthritis

   c. Postoperative pain

   d. On anticoagulant drugs

10. A patient has been prescribed acetaminophen. Which of the following are signs of acetaminophen toxicity?

    a. Malaise

    b. Increased anxiety

    c. Hyperglycemia

    d. Bradycardia

Nonopioid Analgesics: Nonsteroidal Anti-Inflammatory Drugs (NSAIDs)

SECTION I: ASSESSING YOUR UNDERSTANDING

Activity A MATCHING

1. Match the discomforts faced by patients in Column B with related nursing diagnoses in Column A.

Column A

___ 1. Impaired Physical Mobility

___ 2. Disturbed Sensory Perception

___ 3. Acute or Chronic Pain

Column B

A. Visual disturbance

B. Peripheral tissue damage

C. Muscle and joint stiffness

2. Match the drug that interacts with NSAIDs in Column A with its interacting effects in Column B.

Column A

___ 1. Anticoagulants

___ 2. Hydantoins

___ 3. Acetaminophen

___ 4. Diuretics

Column B

A. Increased risk of renal impairment

B. Increased excretion of extracellular fluid

C. Increased effectiveness of the anticonvulsant

D. Increased risk of bleeding

Activity B FILL IN THE BLANKS

1. NSAIDs act by inhibiting prostaglandin synthesis by inhibiting the action of the enzyme _____.

2. _____ is associated with an increased risk of serious cardiovascular thrombosis, myocardial infarction (MI), and stroke.

3. _____, a drug for pain relief, is available over the counter without a prescription.

4. _____ syndrome is an adverse effect of aspirin.

5. NSAIDs are prescribed for the pain and _____ associated with arthritis.

SECTION II: APPLYING YOUR KNOWLEDGE

Activity C SHORT ANSWERS

A nurse's role in managing patients who are being administered NSAIDs involves monitoring them and implementing interventions that aid in their recovery. Answer the following questions, which involve the nurse's role in the management of such situations.

1. What do NSAIDs treat?

_____

_____

_____

2. A nurse is caring for a patient receiving an NSAID drug for moderate pain. What adverse reactions should the nurse monitor for regarding the drug's effect on the sensory organs?

_____

_____

_____

Activity D DOSAGE CALCULATION

1. A patient has been prescribed 150 mg of Cataflam for oral administration each day. Cataflam is available as 50-mg tablets. How many tablets will the nurse administer to the patient each day? _____

2. A patient has been prescribed 1 g of Lodine per day for oral administration. The drug is available in tablets of 200 mg. How many tablets will the nurse administer to the patient per day? _____

3. A patient has been prescribed 1.2 g of Nalfon for oral administration in four doses a day. The drug is available in 200-mg tablets. How many tablets will the nurse administer to the patient each time? _____

4. A patient has been prescribed 200 mg of Ansaid for oral administration in two equally divided doses. The drug is available in tablets of 100 mg. How many tablets will the nurse administer to the patient daily? _____

5. A patient has been prescribed 400 mg of meclofenamate sodium for oral administra-

tion in four divided doses. The drug is available as 100-mg tablets. How many tablets will the nurse administer to the patient per day?

_____

SECTION III: PRACTICING FOR NCLEX

Activity E

Answer the following questions.

1. A patient with rheumatoid arthritis has been administered an NSAID. For which of the following adverse reactions should the nurse monitor the patient, concerning the effects of NSAIDs on the gastrointestinal system? Select all that apply.
   a. Epigastric pain
   b. Appendicitis
   c. Abdominal distress
   d. Indigestion
   e. Intestinal ulceration

2. Why is celecoxib not used to relieve postoperative pain for a patient who has undergone coronary artery bypass graft (CABG) surgery?
   a. Increased risk of duodenal ulcer
   b. Increased risk of gastric bleeding
   c. Increased risk of myocardial infarction
   d. Increased risk of diarrhea

3. A nurse is documenting the history of a patient who is to be initiated on NSAID therapy. In which of the following conditions is ibuprofen contraindicated?
   a. Patients with sulfonamide allergy
   b. Patients with peptic ulceration
   c. Patients with cardiac disease
   d. Patients with history of stroke

4. A nurse is assigned to care for a patient who has to be administered an NSAID. What should the nurse monitor for before administering the NSAID to the patient?
   a. Visual disturbances
   b. Skin reactions
   c. Dizziness
   d. Bleeding disorders

5. A patient is prescribed an NSAID for osteoarthritis. What assessments should the nurse perform before the administration of NSAIDs?

a. Document limitations in mobility

b. Examine the patient's level of consciousness

c. Check the mental stability of the patient

d. Examine the patient's body temperature

6. A nurse is caring for a patient undergoing NSAID treatment. Which of the following should the nurse suggest to the patient to promote an optimal response to therapy?

a. Avoid exercises

b. Restrict intake to a liquid diet

c. Take medication with food

d. Restrict mobility

7. A patient has been prescribed indomethacin for rheumatoid disorders. For which of the following adverse conditions should the nurse monitor the patient?

a. Tinnitus

b. Diarrhea

c. Rash

d. Gastrointestinal bleeding

8. A 68-year-old patient is prescribed an NSAID for arthritis. Why should treatment for the elderly begin with a reduced dosage that is increased slowly?

a. Increased risk of inflammation

b. Increased risk of erythema

c. Increased red blood cell count

d. Increased risk of serious ulcer diseases

9. A patient has been prescribed 1 g of oral nabumetone in two equal doses per day. The drug is available in tablets of 500 mg. How many tablets should the nurse administer to the patient per day?

a. 2

b. 1

c. 2.5

d. 1.5

10. A patient under treatment for arthritis is to be discharged. Which of the following instructions should the nurse include in the patient's teaching plan? Select all that apply.

a. Avoid physical activities during drug therapy

b. Do not use the drugs on a regular basis unless the primary health care physician is notified

c. Keep towels separate from those of other family members

d. Avoid use of aspirin

e. Take the drug with a full glass of water or with food

CHAPTER 19

Opioid Analgesics

SECTION I: ASSESSING YOUR UNDERSTANDING

Activity A MATCHING

1. Match the adverse reaction in Column A with the associated drug names in Column B.

Column A

____ 1. Vertigo

____ 2. Dry mouth

____ 3. Constipation

____ 4. Skeletal muscle rigidity

Column B

A. Demerol

B. Dilaudid

C. Ultiva

D. Levo Dromoran

2. Match the discomforts faced by patients in Column A with their nursing diagnoses in Column B.

Column A

____ 1. Decreased gastrointestinal motility caused by opioids

____ 2. Anorexia caused by opioids

____ 3. Effects on breathing

____ 4. Dizziness or light-headedness from opioid administration

Column B

A. Ineffective Breathing Pattern

B. Constipation

C. Risk for Injury

D. Imbalanced Nutrition

Activity B FILL IN THE BLANKS

1. The most widely used opioid, _____ sulfate, is an effective drug for moderately severe to severe pain.

2. All opioid analgesics are contraindicated in patients with _____ to the drugs.

3. Opioid analgesics are the analgesics obtained from the _____ plant.

4. _____ is an illegal narcotic substance in the United States and is not used in medicine.

5. Elderly, _____, or debilitated patients may have a reduced initial opioid dose until their response to the drug is known.

SECTION II: APPLYING YOUR KNOWLEDGE

Activity C SHORT ANSWERS

A nurse's role in managing patients who are prescribed opioid analgesics involves helping the patients deal with chronic pain. The nurse also assists patients in coping with their drug regimens and helps them in the event of opiate addiction. Answer the following questions, which involve the nurse's role in managing such situations.

1. A patient who has cancer is prescribed morphine through an intravenous (IV) infusion pump. What information should the nurse offer the patient about the use of the patient-controlled analgesia (PCA) infusion pump?

_____

_____

_____

2. What factors should the nurse evaluate to determine the success of an opioid treatment plan?

_____

_____

_____

Activity D   DOSAGE CALCULATION

1. A physician prescribes 30 mg of aspirin-codeine orally four times a day for a patient. The available tablets are 60 mg. How many tablets will the nurse need to administer to the patient daily? _____

2. A physician prescribes 60 mg of methadone, to be spread over six doses per day. Each available tablet of methadone contains 10 mg of the drug. How many tablets will the nurse need to administer to the patient in each dose? _____

3. A physician prescribes butorphanol to a patient. The standard dose is 4 mg/70 kg. The patient weighs 110 kg. The drug has to be taken three times a day. Assuming that the physician prescribes the standard dose, how much butorphanol is prescribed? How much should the nurse administer to the patient in 1 day? _____

4. A patient is prescribed 50 mcg of fentanyl intramuscularly (IM) 30 minutes before surgery. The available vial has a strength of 0.05 mg/1 mL. How much fentanyl will the nurse need to administer to the patient?

_____

5. A physician prescribes 250 mg of morphine sulfate daily to a patient. Each 5 mL of Roxanol 100 contains 100 mg of morphine sulfate. How much Roxanol 100 will the nurse need to administer daily to the patient?

_____

6. A physician prescribes 100 mg of tramadol hydrochloride daily to a patient. Tramadol hydrochloride (Ultram) is available in 50-mg tablets. How many tablets will the nurse need to administer daily to the patient?

_____

SECTION III: PRACTICING FOR NCLEX

Activity E

Answer the following questions.

1. A nurse is caring for a patient who is prescribed opioid analgesics. Which of the following allergic reactions of opioid analgesics should the nurse monitor for in the patient?
   a. Constipation
   b. Urticaria
   c. Palpitations
   d. Facial flushing

2. A patient is prescribed an opioid analgesic for the treatment of pain. What preadministration assessments should the nurse conduct before administration of an opioid analgesic?
   a. Obtain patient's blood pressure
   b. Assess the intensity and location of pain
   c. Monitor patient's pulse rate
   d. Assess patient's respiratory rate

3. A nurse is caring for a patient who would like to use herbal doses of passion flower. Which of the following should the nurse confirm to ensure that the use of passion flower is not contraindicated in the patient?
   a. Patient is not taking monoamine oxidase inhibitors
   b. Patient is not taking opioid analgesics
   c. Patient does not have acute ulcerative colitis
   d. Patient does not have a history of asthma

4. A patient is prescribed an opioid analgesic for pain caused by a terminal illness. The nurse notices that the patient has developed severe anorexia from the opioid treatment. What interventions should the nurse perform for a patient with Imbalanced Nutrition: Related to prolonged administration of an opioid?
   a. Ensure the patient's fluid intake increases
   b. Assess the patient's food intake after each meal
   c. Complement the patient's meal with protein supplements
   d. Record the patient's bowel movements daily

5. A nurse is caring for a patient who has delivered a baby. The patient was opioid dependent during her pregnancy. Which of the following withdrawal symptoms should the nurse monitor for in the newborn?

   a. Excessive crying
   b. Vomiting
   c. Yawning
   d. Coughing
   e. Sneezing

6. Which of the following reinforces a cautious use of naloxone for a patient experiencing a decrease in respiratory rate?

   a. Naloxone leads to withdrawal symptoms
   b. Naloxone leads to vomiting
   c. Naloxone leads to dizziness
   d. Naloxone leads to headache

7. A patient is being prescribed opioid analgesics in a local health care facility. Which of the following is the nurse most likely to observe in this patient that would require immediate attention by the physician?

   a. Decrease in respiratory rate
   b. Change in pulse quality
   c. Decrease in blood pressure
   d. Increase in body weight
   e. Increase in body temperature

8. A nurse is assigned to care for a patient who has to be prescribed opioid therapy. Which of the following statements in the patient's health history will require cautious use of opioid analgesics by the nurse? Select all that apply.

   a. Patient has undiagnosed abdominal pain
   b. Patient is 13 years old
   c. Patient has hepatic or renal impairment
   d. Patient has hypoxia
   e. Patient has fungal infections

9. A nurse is caring for a patient on opioid therapy. The patient is also prescribed barbiturates—under close supervision. The nurse knows that which of the following risks is likely to occur in this patient?

   a. Bacterial infections
   b. Hypertension
   c. Respiratory depression
   d. Hypoxia

10. A patient who was being treated for severe diarrhea with opioid analgesics has recovered and is to be discharged. Which of the following instructions should the nurse include in the patient's teaching plan?

   a. Avoid traveling
   b. Avoid alcohol
   c. Avoid exercising
   d. Avoid starchy food

CHAPTER 20

Opioid Antagonists

SECTION I: ASSESSING YOUR UNDERSTANDING

Activity A FILL IN THE BLANKS

1. A drug that is a(n) _____ has a greater affinity for a cell receptor than an opioid drug, and by binding to the cell it prevents a response to the opioid.

2. _____ antagonists reverse the actions of an opioid.

3. _____ is capable of restoring respiratory function within 1 to 2 minutes of administration.

4. Antagonists are contraindicated in patients with _____ to opioid antagonists.

5. Naloxone is used within the controlled settings of the _____ recovery unit.

6. Opioid antagonists are used for the treatment of postoperative acute _____ depression.

7. The trade name for naloxone is _____.

SECTION II: APPLYING YOUR KNOWLEDGE

Activity B SHORT ANSWERS

A nurse's role in managing respiratory depression in patients involves assisting the patients with the administration of opioid antagonists. The nurse is also expected to monitor and assess the patients' needs. Answer the following questions, which involve the nurse's role in managing such situations.

1. A patient with respiratory depression is administered an opioid antagonist in a health care facility. What preadministration assessments should a nurse perform when caring for the patient?

_____

_____

_____

2. What circumstances should a nurse be aware of that enforce the use of opioid antagonists?

_____

_____

_____

Activity C DOSAGE CALCULATION

1. A patient is prescribed naloxone for a narcotic overdose. A total of 3 mg has to be given to the patient, and the available dosage is in the form of 0.5-mg tablets. Considering that one tablet has already been administered, how many more tablets should the patient take to complete the dosage?_____

2. A patient is prescribed 15 mg of intramuscular nalmefene. The available drug concentration is 2.5 mg/mL. How much drug will the nurse have to administer to the patient?_____

3. A patient has been prescribed 10 mg of buprenorphine intravenously. How much buprenorphine should the nurse administer to

the patient when the available dose is 2 mg/mL?_____

SECTION III: PRACTICING FOR NCLEX

Activity D

Answer the following questions.

1. A patient is administered a postoperative opioid antagonist for pain management. Which of the following should the nurse identify as the action of the opioid antagonist in the patient's body?

   a. Opioid antagonists instantly relieve pain

   b. Opioid antagonists reverse the effect of pain medication

   c. Opioid antagonists neutralize the effect of opioid drugs

   d. Opioid antagonists decrease pain

2. A nurse has been caring for a patient with respiratory depression. The nurse knows that which of the following critical factors are used to evaluate the treatment of a patient receiving an opioid antagonist for respiratory depression? Select all that apply.

   a. Positive response to therapeutic treatment

   b. Normal blood pressure

   c. Normal respiratory rate

   d. Resumption of pain

   e. Normal heart rate

3. A patient has been prescribed naloxone for respiratory depression. Which of the following interventions should the nurse perform to promote an optimal response in the patient?

   a. Monitor for an increase in the patient's body temperature

   b. Monitor for any signs of dehydration and water loss in the patient

   c. Balance the need for continued pain relief with patient's ability to breathe

   d. Administer the drug through a rapid intravenous (IV) push

4. A patient in a health care facility is prescribed a postoperative dose of naloxone. Which of the following interventions should the nurse perform during and after naloxone administration when caring for this patient? Select all that apply.

   a. Monitor the patient for symptoms of hypotension

   b. Make the suction equipment available

   c. Turn and suction the patient when needed

   d. Provide artificial ventilation

   e. Monitor hematologic changes

5. A patient in a health care facility is prescribed an opioid antagonist. The nurse knows that which of the following statements in the patient's health records will require a cautious use of the opioid antagonist in this patient?

   a. Patient has liver impairment

   b. Patient is lactating

   c. Patient has renal failure

   d. Patient is hypersensitive to the drug

6. Which of the following interventions should a nurse perform when caring for patients with respiratory depression to ensure an expected outcome from the treatment?

   a. Provide adequate ventilation of patient's body

   b. Provide patients with controlled analgesic pumps

   c. Administer prescribed sedatives through IV route

   d. Ensure that the patients' rooms are odor free

CHAPTER 21

Anesthetic Drugs

SECTION I: ASSESSING YOUR UNDERSTANDING

Activity A MATCHING

1. Match the various types of local anesthesia in Column A with their applications in Column B.

Column A	Column B
____ 1. Spinal	A. Injection of anesthetic around nerves
____ 2. Local infiltration	B. Application of anesthetic to surface of the skin
____ 3. Regional	C. Injection of local anesthetic into the subarachnoid space
____ 4. Topical	D. Injection of local anesthetic into tissues

2. Match the drugs used for general anesthesia in Column A with their uses in Column B.

Column A	Column B
____ 1. Methohexital	A. Surgical procedures that do not require relaxation of skeletal muscles
____ 2. Midazolam	B. Continuous sedation of intubated or respiratory-controlled patients in intensive care units
____ 3. Propofol	
____ 4. Ketamine	

C. Conscious sedation before minor procedures

D. Short surgical procedures with minimal painful stimuli

Activity B FILL IN THE BLANKS

1. A _____ block is a type of regional anesthesia produced by injection of a local anesthetic drug into or near a nerve trunk.

2. _____ anesthesia is the provision of a pain-free state for the entire body.

3. _____ is a loss of feeling or sensation.

4. A nurse _____ is a nurse with a master's degree and special training who is qualified to administer anesthetics.

5. A _____ is a physician with special training in administering anesthesia.

6. _____ liquid anesthetics produce anesthesia when their vapors are inhaled.

SECTION II: APPLYING YOUR KNOWLEDGE

Activity C SHORT ANSWERS

A nurse is required to care for patients who will receive anesthesia. A number of nursing interventions are associated with the administration of anesthesia. Answer the following questions, which involve the nurse's role in managing such situations.

1. A nurse observes that an abnormal laboratory test finding was included in the patient's chart shortly before surgery. What should be the nurse's immediate reaction?

_____

_____

_____

2. What are the postoperative nursing interventions that a nurse has to perform when caring for a patient?

_____

_____

_____

3. What factors should a nurse be aware of that influence the choice of anesthetic drug?

_____

_____

_____

Activity D   DOSAGE CALCULATION

1. A patient is to be administered 0.6 mg of Robinul. The dose is available as 0.2 mg/mL and is to be administered intramuscularly. How much Robinul should the nurse prepare to be administered as a preanesthetic? _____

2. A patient is to be administered 30-mg of chlordiazepoxide a day. Chlordiazepoxide is available in 15-mg tablets. How many tablets should the nurse administer to the patient?

_____

3. A patient is to be administered 25 mL of Marcaine HCl over 5 days. Each dose of Marcaine HCl contains 5 mL. How many doses should the nurse administer if one dose is to be administered each day?_____

4. A patient is to be administered 240 mg of fentanyl, available as 80-mg tablets. How many tablets should be administered to the patient?_____

5. A patient is prescribed Ultiva. The normal dosage of this drug is 0.5 mcg/kg, and the patient weighs 90 kg. If the rate of infusion of the drug is 0.5 mcg/30 seconds, calculate the time taken—in minutes—for the infusion of the entire dose of the drug. _____

SECTION III: PRACTICING FOR NCLEX

Activity E

Answer the following questions.

1. The physician prescribes the drug methohexital to a patient. The nurse knows that which of the following are the effects of methohexital?
   a. Produces mild stimulation of respiratory and bronchial secretions
   b. Brings about moderate muscle relaxation
   c. Depresses the central nervous system (CNS) to produce hypnosis and anesthesia
   d. Decreases secretions in the upper respiratory tract

2. Which of the following stages of general anesthesia begins with a loss of consciousness?
   a. Analgesia
   b. Delirium
   c. Surgical analgesia
   d. Respiratory paralysis

3. Which of the following are the effects of topical anesthesia that a nurse should know?
   a. Decrease anxiety and apprehension
   b. Desensitize skin or mucous membranes
   c. Cause loss of feeling in the lower extremities
   d. Cause cardiovascular stimulation

4. Which of the following activities should the nurse perform as postoperative interventions after anesthesia administration?
   a. Review patient's laboratory test records
   b. Administer a hypnotic agent to the patient
   c. Position the patient to prevent aspiration of vomitus
   d. Monitor patient's blood pressure every 12 hours

5. A patient who was administered a preanesthetic drug is experiencing an increase in his respiratory secretions. The nurse knows that which of the following has occurred during administration of the preanesthetic drug?
   a. Patient's anesthesia records were not reviewed
   b. The drug was not administered on time
   c. Patient's respiratory status was not assessed

d. Patient's intravenous (IV) lines were not well assessed

6. A nurse is caring for a patient who is to receive local anesthesia for wound suturing. Which of the following interventions should the nurse perform when caring for this client? Select all that apply.

a. Observe if there is any oozing

b. Apply dressing to the surgical areas

c. Observe the patient for any signs of bleeding

d. Assess the patient's pulse every 5 to 15 minutes

e. Exercise caution in administering opioids

7. A nurse is assigned to care for a patient who is to receive anesthesia. Which of the following should the nurse confirm to ensure that the use of preanesthetic drugs is not contraindicated in this patient?

a. Patient is not older than 60 years of age

b. Patient does not need anesthesia on his or her extremities

c. Patient is not younger than 13 years of age

d. Patient does not have a low body weight

8. A patient is admitted to a local health care facility for a kidney operation. The nurse knows that which of the following preanesthetic drugs should be administered to reduce the incidence of upper respiratory tract secretions in the patient?

a. Cholinergic blocking drug

b. Scopolamine and glycopyrrolate

c. Opioid or antianxiety drug

d. Diazepam or Valium

9. A pregnant patient is admitted to a local health care facility for a C-section delivery. The primary health care provider decides to administer a trans-sacral block as anesthesia. Where is the trans-sacral block injected in a patient?

a. Epidural space at the level of the sacrococcygeal notch

b. Space surrounding the dura of spinal cord

c. Subarachnoid space of the spinal cord

d. Brachial plexus

10. A nurse is assigned to care for a patient who is to be administered local anesthesia. Which of the following should the nurse confirm to ensure that the use of epinephrine along with the local anesthesia is not contraindicated in the patient?

a. Patient does not have anemia

b. Patient does not have a low blood pressure

c. Patient is not older than 60 years of age

d. Patient does not need anesthesia for his or her extremities

CHAPTER 22

Antianxiety Drugs

SECTION I: ASSESSING YOUR UNDERSTANDING

Activity A MATCHING

1. Match the drug interacting with an anxiolytic in Column A with its interacting effect in Column B.

Column A

____ 1. Alcohol

____ 2. Digoxin

____ 3. Antipsychotic

____ 4. Analgesic

Column B

A. Increased risk for central nervous system (CNS) depression

B. Increased risk for convulsions

C. Increased risk for digitalis toxicity

D. Increased risk for sedation and respiratory depression

2. Match the generic drugs (with trade names in parentheses) in Column A with their actions in Column B.

Column A

____ 1. Buspirone (BuSpar)

____ 2. Hydroxyzin (Atarax, Vistaril)

____ 3. Chlordiazepoxide (Librium)

Column B

A. Acts on the hypothalamus and brain stem reticular formation

B. Acts by enhancing the actions of a natural brain chemical gamma-aminobutyric acid (GABA)

C. Acts on the brain's serotonin receptors

Activity B FILL IN THE BLANKS

1. Drugs used to treat anxiety are called _____ .

2. _____ drugs are used for the management of cardiac problems.

3. Antianxiety drugs are used as _____ sedatives and muscle relaxants.

4. _____ administration is indicated primarily in acute states when it is difficult to have the patient take the medication by mouth.

5. _____ symptoms occur if benzodiazepines are taken for more than 3 months and discontinued abruptly.

SECTION II: APPLYING YOUR KNOWLEDGE

Activity C SHORT ANSWERS

A nurse's role in managing patients who are being administered antianxiety drugs involves monitoring them and implementing interventions that aid in their recovery. Answer the following questions, which involve the nurse's role in managing such situations.

1. A patient with anxiety has been prescribed alprazolam. What should a nurse assess for in this patient before administering the first dose of alprazolam?

_____

_____

_____

2. A patient receiving alprazolam complains of constipation. What effective interventions should the nurse perform to ensure the patient's well-being?

_____

_____

_____

Activity D DOSAGE CALCULATION

1. A patient is prescribed 0.25 mg of alprazolam orally three times a day. The drug is available in tablets of 0.5 mg. How many tablets should the nurse administer to the patient daily?

_____

2. A patient is prescribed 30 mg of oxazepam orally four times a day. At what interval should the nurse administer the drug, which is available in tablets of 15 mg?

_____

3. A patient is prescribed 15 mg of BuSpar daily. The tablet is available in doses of 5 mg. How many tablets are needed daily to meet the prescribed drug level? _____

4. A physician prescribes 25 mg of chlordiazepoxide orally four times a day for a patient. The drug is available in tablets of 10 mg. How many tablets will the nurse administer to the patient daily? _____

5. A physician prescribes 0.25 mg of clonazepam every 12 hours for the first 3 days. How many milligrams of the drug would the nurse administer to the patient over 3 days?

_____

6. A patient has been prescribed 150 mg of doxepin HCl daily. The drug is available in tablets of 25 mg. How many tablets are needed daily to meet the prescribed drug level?

_____

SECTION III: PRACTICING FOR NCLEX

Activity E

Answer the following questions.

1. A nurse is caring for a patient who is receiving antianxiety drugs. Which of the following is an adverse reaction that the nurse should monitor for in the patient?
   a. Seizures
   b. Diarrhea
   c. Abdominal cramps
   d. Bradycardia

2. A patient who was on benzodiazepine therapy for 4 weeks visits a health care facility. The patient exhibits benzodiazepine withdrawal symptoms. Which of the following should the nurse assess for in the patient?
   a. Increased red blood cell (RBC) count
   b. Decreased pulse rate
   c. Increased anxiety
   d. Increased appetite

3. A patient undergoing digoxin therapy for cardiac problems is prescribed diazepam for anxiety disorders. Which of the following effects should the nurse monitor for in the patient that results from interaction between the two drugs?
   a. Increased risk for CNS depression
   b. Increased risk for respiratory depression
   c. Increased risk for sedation
   d. Increased risk for digitalis toxicity

4. A patient visits a health care facility with symptoms of anxiety. The primary health care provider has prescribed hydroxyzine. For patients with which of the following conditions should the nurse take precautions when administering hydroxyzine? Select all that apply.
   a. Impaired liver function
   b. Impaired pancreas function
   c. Impaired kidney function
   d. Bone marrow depression
   e. Debilitation

5. The primary health care provider has diagnosed a patient with anxiety caused by withdrawal of alcohol. Which of the following should the nurse relate to alcohol withdrawal?

a. Diarrhea

b. Acute panic

c. Dry mouth

d. Light-headedness

6. A nurse is caring for a patient with anxiety who is to be administered lorazepam. Which of the following should the nurse ensure to confirm that lorazepam is not contraindicated in the patient?

a. Patient is not younger than 18 years of age

b. Patient is not hypersensitive

c. Patient does not have myasthenia gravis

d. Patient does not have parkinsonism

7. A patient is prescribed a chlordiazepoxide drug for anxiety. Which of the following interventions should the nurse perform to prevent the occurrence of constipation in the patient?

a. Provide vitamin supplements

b. Restrict patient's diet to fluids only

c. Provide patient with a fiber-rich diet and plenty of fluids

d. Restrict patient to a strict vegetarian diet

8. A patient being treated for anxiety is to be discharged. Which of the following instructions should the nurse include in the patient's teaching plan?

a. Avoid sunlight

b. Avoid alcohol

c. Avoid yogurt

d. Avoid sour cream

9. A nurse is assigned to care for an elderly patient who has to be administered doxepin. Which of the following safety measures should the nurse take while administering doxepin?

a. Administer the drug intramuscularly in the gluteus muscle

b. Monitor for hearing or kidney problems

c. Administer the drug intramuscularly in the arms

d. Monitor for secondary bacterial or fungal infections

10. A patient on alprazolam therapy has discontinued treatment for a week. Which of the following is a withdrawal symptom that the nurse should monitor for in the patient?

a. Diarrhea

b. Dizziness

c. Metallic taste

d. Dry mouth

23

Sedatives and Hypnotics

SECTION I: ASSESSING YOUR UNDERSTANDING

Activity A MATCHING

1. Match the type of drug in Column A with its common uses in Column B.

Column A	Column B
____ 1. Antidepressants	A. Pain relief
____ 2. Opioid analgesics	B. Management of gastric upset
____ 3. Antihistamines	C. Management of depression
____ 4. Phenothiazines	D. Relief of allergy symptoms
____ 5. Cimetidine	E. Management of agitation and psychotic symptoms

2. Match the key terms in Column A with their definitions in Column B.

Column A	Column B
____ 1. Ataxia	A. Agents that produce a relaxing, calming effect
____ 2. Hypnotics	B. An unsteady gait
____ 3. Sedatives	C. Agents that induce drowsiness or sleep

Activity B FILL IN THE BLANKS

1. Sleep deprivation may interfere with the _____ process of a patient.

2. Sedatives and hypnotics are primarily used to treat _____ and convulsions or seizures.

3. The herb _____ was originally used in Europe for its sedating effects in conditions of mild anxiety or restlessness.

4. Drinking beverages containing caffeine contribute to _____.

5. _____ is a hormone produced by the pineal gland in the brain.

6. _____, when given in the presence of pain, may cause restlessness, excitement, and delirium.

SECTION II: APPLYING YOUR KNOWLEDGE

Activity C SHORT ANSWERS

A nurse's role in managing patients who are being administered sedatives and hypnotic drugs involves monitoring the patients and implementing interventions that aid in their recovery. Answer the following questions, which involve the nurse's role in managing such situations.

1. A patient is prescribed a sedative. What assessments should the nurse perform before administering the drug?

   _____

   _____

   _____

2. List nursing diagnoses specific to a patient taking a sedative or hypnotic.

   _____

   _____

   _____

Activity D DOSAGE CALCULATION

1. A patient is prescribed 2 mg of estazolam twice a day. Estazolam is available in the form of 1-mg tablets. How many tablets will the nurse have to administer to the patient in a day? _____

2. A patient is prescribed 15 mg of temazepam per day. The available tablet of temazepam contains 5 mg of the drug. How many tablets will the nurse have to administer to the patient at one time? _____

3. A patient is prescribed 10 mg of zaleplon at bedtime. The available zaleplon tablet contains 5 mg of the drug. How many tablets of zaleplon will the nurse have to administer to the patient? _____

4. A patient is prescribed 0.25 mg of triazolam (Halcion) orally at bedtime. Triazolam is available in the form of 0.125-mg tablets. How many tablets will the nurse have to administer to the patient? _____

5. A patient is prescribed 10 mg of zolpidem tartrate orally at bedtime. Zolpidem tartrate is available in tablets of 5 mg. How many tablets of the drug will the nurse have to administer to the patient? _____

SECTION III: PRACTICING FOR NCLEX

Activity E

Answer the following questions.

1. A nurse is caring for a patient who has been prescribed a sedative. Which of the following measures can ensure an optimal response to sedative therapy? Select all that apply.
   a. Back rubs
   b. Alcohol intake
   c. Night-lights
   d. Darkened room
   e. Bedtime coffee

2. A nurse is caring for a patient who has received sedatives for insomnia. Which of the following is a criterion for evaluating the effectiveness of the treatment?
   a. Decreased level of consciousness
   b. Normal respiration rate
   c. Improved sleep pattern
   d. Decrease in restlessness

3. A patient is admitted to a health care facility with convulsions and is prescribed a sedative. Which of the following should the nurse record before administration of the drug?
   a. Platelet count
   b. Blood pressure
   c. Hematocrit
   d. Blood sugar

4. A nurse is caring for a patient who is to undergo surgery. The patient is prescribed a preoperative sedation. What adverse reactions should the nurse monitor for in this patient?
   a. Nausea
   b. Headache
   c. Restlessness
   d. Anxiety

5. Which of the following types of patients should a nurse identify as candidates for cautious use of sedatives and hypnotics?

    a. Patients with hearing impairment

    b. Patients with hyperglycemia

    c. Patients with glucose intolerance

    d. Patients with renal impairment

6. A patient undergoing allergy treatment is prescribed sedatives for anxiety. Which of the following should the nurse monitor the patient for as a possible effect of the interaction between antihistamines and sedatives?

    a. Restlessness

    b. Increased sedation

    c. Headache

    d. Chronic pain

7. A nurse is caring for a patient who has been prescribed barbiturates. Which of the following is a symptom of acute drug toxicity?

    a. Increased blood pressure

    b. Respiratory depression

    c. Lowered blood sugar

    d. Frequent micturition

8. A patient is admitted to the local health care facility for the treatment of insomnia caused by pain. Why would the primary health care provider not prescribe barbiturates for the patient?

    a. They cause an allergic reaction

    b. They cause an increase in temperature

    c. They cause delirium

    d. They cause an increase in blood sugar

9. A patient who was prescribed a barbiturate has abruptly discontinued use of the drug. The nurse expects withdrawal symptoms. Which of the following are withdrawal symptoms of barbiturates? Select all that apply.

    a. Restlessness

    b. Euphoria

    c. Seizures

    d. Confusion

    e. Convulsions

10. A patient is admitted to the health care facility with insomnia related to chronic headache and has been prescribed a sedative. Which of the following are benefits of sedatives? Select all that apply.

    a. Relaxing effect

    b. Nausea

    c. Calming effect

    d. Dizziness

    e. Drowsiness

Antidepressant Drugs

SECTION I: ASSESSING YOUR UNDERSTANDING

Activity A MATCHING

1. Match the key terms in Column A with their meanings in Column B.

Column A

____ 1. Depression

____ 2. Dysphoric mood

____ 3. Priapism

____ 4. Tardive dyskinesia

Column B

A. Syndrome of involuntary movement that may be irreversible

B. A persistent erection of the penis

C. Extreme sadness, anxiety, or unhappiness that interferes with daily functioning

D. Feeling sad, unhappy, or "down in the dumps"

2. Match the key terms in Column A with their meanings in Column B.

Column A

____ 1. Endogenous

____ 2. Hypertensive crisis

____ 3. Tyramine

____ 4. Strokes

Column B

A. Extremely high blood pressure

B. An amino acid present in some foods

C. Cerebrovascular accidents

D. Produced within the body

Activity B FILL IN THE BLANKS

1. _____ is used with antidepressants in treating major depressive episodes.

2. Patients receiving monoamine oxidase (MAO) inhibitors should not eat foods containing _____.

3. Injection of alpha-adrenergic stimulants may be helpful in treating _____.

4. Older men with prostatic enlargement are at increased risk for urinary retention when they take _____ antidepressants.

5. Parenteral administration of antidepressants is given intramuscularly in a large muscle mass, such as the _____ muscle.

SECTION II: APPLYING YOUR KNOWLEDGE

Activity C SHORT ANSWERS

A nurse's role in administering antidepressant drugs involves assisting patients in managing the common adverse reactions of the drugs. The nurse also educates patients about the use of these drugs. Answer the following questions, which involve the nurse's role in managing such situations.

1. How is clinical depression treated?

_____

_____

_____

2. What are the different types of antidepressants?

_____

_____

_____

3. What are the effects of antidepressants?

_____

_____

_____

4. What are the uses of tricyclic antidepressants?

_____

_____

_____

Activity D **DOSAGE CALCULATION**

1. A physician prescribes 150 mg of amitriptyline per day for a patient. The available tablets are 50 mg each. How many tablets should the nurse administer to the patient daily?

   _____

2. A patient is prescribed 50 mg of amoxapine three times a day. The drug is available in 25-mg tablets. How many tablets should the nurse administer to the patient daily?

   _____

3. A patient is prescribed 25 mg of clomipramine (Anafranil) daily. The available tablet contains 10 mg of clomipramine. How many tablets are needed each day to meet the prescribed drug level? _____

4. A patient is prescribed 25 mg of nortriptyline four times a day. The drug is available in 25-mg tablets. To give the drug equally, how much time should pass between consecutive administrations? _____

5. A physician has prescribed 90 mg of phenelzine (Nardil) per day for a patient. The available tablets contain 15 mg of drug. How many tablets should the nurse administer to the patient daily? _____

6. A patient has been prescribed 80 mg of fluoxetine (Prozac) per day to be administered in two equal doses, once in the morning and once at noon. The drug is available in 20-mg tablets. How many tablets should the nurse administer to the patient each time? _____

SECTION III: PRACTICING FOR NCLEX

Activity E

Answer the following questions.

1. A nurse is caring for a patient whose physician prescribed a tricyclic antidepressant drug for depression. Which of the following is an adverse reaction to the drug?

   a. Photosensitivity

   b. Hypertensive episodes

   c. Severe convulsions

   d. Nervous system depression

2. A patient undergoing psychotherapy in a local health care facility is prescribed MAO inhibitors. Which of the following contraindications should the nurse screen the patient for when administering MAO inhibitors?

   a. Urinary retention

   b. Seizure disorder

   c. Myocardial infarction

   d. Cerebrovascular disease

3. A nurse is caring for a patient undergoing antidepressant therapy. The patient is also receiving warfarin for circulatory disorders. Which of the following risks should the nurse monitor for in the patient?

   a. Increased risk for bleeding

   b. Increased risk for hypotension

   c. Increased anticholinergic symptoms

   d. Increased risk for nervous system depression

4. A nurse is caring for a patient with bulimia nervosa. The patient receives a prescription for fluoxetine, an SSRI. Which of the following is an adverse reaction of this type of drug that the nurse should monitor for in the patient?

   a. Vertigo

   b. Blurred vision

   c. Somnolence

   d. Tremor

5. A patient under treatment with MAO inhibitor antidepressants shows symptoms including a headache followed by a sore neck, nausea, vomiting, sweating, fever, chest

pain, dilated pupils, and bradycardia indicative of hypertensive crisis. Which of the following factors needs immediate attention?

a. Blood pressure

b. Blood sugar

c. Temperature

d. Respiration rate

6. A nurse is caring for a patient under treatment with trazodone. Which of the following is a major adverse reaction that the nurse should ask the patient to report immediately?

a. Priapism

b. Orthostatic hypotension

c. Insomnia

d. Diarrhea

7. A nurse is required to administer antidepressant therapy to an outpatient. Which of the following activities should the nurse perform as a part of preadministration assessment? Select all that apply.

a. Obtain a complete medical history

b. Obtain blood pressure measurements

c. Obtain a complete blood count

d. Obtain blood sugar levels

e. Obtain pulse and respiratory rates

8. A nurse is caring for a patient receiving MAO inhibitor antidepressants. The nurse instructs the patient to avoid foods containing tyramine. Which of the following can result from tyramine interacting with a MAO inhibitor antidepressant?

a. Blurred vision

b. Hypertensive crisis

c. Orthostatic hypotension

d. Photosensitivity

9. A nurse is caring for a patient undergoing antidepressant therapy. The nurse observes the patient showing signs of orthostatic hypotension. What intervention should the nurse perform in this case?

a. Instruct the patient to change positions slowly

b. Instruct the patient to drink plenty of fluids

c. Monitor the patient for hyperglycemia

d. Monitor the patient's vital signs frequently

10. A nurse is caring for a patient with bulimia nervosa who has been prescribed fluoxetine. Which of the following should the nurse identify as the best time to administer an SSRI?

a. At bedtime

b. With dinner

c. In the morning

d. With lunch

Central Nervous System Stimulants

SECTION I: ASSESSING YOUR UNDERSTANDING

Activity A MATCHING

1. Match the interactant drug in Column A with the likely effect of interaction in Column B when the drug is combined with a central nervous system (CNS) stimulant.

Column A

___ 1. Anesthetics

___ 2. Theophylline

___ 3. Modafinil

Column B

A. Decreases effect of oral contraceptives

B. Increases risk of cardiac arrhythmias

C. Increases risk of hyperactive behaviors

Activity B FILL IN THE BLANKS

1. Analeptics increase the depth of respirations by stimulating special receptors located in the _____ arteries and upper aorta.

2. Modafinil analeptic is used to treat _____.

3. Amphetamines are _____ drugs that stimulate the CNS.

4. The doxapram drug increases the respiratory rate by stimulating the _____.

5. When a CNS stimulant is administered with anesthetics, there is an increased risk of cardiac _____.

SECTION II: APPLYING YOUR KNOWLEDGE

Activity C SHORT ANSWERS

A nurse's role in managing patients who are administered CNS stimulants involves understanding the effects of the drugs and performing appropriate interventions depending on the type of drugs administered. Answer the following questions, which involve the nurse's role in managing such situations.

1. A nurse is caring for a patient undergoing CNS stimulant treatment. What are the nursing interventions while caring for a patient with an ineffective breathing pattern and being administered CNS stimulants?

_____

_____

_____

2. A nurse is caring for a patient undergoing CNS stimulant treatment. What are the nursing interventions for a patient experiencing nausea and vomiting from an analeptic?

_____

_____

_____

Activity D DOSAGE CALCULATION

1. A patient has been prescribed 400 mg of modafinil per day. The available tablets consist of 100 mg of drug each. How many tablets will the nurse administer to the patient daily?

   _____

2. A patient has been prescribed 80 mg of doxapram HCl to be administered intravenously. The drug is available in 20-mL vials containing 400 mg of the drug. How many milliliters of the available solution should be administered to the patient? _____

3. A patient has been prescribed 20 mg of Focalin twice a day. The available tablets are 10 mg each. How many tablets will the nurse administer to the patient daily? _____

4. A patient has been prescribed 15 mg of Meridia once daily. The available tablets are 5 mg each. How many tablets will the nurse administer to the patient daily? _____

5. A patient has been prescribed 90 mg of Meridia, to be taken over a period of 6 days. The available tablets are 15 mg each. How many tablets will the nurse administer to the patient each day? _____

SECTION III: PRACTICING FOR NCLEX

Activity E

Answer the following questions.

1. A nurse is caring for a patient who is receiving CNS stimulants. Which of the following adverse reactions should the nurse monitor for in this patient?
   a. Bradycardia
   b. Hyperactivity
   c. High blood pressure
   d. Elevated temperature

2. Which of the following points should the nurse include in the teaching plan for patients who are being administered CNS stimulants for attention deficit hyperactivity disorder (ADHD)?
   a. Administer drug ½ hour before breakfast
   b. Administer drug in the late afternoon

   c. Administer drug with milk, not water
   d. Dissolve drug in milk or water before consuming

3. With which of the following conditions is the use of CNS stimulants contraindicated?
   a. Liver disorders
   b. Acute ulcerative colitis
   c. Ventilation mechanism disorders
   d. Bone marrow suppression

4. Which of the following reactions could occur if theophylline is combined with CNS stimulants?
   a. Decreased effectiveness of the CNS stimulant
   b. Increased risk of cardiac arrhythmias
   c. Increased risk of hyperactive behaviors
   d. Decreased effectiveness of theophylline

5. Which of the following interventions should the nurse perform as part of the ongoing assessment after administering an analeptic?
   a. Send a blood sample for a platelet count test
   b. Check pulse rate and blood pressure every hour
   c. Monitor consciousness levels every 5 to 15 minutes
   d. Monitor respiratory rate for 5 minutes after administration

6. A nurse is caring for a patient on CNS stimulant therapy. The patient complains of insomnia. Which of the following interventions should the nurse perform to diminish sleep disturbances?
   a. Encourage patient to avoid napping during daytime
   b. Administer the drug in the evening, if possible
   c. Offer stimulants such as coffee or tea
   d. Administer any over-the-counter (OTC) sleeping pills

7. CNS stimulants have been prescribed for a child with ADHD. Which of the following points should the nurse include in the teaching plan? Select all that apply.
   a. Monitor the child's eating patterns
   b. Teach the parents the importance of preparing nutritious meals

c. Provide a light breakfast so that the child stays alert

d. Advise parents to give OTC sleeping pills in case of insomnia

e. Check the child's height and weight measurements to monitor growth

8. A patient is prescribed amphetamines as part of obesity treatment. Which of the following interventions should the nurse perform as part of the preadministration process? Select all that apply.

a. Record blood pressure

b. Observe urinary output

c. Record height

d. Measure blood glucose

e. Record weight

CHAPTER 26

Antipsychotic Drugs

SECTION I: ASSESSING YOUR UNDERSTANDING

MATCHING

1. Match the drugs in Column A with the effects in Column B that are produced when interacting with antipsychotic drugs.

Column A

____ 1. Anticholinergic drugs

____ 2. Immunologic drugs

____ 3. Antacids

____ 4. Loop diuretics

Column B

A. Decreased effectiveness of lithium

B. Increased risk for tardive dyskinesia (TD) and psychotic symptoms

C. Increased risk for lithium toxicity

D. Increased severity of bone marrow suppression

2. Match the conditions in Column A with their manifestations in Column B.

Column A

____ 1. Hallucinations

____ 2. Delusions

____ 3. Flattened affect

____ 4. Anhedonia

Column B

A. False beliefs that cannot be changed with reason

B. Finding no pleasure in activities that are normally pleasurable

C. False perceptions having no basis in reality

D. Absence of an emotional response to any situation or condition

FILL IN THE BLANKS

1. _____ disorder is a psychiatric disorder characterized by severe mood swings, from extreme hyperactivity to depression.

2. Antipsychotic drugs are thought to act by inhibiting or blocking the release of the neurotransmitter _____ in the brain.

3. Atypical antipsychotics act upon _____ receptors as well as the dopamine receptors in the brain.

4. _____ affect is the absence of an emotional response to any situation or condition.

5. The term _____ syndrome refers to a group of adverse reactions occurring in the extrapyramidal portion of the nervous system as a result of antipsychotic drugs.

SECTION II: APPLYING YOUR KNOWLEDGE

SHORT ANSWERS

A nurse's role in managing patients being administered antipsychotic drugs involves monitoring and performing interventions for serious manifestations of acute psychosis. Answer the following questions, which involve the nurse's role in managing such situations.

1. What should a nurse assess for in the patient before administering the first dose of an antipsychotic drug?

_____

_____

_____

2. A patient receiving Risperdal is showing signs of hallucinations. What should the nurse closely monitor for in this patient?

_____

_____

_____

Activity D DOSAGE CALCULATION

1. A physician prescribes 400 mg of Thorazine daily for a patient with psychiatric disorders. The available Thorazine tablet is 100 mg. How many tablets will the nurse administer to the patient? _____

2. A physician prescribes 5 mg of haloperidol daily to be administered intramuscularly. After reconstitution, the concentration of the drug is 2 mg/mL. How many milliliters should the nurse administer to the patient? _____

3. A physician prescribes 1200 mg of lithium per day in divided doses for a patient having manic episodes of bipolar disorder. The available lithium tablet is 300 mg. How many total tablets will the nurse administer to the patient? _____

4. A physician prescribes 100 mg of Moban in two doses to a patient with schizophrenia. Moban is available as syrup in 120-mL bottles with a concentration of 20 mg/mL. How many milliliters should the nurse administer to the patient in a single dose? _____

5. A physician prescribes 5 mg of Compazine three times a day for a patient with anxiety. Compazine is available as 120-mL syrup. 5 mL of Compazine is equivalent to 5 mg. How many milliliters should the nurse administer to the patient? _____

SECTION III: PRACTICING FOR NCLEX

Activity E

Answer the following questions.

1. A patient who received Haldol has developed photosensitivity. What should the nurse include in patient teaching?

a. Ask the patient to minimize alcohol use

b. Ask the patient to avoid natural sunlight

c. Suggest the patient use tanning beds

d. Suggest the patient drink at least 5 five glasses of water per day

2. A nurse has administered lithium carbonate to a patient. Which of the following adverse reactions should the nurse monitor in the patient?

a. Rashes

b. Polyuria

c. Dystonia

d. Insomnia

3. Before beginning antipsychotic drug therapy, a nurse is required to assess a patient. Which of the following should the nurse record as deviations from normal behavior?

a. Shy or timid behavior

b. Brief replies to questions

c. Frequent laughter

d. Poor eye contact

4. A patient is displaying violent behavior, and antipsychotic drugs have to be given parenterally. Which of the following interventions should the nurse perform while administering the drug?

a. Administer the drug intravenously to the patient

b. Ensure the injection site has minimal muscle mass

c. Ensure the patient remains upright after the injection

d. Ensure that assistance is available for securing the patient

5. A nurse is required to give antipsychotic drugs to a patient orally. Which of the following interventions should the nurse perform during the drug regimen?

a. Give the drugs in one single daily dose only, not in divided doses

b. Confirm whether the drug has been swallowed by asking the patient

c. Mix the drug in liquids such as fruit juice, tomato juice, or milk

d. Compel the patient to swallow the drug if he or she refuses to do so

6. Which of the following are symptoms of TD that the nurse should report immediately?

    a. Dry feeling in mouth

    b. Rhythmic face movements

    c. Orthostatic hypotension

    d. Lethargy or drowsiness

7. A schizophrenic patient has been prescribed clozapine. Which of the following points should the nurse include in the teaching program?

    a. Purchase a month's supply of the drug

    b. Schedule white blood cell (WBC) count tests every 2 weeks

    c. Continue WBC test for 1 week after the end of therapy

    d. Monitor the patient for bone marrow suppression

8. A nurse is required to obtain a blood sample from a patient in the acute phase to test serum lithium levels. Which of the following interventions should the nurse perform?

    a. Obtain a sample at least 5 hours after the last dose

    b. Monitor patient for muscular weakness

    c. Monitor serum lithium levels every 2 weeks

    d. Obtain sample 1 hour before next dose

9. A patient with schizophrenia has been prescribed chlorpromazine. If symptoms of hypotension and sedation are observed after administration of the drug, which of the following interventions should the nurse perform to minimize the risk of injury to the patient?

    a. Administer the drug with food

    b. Administer the drug with a calcium supplement

    c. Administer the drug every 8 hours

    d. Administer the drug at bedtime

10. A patient who has undergone antipsychotic drug therapy is being discharged from a health care facility. Which of the following points should the nurse include in the teaching plan? Select all that apply.

    a. Report any unusual changes or physical effects

    b. Inform the patient about the risks of extrapyramidal symptoms and TD

    c. Decrease dosage if the symptoms increase

    d. Take the drug on an empty stomach

    e. Avoid exposure to the sun

Adrenergic Drugs

SECTION I: ASSESSING YOUR UNDERSTANDING

Activity A MATCHING

1. Match the drug names in Column A with their corresponding contraindications in Column B.

Column A

B 1. Isoproterenol

C 2. Dopamine

D 3. Midodrine

A 4. Epinephrine

Column B

A. Narrow-angle glaucoma

B. Tachyarrhythmias

C. Ventricular fibrillation

D. Severe hypertension

2. Match the drugs in Column A with their effects when mixed with adrenergic drugs in Column B.

Column A

C 1. Antidepressants

A 2. Oxytocin

D 3. Bretylium

B 4. Dilantin

Column B

A. Increased risk of hypertension

B. Increased risk of bradycardia

C. Increased sympathomimetic effect

D. Increased risk of arrhythmias

Activity B FILL IN THE BLANKS

1. Adrenergic drugs are useful in improving hemodynamic status by improving **myocardial** contractility and increasing heart rate.

2. The autonomic nervous system is divided into the sympathetic and the **parasympathetic** nervous branches.

3. Supine **hypertension** is a potentially dangerous adverse reaction that can occur when a patient is taking midodrine.

4. Adrenergic drugs are classified as pregnancy category **C** and are used with extreme caution during pregnancy.

5. **Vasopressors** are drugs that raise the blood pressure because of their ability to constrict blood vessels.

SECTION II: APPLYING YOUR KNOWLEDGE

Activity C SHORT ANSWERS

A nurse's role in managing patients who are being administered adrenergic drugs involves monitoring and interventions. Answer the following questions, which involve the nurse's role in managing such situations.

1. A patient is admitted to a health care facility after receiving a shock. The primary care provider has recommended an adrenergic drug. What should a nurse assess for in the patient before administering the first dose?

    Mental status + Past Med Hx.
    V/s, s/s, probs. needs any
    subjective/objective data documented

2. A nurse is monitoring a patient receiving metaraminol. What are the appropriate nursing interventions involved during the ongoing administration of metaraminol?

Monitor effect of drug, V/s, compare c̄ pre assessment, report Adv. Rt to MD

Activity D DOSAGE CALCULATION

1. A patient is prescribed 20 mg of midodrine HCl per day. The available tablet contains 10 mg of midodrine HCl. How many tablets are needed daily to meet the prescribed drug level? _____

2. A primary health care provider has prescribed 15 mg of ProAmatine to be taken orally three times a day. The available tablets contain ProAmatine equivalent to 5 mg. The nurse should administer how many tablets in a day? _____

3. A primary health care provider prescribes 2.5 mg of Requip, a dopamine agonist, to be taken orally four times a day. The available tablets are 5 mg. How many tablets will the nurse administer to the patient daily? _____

4. A patient is prescribed 10 mg of Aramine to be administered intramuscularly. Aramine is available as a solution in 10-mL vials with a concentration of 100 mg of the drug. How many milliliters of Aramine should the nurse administer to the patient? _____

5. A primary health care provider prescribes 2 mg of Requip, a dopamine agonist, to be taken orally four times a day. The available tablets are 4 mg. How many tablets will the nurse administer to the patient daily? _____

SECTION III: PRACTICING FOR NCLEX

Activity E

Answer the following questions.

1. A nurse is required to administer metaraminol for a patient who is taking digoxin. The patient is at an increased risk for which of the following adverse reactions?

a. Epigastric distress
b. Pheochromocytoma
c. Cardiac arrhythmias
d. Decrease in blood pressure

2. For which of the following patients is isoproterenol contraindicated?

a. Patients with narrow-angle glaucoma
b. Patients with tachycardia
c. Patients with hypotension
d. Patients with pheochromocytoma

3. A 65-year-old patient has been prescribed isoproterenol. Which of the following should the nurse report immediately to the primary care provider?

a. Feelings of nausea
b. Changes in pulse rate
c. Severe headache
d. Urinary urgency

4. A patient has been prescribed midodrine. Which of the following is an adverse effect of midodrine that the nurse should monitor in the patient?

a. Supine hypertension
b. Tachycardia
c. Orthostatic hypotension
d. Respiratory distress

5. A nurse is required to administer dopamine to a patient. Which of the following nursing interventions should the nurse perform when caring for the client? Select all that apply.

a. Administer dopamine only through the intravenous route
b. Mix dopamine with alkaline solutions before administering
c. Use an electronic infusion pump to administer these drugs
d. Monitor blood pressure every 30 minutes
e. Inspect needle site and surrounding tissues at frequent intervals

6. A nurse is caring for a patient who has received metaraminol. Which of the following changes should the nurse immediately report to the primary care provider?

a. Consistent fall in blood pressure
b. Rise in blood glucose levels

c. Decrease in gastric motility

d. Increase in heart rate

7. A patient is experiencing insomnia during epinephrine therapy. Which of the following interventions should the nurse perform while caring for the client? Select all that apply.

a. Identify circumstances that disturb sleep

b. Draw curtains over windows

c. Provide bedtime snacks to the patient

d. Give frequent sips of tea and coffee

e. Administer drugs only during daytime

8. A nurse observes leakage of norepinephrine from the intravenous (IV) line. Which of the following interventions should the nurse perform to minimize tissue perfusion?

a. Discontinue old IV line immediately

b. Do not add another IV line unless instructed

c. Move the head of the bed to an elevated position

d. Mix alkaline solutions with norepinephrine

CHAPTER 28

Adrenergic Blocking Drugs

SECTION I: ASSESSING YOUR UNDERSTANDING

Activity A MATCHING

1. Match the drugs in Column A with the effect of their interaction with beta-adrenergic blockers in Column B.

Column A

B 1. Clonidine

D 2. Lidocaine

A 3. Antidepressants (monoamine oxidase inhibitors [MAOIs], selective serotonin reuptake inhibitors [SSRIs])

C 4. Loop diuretics

Column B

A. Increased effect of the beta-blocker and bradycardia

B. Increased risk of paradoxical hypertensive effect

C. Increased risk of hypotension

D. Increased serum level of the beta-blocker

2. Match the drugs in Column A with their common uses in Column B.

Column A

C 1. Adrenergics

D 2. Levodopa

B 3. Lithium

A 4. Anesthetic agents

Column B

A. Surgery

B. Treatment of psychosis

C. Management of cardiovascular problems

D. Management of Parkinson's disease

Activity B FILL IN THE BLANKS

1. **Norepinephrine** is the substance that transmits nerve impulses across the sympathetic branch of the autonomic nervous system.

2. **Sympatholytic** drugs block the transmission of norepinephrine in the sympathetic system.

3. When **Phentolamine** is administered with epinephrine, vasoconstrictor and hypertensive action decreases.

4. Beta-adrenergic blocking drugs are also called beta-**blockers**

5. **Glaucoma** is a narrowing or blockage of the drainage channels between the anterior and posterior chambers of the eye.

6. **Sotalol** is given on an empty stomach because food may reduce absorption of the drug.

SECTION II: APPLYING YOUR KNOWLEDGE

Activity C SHORT ANSWERS

A nurse's role in managing a patient who is prescribed adrenergic blocking drugs involves assisting the patient by conducting a preadministration assessment and monitoring. Answer the following questions, which involve the nurse's role in managing patients on adrenergic blocking drug therapy.

1. A patient is prescribed an adrenergic blocking drug. What preadministration assessments should the nurse follow before administering the adrenergic blocking drug?

_____

_____

_____

2. What are the nursing interventions for a patient receiving adrenergic blocking drug therapy for hypertension?

_____

_____

_____

Activity D DOSAGE CALCULATION

1. A patient has received a prescription for 20 mg of bisoprolol every 24 hours. The available drug is in a 5-mg tablet. To meet the prescribed dose, how many tablets should the nurse administer each day? _____

2. A patient with hypertension has been prescribed 30 mg of pindolol twice daily. The drug is available in 10-mg tablets at the local pharmacy. The patient would like to know the total number of tablets he should buy to meet the prescribed dose for a 3-day course. What is the total number of tablets required for this patient? _____

3. A patient has been prescribed 10 mg of alfuzosin daily. The available drug is in the form of a 10-mg tablet. The patient would like to know the total number of tablets he should buy to meet the prescribed dose for a 9-day course. What is the total number of tablets required for this patient? _____

4. A patient with hypertension has been prescribed 5 mg of doxazosin daily. The drug is available in 1-mg tablets at the local pharmacy. The patient would like to know the total number of tablets he should buy to meet the prescribed dose for a 10-day course. What is the total number of tablets required for this patient? _____

5. A patient has been prescribed 10 mg of prazosin every 24 hours. The available drug is in the form of a 5-mg tablet. To meet the pre-

scribed dose, how many tablets should the nurse administer each day? _____

SECTION III: PRACTICING FOR NCLEX

Activity E

Answer the following questions.

1. A patient with pheochromocytoma is admitted to a health care facility. The physician prescribes phentolamine, an alpha-adrenergic blocking drug, to the patient. Which of the following reactions should the nurse monitor for in the patient?
   a. Diarrhea
   b. Orthostatic hypotension
   c. Bradycardia
   d. Bronchospasm

2. The nurse is documenting the history of a patient who is beginning alpha-adrenergic blocking drug therapy. In which of these conditions are alpha-adrenergic blocking drugs contraindicated?
   a. Sinus bradycardia
   b. Heart failure
   c. Coronary artery disease
   d. Emphysema

3. A nurse is caring for a patient receiving adrenergic blocking drugs. Which of the following actions should the nurse perform when the patient receiving adrenergic blocking drugs shows a decrease in blood pressure?
   a. Monitor for excessive perspiration
   b. Monitor for confusion
   c. Adjust into a more conducive position
   d. Discontinue the drug

4. A nurse is caring for an elderly patient. The physician has prescribed a beta-adrenergic blocking drug to the patient. What should the nurse monitor for in the elderly patient when administering a beta-adrenergic blocking drug?
   a. Vascular insufficiency
   b. Occipital headache
   c. Dizziness
   d. Central nervous system (CNS) depression

5. A nurse is caring for a patient on beta-adrenergic blocker therapy. The patient is also to be administered lidocaine. Which of the following risks will this maximize?

   a. Increased risk of hypotension

   b. Increased serum level of the beta-blocker

   c. Increased risk of paradoxical hypertensive effect

   d. Increased effect of the beta-blocker

6. A nurse is caring for a patient who has been administered prazosin. For which of the following adverse reactions should the nurse monitor the patient who is receiving peripherally acting antiadrenergic drugs?

   a. Dry mouth

   b. Drowsiness

   c. Malaise

   d. Light-headedness

7. A nurse is caring for a patient whose physician has prescribed the sympatholytic drug propranolol for him. What nursing interventions should the nurse perform when the patient is administered this sympatholytic drug?

   a. Measure the apical pulse rate

   b. Measure the body temperature

   c. Measure the heart rate

   d. Measure the respiration rate

8. A nurse at a health care center is assigned to prepare a teaching plan for a patient undergoing adrenergic blocking drug ther-apy for glaucoma. Which of the following should the nurse include in the patient's teaching plan?

   a. Monitor his or her own pulse and blood pressure

   b. Take drugs as directed, with food or on an empty stomach

   c. Contact the primary health care provider if vision changes occur

   d. Keep ambulating often

9. A nurse is caring for a patient with glaucoma. The patient is administered a beta-adrenergic blocking ophthalmic preparation, such as timolol. What is the role of the nurse in determining the effect of drug therapy?

   a. Measure intraocular pressure of the patient

   b. Monitor blood pressure of the patient

   c. Monitor respiratory rate of the patient

   d. Measure the pulse rate of the patient

10. A patient has been administered an anti-adrenergic drug. The patient has also been taking haloperidol for the treatment of psychosis. Which of the following interactions should the nurse monitor for in the patient?

   a. Increased risk of lithium toxicity

   b. Increased risk of psychotic behavior

   c. Increase risk of hypertension

   d. Increased anesthetic effects

CHAPTER 29

Cholinergic Drugs

SECTION I: ASSESSING YOUR UNDERSTANDING

Activity A MATCHING

1. Match the disorders in Column A with the treatment effect with cholinergic drugs in Column B.

Column A

B 1. Myasthenia gravis

C 2. Urinary retention

A 3. Glaucoma

Column B

A. Produces constriction of the iris

B. Inhibits the activity of acetylcholinesterase

C. Contracts the bladder smooth muscles

2. Match the cholinergic drugs in Column A with their uses in Column B.

Column A

B 1. Edrophonium

C 2. Bethanechol chloride

A 3. Carbachol

Column B

A. Treats glaucoma

B. Diagnoses myasthenia gravis

C. Treats acute nonobstructive urinary retention

Activity B FILL IN THE BLANKS

1. **Muscarinic** receptors stimulate the smooth muscle.

2. Cholinergic drugs mimic the activity of the **Parasympathetic** nervous system.

3. **Acetylcoline** is the substance that transmits nerve impulses across the parasympathetic branch of the autonomic nervous system.

4. Drugs that inhibit the enzyme acetylcholinesterase are called **anticholinesterase**

5. **Nicotinic** receptors stimulate the skeletal muscles in the parasympathetic nerve branch of the autonomic nervous system.

SECTION II: APPLYING YOUR KNOWLEDGE

Activity C SHORT ANSWERS

A nurse's role in managing patients with myasthenia gravis involves monitoring them and implementing interventions that aid in their recovery. Answer the following questions, which involve the nurse's role in the management of such situations.

1. A patient with myasthenia gravis has been prescribed ambenonium. What should a nurse assess for in the patient before administering the first dose?

_____

_____

_____

2. A patient is undergoing treatment for myasthenia gravis. What should the nurse explain to the patient about the disorder and the drug to be administered for myasthenia gravis?

_____

_____

_____

Activity D DOSAGE CALCULATION

1. A physician prescribes 70 mg of Mytelase four times a day for the treatment of myasthenia gravis. Mytelase is available as 10-mg tablets. How many tablets should the nurse administer to the patient for the whole day?

   _____

2. A patient has been prescribed 30 mg of bethanechol chloride three times a day for the treatment of urinary retention. Bethanechol chloride is available as 5-mg tablets. How many tablets should the nurse administer to the patient in a single dose? _____

3. A patient has been prescribed 0.2 mL of carbachol five times a day. Carbachol is available as 1.0-mL sterile glass vials. How many vials should the patient be administered in a single day? _____

4. A physician has prescribed 240 mg of Mestinon over two doses for myasthenia gravis. Mestinon is available as 60-mg tablets. How many tablets should the nurse administer to the patient for each dose? _____

5. A patient has been prescribed 5 mg of edrophonium intravenously. Edrophonium is available as 15-mL vials. One mL of edrophonium is equivalent to 10 mg. How many milliliters should the nurse administer to the patient? _____

SECTION III: PRACTICING FOR NCLEX

Activity E

Answer the following questions.

1. A nurse is caring for a patient with urinary retention. Which of the following adverse effects should the nurse monitor for during the topical administration of cholinergic drugs?

   a. Temporary reduction of visual acuity
   b. Increased ocular tension
   c. Decreased sweat production
   d. Anaphylactic shock

2. A patient has been prescribed the pilocarpine ocular system. What should the nurse instruct the patient about the system?

   a. Remove and replace the system every 7 days
   b. Instruct the patient that replacement is best during daytime
   c. Change the system every day if eye secretions are excessive
   d. Instruct the patient to carry identification about the disorder

3. A physician has prescribed bethanechol to a patient for acute nonobstructive urinary retention. What should the nurse check in the patient before administration of bethanechol?

   a. Tachyarrhythmias
   b. Myocardial infarction
   c. Coronary occlusion
   d. Mechanical obstruction of the gastrointestinal tract

4. A patient with myasthenia gravis has been prescribed ambenonium. The patient informs the nurse that he has respiratory problems and is under corticosteroid treatment. Which of the following effects of interactions between the two drugs should the nurse anticipate in the patient?

   a. Increased neuromuscular blocking effect
   b. Decreased effect of the cholinergic
   c. Increased absorption of the cholinergic
   d. Decreased serum level of corticosteroids

5. A nurse is caring for a patient undergoing Pilopine drug therapy for glaucoma. Which of the following should be the ongoing assessments for the patient after instilling the drug?

   a. Assess for signs of muscle weakness in the patient
   b. Dry the upper respiratory and oral secretions
   c. Remove excessive secretions with a cotton ball soaked in normal saline solution
   d. Measure and record the fluid intake and output

6. A patient is undergoing cholinergic drug therapy. The nurse knows that which other drug needs to be used cautiously if it has to be administered along with cholinergic drugs?

   a. Salicylates
   b. Analgesics

c. Aminoglycoside antibiotics
d. Antidiabetics

7. What interventions should the nurse perform when caring for a patient who has been prescribed Miostat? Select all that apply.
a. Instill drug in lower conjunctival sac
b. Avoid tip of dropper touching the eye
c. Support hand by holding dropper against patient's forehead
d. Allow patient to instill his or her own eye drops
e. Instruct the patient to wear or carry identification

8. A nurse is caring for a patient with myasthenia gravis. The patient has been administered pyridostigmine bromide. What symptoms of drug overdose should the nurse monitor in the patient to make frequent dosage adjustments? Select all that apply.
a. Drooping of the eyelids
b. Rapid fatigability of the muscles
c. Salivation
d. Clenching of the jaw
e. Muscle rigidity and spasm

9. A patient has been admitted for urinary retention. What is the role of the nurse when caring for the patient receiving cholinergic therapy?
a. Instruct the patient to void before the drug is administered
b. Encourage the patient to take the drug with milk to enhance absorption
c. Place the call light and items that patient might need within easy reach
d. Encourage the patient to have five to seven glasses of water after drug administration

10. Which of the following interventions should the nurse perform if the patient develops diarrhea after taking Urecholine orally? Select all that apply.
a. Ensure that the bedpan or bathroom is readily available
b. Check for bloodstains in the stool
c. Encourage the patient to ambulate to assist the passing of flatus
d. Encourage the patient to increase fibrous food intake
e. Record the number, consistency, and frequency of stools

Cholinergic Blocking Drugs

SECTION I: ASSESSING YOUR UNDERSTANDING

Activity A MATCHING

1. Match the cholinergic blocking drugs in Column A with their uses in Column B.

Column A	Column B
D 1. Atropine	A. Treatment of irritable bowel syndrome
C 2. Belladonna alkaloids	B. Adjunctive treatment of peptic ulcer
A 3. Dicyclomine HCl	C. Adjunctive therapy for diverticulitis
B 4. Mepenzolate bromide	D. Treatment of pylorospasm

2. Match the adverse reactions associated with cholinergic blocking drugs in Column A with the measures to lessen their intensity in Column B.

Column A	Column B
C 1. Photophobia	A. Chew gum or dissolve hard candy in mouth
A 2. Dry mouth	B. Schedule tasks requiring alertness before the first dose of the drug is taken
D 3. Constipation	
B 4. Drowsiness	

C. Schedule outdoor activities before the first dose of the drug is taken

D. Eat foods high in fiber

Activity B FILL IN THE BLANKS

1.  Acetylcholine is the primary neurotransmitter in the parasympathetic branch of the autonomic nervous system.

2. Cholinergic blocking drugs inhibit the activity of acetylcholine at the Parasympathetic nerve synapse.

3. Cycloplegia is a type of visual impairment occurring due to the use of cholinergic blocking drugs, which is characterized by a difficulty in focusing, resulting from paralysis of the ciliary muscle.

4. The nurse should use Atropine with caution in patients with asthma.

5. An unexpected or unusual reaction to cholinergic blocking drugs is known as drug Idiosyncrasy

SECTION II: APPLYING YOUR KNOWLEDGE

Activity C SHORT ANSWERS

A nurse's role in caring for patients receiving cholinergic blocking drugs involves monitoring and managing patients' needs and helping them in their recovery. Answer the following questions, which involve the nurse's role in the management of such situations.

1. A nurse has been caring for a patient with a peptic ulcer. Which of the following points should the nurse include when evaluating the patient's treatment plan?

_____

_____

_____

2. What instructions should the nurse offer an elderly patient's family when monitoring the patient receiving cholinergic blocking drugs?

_____

_____

_____

Activity D   DOSAGE CALCULATION

1. A patient with an overactive bladder receives 60 mg of trospium per day. The drug is available in 20-mg tablets. How many tablets should the nurse administer per day to meet the recommended dose?_____

2. The physician has prescribed 800 mg of flavoxate for a patient to be administered four times a day. The available drug is in 100-mg tablets. How many tablets should the nurse administer each time to meet the recommended dose?_____

3. A patient with peptic ulcers is prescribed 0.25 mg of glycopyrrolate to be injected in a patient intramuscularly. The available drug is in a 0.2 mg/mL solution. How much glycopyrrolate should the nurse prepare to be administered to the patient?_____

4. A patient with irritable bowel syndrome is prescribed 120 mg of dicyclomine HCl, to be administered four times per day. The available drug is in 10-mg tablets. How many tablets should the nurse administer to the patient each time?_____

SECTION III: PRACTICING FOR NCLEX

Activity E

Answer the following questions.

1. In which of the following patients should a nurse use atropine cautiously?
   a. Patients with tachyarrhythmias
   b. Patients with myasthenia gravis
   c. Patients with glaucoma
   d. Patients with asthma

2. A patient is being administered propantheline bromide for the treatment of a peptic ulcer. After administration of the drug, the patient complains of constipation. Which of the following instructions should the nurse provide this patient to help relieve constipation?
   a. Consume an antacid after meals for severe constipation
   b. Increase the consumption of food rich in fiber
   c. Increase the consumption of citrus fruits
   d. Restrict fluid consumption to prevent urinary frequency

3. Which of the following interventions should a nurse perform when caring for a patient receiving atropine for third-degree heart block?
   a. Place the patient on a cardiac monitor before drug administration
   b. Provide oxygen support to the patient every hour
   c. Monitor for symptoms of mydriasis and cycloplegia
   d. Monitor for a change in pulse rate or rhythm

4. A patient with bladder overactivity is admitted to a health care facility. The nurse administers a cholinergic blocking drug to the patient, as prescribed by the physician. The drug is known to cause heat prostration. What instructions should the nurse offer the patient to help lessen the intensity of heat prostration? Select all that apply.

a. Wear loose-fitting clothes
b. Sponge the skin with cool water
c. Apply sunscreen when outside
d. Use fans to cool the body
e. Wear sunglasses when outdoors

5. A patient with excessive vagal-induced brady-cardia has been prescribed atropine. The patient informs the nurse that he is receiving tricyclic antidepressants to treat depression. What effect of this drug interaction should the nurse assess for in the patient?
   a. Decreased effectiveness of the antidepressant
   b. Increased respiratory rate
   c. Increased effect of atropine
   d. Decreased blood pressure

6. A nurse is administering glycopyrrolate to a patient through the parenteral route to reduce bronchial and oral secretions. Which of the following adverse reactions of the drug should the nurse monitor for in this patient? Select all that apply.
   a. Nausea
   b. Altered taste perception
   c. Tachycardia
   d. Mydriasis
   e. Dysphagia

7. A nurse is caring for a 65-year-old patient with pylorospasm. Which of the following interventions should the nurse perform when caring for this patient as a part of pre-operative interventions?
   a. Ensure that a cholinergic drug is not administered preoperatively
   b. Monitor for changes in the patient's pulse rate or rhythm

c. Ensure that the patient has not received antibiotics recently
d. Position the patient in Fowler's position

8. A nurse needs to administer a cholinergic blocking drug preoperatively to a patient. Why should the nurse administer the drug to the patient at the exact time prescribed by the physician?
   a. To avoid abdominal cramping in the patient after drug administration
   b. To ensure effectiveness of the drug after administration of the anesthetic
   c. To allow the drug to produce its greatest effect before administration of the anesthetic
   d. To avoid excessive salivation and make the patient feel comfortable

9. A nurse is caring for a patient with bladder overactivity. The physician has prescribed oxybutynin to the patient. Which of the following conditions should the nurse monitor for in the patient if the drug is administered on a daily basis?
   a. Mydriasis
   b. Mouth dryness
   c. Blurred vision
   d. Hesitancy

10. A nurse is caring for a patient who has been administered atropine preoperatively to reduce the production of secretions in the respiratory tract. Which of the following drug reactions should the nurse identify as a part of the desired response?
    a. Vomiting
    b. Elevated temperature
    c. Low pulse rate
    d. Drowsiness

Anticonvulsants

SECTION I: ASSESSING YOUR UNDERSTANDING

Activity A MATCHING

1. Match the anticonvulsant drugs in Column A with their uses in Column B.

Column A	Column B
C 1. Diamox	A. Neuropathic pain
A 2. Lyrica	B. Preanesthetic
D 3. Diastat	C. Altitude sickness
B 4. Ativan	D. Anxiety disorders

2. Match the anticonvulsant drugs in Column A with their adverse reactions in Column B.

Column A	Column B
C 1. Epitol	A. Urinary frequency, pruritus, urticaria
D 2. Peganone	B. Ataxia, visual disturbances, rash
B 3. Klonopin	C. Unsteady gait, aplastic anemia, and other blood cell abnormalities
A 4. Zarontin	D. Hypotension, nystagmus, slurred speech

Activity B FILL IN THE BLANKS

1. Sudden involuntary contraction of the muscles of the body, often accompanied by loss of consciousness, is termed as a *convulsion*

2. *Hydantoins* stabilize hyperexcitability post-synaptically in the motor cortex of the brain.

3. *Oxa* _____ decrease the repetitive synaptic transmission of nerve impulses.

4. The *succinides* are contraindicated in patients with bone marrow depression or hepatic or renal impairment.

5. The *barbiturates* are used with caution in patients with pulmonary disease and in hyperactive children.

SECTION II: APPLYING YOUR KNOWLEDGE

Activity C SHORT ANSWERS

A nurse's role in managing a patient who has been prescribed an anticonvulsant drug involves assisting the patient with preadministration assessment. The nurse also helps in monitoring patients who are receiving anticonvulsant drugs. Answer the following questions, which involve the nurse's role in the management of patients on anticonvulsant therapy.

1. A patient with seizures visits a health care facility and has been prescribed an anticonvulsant drug. What assessments should the nurse perform before the administration of an anticonvulsant drug?

_____

_____

_____

2. After the preadministration assessment, the nurse administers an anticonvulsant drug for seizure disorders. What is the nurse's role when caring for this patient?

_____

_____

_____

Activity D   DOSAGE CALCULATION

1. A patient has been prescribed 400 mg of Zonegran daily. The available drug is in the form of 50-mg capsules. The patient would like to know the total number of capsules he should buy for a 3-day course to meet the prescribed dose. What is the total number of capsules required for this patient?

_____

2. A patient has been prescribed 200 mg of Topamax daily. It is available in 100-mg capsules. The patient has to continue the drug therapy for 2 days. What is the total number of capsules required for this client?

_____

3. A patient is prescribed 500 mg of Depakote to be taken in equal doses two times a day orally. On-hand are 125-mg tablets. How many tablets should the nurse administer to the patient each time? _____

4. A patient has been prescribed 48 mg of Gabitril once a day orally. The drug is available in 12-mg tablets in a pharmacy store. How many tablets should the nurse administer to the client? _____

5. A patient has been prescribed 400 mg of Mysoline to be taken in four divided doses. The drug is available in 50-mg tablets. How many tablets should the nurse administer to the patient each time? _____

6. A patient has been prescribed 1200 mg of Trileptal to be taken in two divided doses. The drug is available in 300-mg tablets. How many tablets should the nurse administer to the patient each time? _____

SECTION III: PRACTICING FOR NCLEX

Activity E

Answer the following questions.

1. A physician has prescribed trimethadione to a patient with epilepsy at a health care facility. Which of the following should the nurse monitor for in the patient while administering trimethadione?
   a. Eye disorders
   b. Bone marrow depression
   c. Hypotension
   d. Myocardial insufficiency

2. A patient with anxiety disorders visits a health care facility. A physician prescribes tranxene to the patient. Which of the following adverse drug reactions should the nurse monitor in the patient?
   a. Dyspepsia
   b. Vomiting
   c. Fatigue
   d. Palpitations

3. A nurse at a health care center is assigned to prepare a teaching plan for a patient undergoing hydantoin drug therapy. Which of the following should the nurse include in the teaching plan of the patient? Select all that apply.
   a. Avoid taking the drugs during pregnancy
   b. Brush and floss teeth after each meal
   c. Avoid consumption of discolored capsules
   d. Notify primary health care provider if blurred vision occurs
   e. Take medication with food

4. A nurse is caring for a patient with tonic-clonic seizures in a health care facility. The physician has prescribed Dilantin to the patient. For which of the hematologic changes in the patient should the nurse immediately report to the primary health care provider?
   a. Sinus bradycardia
   b. Sinoatrial block
   c. Thrombocytopenia
   d. Adams-Stokes syndrome

5. A nurse is caring for a patient with disturbed sensory perception. The physician has prescribed Lamictal. What instructions should the nurse provide the patient receiving Lamictal? Select all that apply.

   a. Stay out of sun

   b. Wear sunscreen

   c. Wear protective clothes

   d. Wear light-colored clothes

   e. Place cotton pads soaked in rose water on the eyes

6. A nurse is assigned to care for a patient who has been prescribed phenytoin. In which of the following cases is the use of phenytoin contraindicated?

   a. History of asthma

   b. Cardiac problems

   c. Hepatic abnormalities

   d. Liver dysfunction

7. A nurse is caring for an elderly patient undergoing diazepam therapy. Which of the following interventions should the nurse perform for the patient?

   a. Examine the mouth and gums of the patient

   b. Examine the skin frequently

   c. Observe the patient for throat irritation

   d. Observe the patient for apnea and cardiac arrest

8. A nurse is caring for a patient on analgesic therapy, who will also receive an anticonvulsant drug. What possible effect should the nurse be aware of concerning the interaction of analgesics with anticonvulsants?

   a. Increased carbamazepine levels

   b. Increased seizure activity

   c. Increased blood glucose levels

   d. Increased depressant effect

9. A patient with seizures has been prescribed phenytoin at a health care facility. Which of the following would indicate drug toxicity?

   a. Plasma levels greater than 20 mcg/mL

   b. Phenytoin plasma levels greater than 20 mcg/mL

   c. Plasma levels greater than 30 mcg/mL

   d. Phenytoin plasma levels between 10 and 20 mcg/mL

10. A nurse is caring for a patient on barbiturate therapy for status epilepticus at a health care facility. What ongoing assessment should the nurse perform on the patient? Select all that apply.

   a. Document vital signs of the patient every 4 hours

   b. Document each seizure's time of occurrence

   c. Measure blood pressure every hour

   d. Measure serum plasma levels of the anticonvulsant

   e. Document each seizure's duration

CHAPTER 32

Antiparkinsonism Drugs

SECTION I: ASSESSING YOUR UNDERSTANDING

Activity A MATCHING

1. Match the dopaminergic agents in Column A with their adverse reactions in Column B.

Column A	Column B
____ 1. Amantadine	A. Dysphagia
____ 2. Bromocriptine	B. Orthostatic hypotension
____ 3. Carbidopa/ levodopa	C. Rhinitis
____ 4. Pergolide	D. Epigastric distress

2. Match the drugs in Column A with their uses in Column B.

Column A	Column B
____ 1. Bromocriptine	A. Treatment of drug-induced extrapyramidal symptoms
____ 2. Benztropine mesylate	B. Treatment of Parkinson's disease "off" episodes
____ 3. Entacapone	C. Treatment of female endocrine imbalances
____ 4. Apomorphine HCl	D. Adjunct to carbidopa/levodopa in Parkinson's disease

Activity B FILL IN THE BLANKS

1. _____ disease is a degenerative disorder of the central nervous system (CNS) caused by an imbalance of dopamine and acetylcholine within the CNS.

2. Failure of the muscles of the lower esophagus to relax, causing difficulty swallowing, is known as _____.

3. The _____ phenomenon occurs in patients taking levodopa in which the patient may suddenly alternate between improved clinical status and loss of therapeutic effect.

4. _____ movements are involuntary muscular twitches of the limbs or facial muscles.

5. _____ is a milder catechol-O-methyl-transferase (COMT) inhibitor used to help manage fluctuations in the response to levodopa in individuals with Parkinson's disease.

SECTION II: APPLYING YOUR KNOWLEDGE

Activity C SHORT ANSWERS

A nurse's role in managing parkinsonism involves assisting the patients with the administration of antiparkinsonism drugs. The nurse also helps in educating patients and their families about the treatment regimen. Answer the following questions, which involve the nurse's role in the management of such situations.

1. A nurse is assigned to care for a patient with Parkinson's disease. Under preadministration assessment, the nurse has to evaluate the patient's neuromuscular status. What should the nurse observe to evaluate the neuromuscular status of the patient?

_____

_____

_____

2. A nurse has been caring for a patient with Parkinson's disease. What factors should the nurse keep in mind when evaluating the treatment plan for the patient?

_____

_____

_____

3. A patient with Parkinson's disease is administered levodopa treatment. The patient's condition is alternating between improved clinical status and loss of therapeutic effect, and the patient is showing an on-off phenomenon. What nursing interventions should the nurse perform when caring for this patient?

_____

_____

_____

4. A patient with Parkinson's disease is vomiting and experiencing gastrointestinal (GI) disturbances. What interventions should the nurse perform when caring for this patient?

_____

_____

_____

5. A nurse has been caring for a patient on antiparkinsonism drugs. What information should the nurse include in her family and patient teaching plan when caring for this patient on an outpatient basis?

_____

_____

_____

Activity D DOSAGE CALCULATION

1. A patient with Parkinson's disease has been prescribed 400 mg of amantadine per day. The available drug is in a 100-mg capsule. To meet the recommended dose, how many capsules should the nurse administer each day?

_____

2. A patient is required to take 25 mg of Lodosyn per day with Sinemet. The ratio of carbidopa/levodopa in Sinemet is 1:10. If 25 mg of Lodosyn has to be taken with 100 mg of levodopa in the Sinemet then how

much Lodosyn should the patient consume if the carbidopa ratio in the Sinemet rises to 25 mg? _____

3. A patient with an off episode of Parkinson's disease has been prescribed 0.2 mL of benztropine mesylate. The dosage-administering mechanism consists of a pen that can deliver doses in increments of 0.02 mL. To meet the recommended dose, how many increments should the nurse administer to the patient each day? _____

4. A physician has prescribed 1000 mg of entacapone to a patient with Parkinson's disease. The available drug is in 200-mg tablets. To meet the recommended dose, how many tablets should the nurse administer to the patient each day? _____

SECTION III: PRACTICING FOR NCLEX

Activity E

Answer the following questions.

1. A nurse is caring for a patient who has been prescribed carbidopa. After administration of the drug, the nurse observes the occurrence of choreiform and dystonic movements in the patient. Which of the following interventions should the nurse perform when caring for this patient?
   a. Monitor vital signs frequently
   b. Withhold the next dose of the drug
   c. Offer frequent sips of water
   d. Observe the patient for nausea and fatigue

2. A nurse is caring for a patient receiving an antiparkinsonism drug. The patient is complaining of constipation. What instructions should the nurse offer the patient to help relieve constipation? Select all that apply.
   a. Decrease intake of carbohydrates
   b. Use a stool softener
   c. Increase intake of fiber in the diet
   d. Increase intake of fluids in the diet
   e. Increase intake of vitamin C

3. A nurse is assigned to care for a patient with neuroleptic malignant syndrome that has occurred because of the abrupt discontinuation of an antiparkinsonism drug. For which

of the following symptoms should the nurse monitor the patient? Select all that apply.

a. Muscular rigidity
b. Elevated body temperature
c. Mental changes
d. Tachycardia
e. Orthostatic hypotension

4. A nurse is caring for a patient who has been prescribed levodopa for the treatment of Parkinson's disease. The patient informs the nurse that he is taking antacids to relieve heartburn. What effect of the interaction of the two drugs should the nurse anticipate in the patient?

a. Increased risk of hypertension
b. Increased risk of dyskinesia
c. Increased effect of levodopa
d. Increased risk of cardiac symptoms

5. A nurse is assigned to care for a patient who has to be administered COMT inhibitors. Which of the following pieces of patient-related information should the nurse obtain to understand that the drug has to be administered cautiously to the patient?

a. Patient has decreased renal function
b. Patient has tachycardia
c. Patient has cardiac arrhythmias
d. Patient has GI tract problems

6. What should the nurse's plan include when a patient receiving antiparkinsonism drugs is discharged? Select all that apply.

a. Instruct the patient to avoid taking vitamin B_6 with levodopa
b. Instruct the patient to contact primary health care provider in case of severe dry mouth
c. Instruct the patient to avoid the consumption of alcohol
d. Instruct the patient to have small and frequent meals

e. Encourage the patient to increase their intake of vitamin C

7. A nurse is caring for a patient undergoing antiparkinsonism drug therapy. The nurse observes that the patient is vomiting frequently. Which of the following nursing interventions should the nurse perform when caring for this patient?

a. Change the antiparkinsonism drug
b. Administer the drug before meals
c. Administer antacids after meals
d. Refrain from giving liquids after meals

8. Which nursing interventions are appropriate when the patient is showing response to therapy with antiparkinsonism drugs?

a. Change the antiparkinsonism drug to another
b. Discontinue the use of antiparkinsonism drugs
c. Observe the patient's behavior at frequent intervals
d. Observe a drug holiday, as prescribed

9. A nurse is caring for a patient with parkinsonism. Which of the following conditions should the nurse observe that may indicate abdominal pain caused by constipation in the patient?

a. Change in facial expression
b. Change in style of walking
c. Change in diet intake
d. Change in sleeping patterns

10. For which category of patient is the use of cholinergic blocking drugs contraindicated?

a. Patients with bone marrow depression
b. Patients with cardiac disorders
c. Patients with visual impairment
d. Patients with prostatic hypertrophy

CHAPTER 33

Cholinesterase Inhibitors

SECTION I: ASSESSING YOUR UNDERSTANDING

Activity A MATCHING

1. Match the cholinesterase inhibitor drugs in Column A with their corresponding adverse reactions in Column B.

Column A	Column B
____ 1. Donepezil	**A.** Vomiting
____ 2. Memantin	**B.** Dyspepsia
____ 3. Rivastigmine	**C.** Confusion
____ 4. Tacrine	**D.** Muscle cramps

2. Match the interactant drugs in Column A with their corresponding uses in Column B.

Column A	Column B
____ 1. Anticholinergics	**A.** Breathing problems
____ 2. Nonsteroidal anti-inflammatory drugs	**B.** Decrease of bodily secretions
____ 3. Theophylline	**C.** Pain relief

Activity B FILL IN THE BLANKS

1. _____ disease is a progressive deterioration of emotional, physical, and cognitive abilities.

2. Acetylcholine is a transmitter in the _____ neuropathway.

3. Disease or injury to the _____ causes alanine aminotransferase (ALT) enzyme to be released into the bloodstream, resulting in elevated ALT levels.

4. In Alzheimer's disease, specific pathologic changes occur in the cortex of the _____.

5. Tacrine is particularly damaging to the liver and can result in _____.

SECTION II: APPLYING YOUR KNOWLEDGE

Activity C SHORT ANSWERS

A nurse's role in managing patients who are being administered cholinesterase inhibitors involves implementing interventions that aid in their recovery and monitoring the patients for occurrences of adverse reactions of the drug administration. Answer the following questions, which involve the nurse's role in managing such situations.

1. A patient is administered a cholinesterase inhibitor for treating mild-to-moderate dementia of Alzheimer's disease. What preadministration assessments should the nurse perform in patients who are prescribed cholinesterase inhibitors?

_____

_____

_____

2. A patient is administered tacrine for treating mild-to-moderate dementia of Alzheimer's disease.

   a. What interventions should a nurse perform when caring for the patient?

   _____

   _____

   _____

   b. What adverse reactions to tacrine administration should the nurse monitor for in the patient?

   _____

   _____

   _____

Activity D   DOSAGE CALCULATION

1. A physician prescribes 15 mg of donepezil hydrochloride per day for a patient with dementia of Alzheimer's disease. Donepezil is available in 5-mg tablets. How many tablets will the nurse have to administer to the patient in 3 days? _____

2. A patient with severe dementia of the Alzheimer's type is prescribed 200 mg of memantine for a period of 10 days. Memantine hydrochloride is supplied in 10-mg tablets. How many tablets should the nurse administer to the patient in 1 day?

   _____

3. A physician prescribes a total of 18 mg of rivastigmine tartrate for a patient with moderate dementia of the Alzheimer's type for a period of 3 days. The drug is to be administered twice a day. Rivastigmine tartrate is supplied in 1.5-mg capsules. How many capsules should the nurse administer to the patient each time? _____

4. A patient with mild-to-moderate dementia of the Alzheimer's type is prescribed a total of 120 mg of tacrine HCl for 4 days. Tacrine HCl is supplied in 10-mg capsules. How many capsules should the nurse administer to the patient per day? _____

SECTION III: PRACTICING FOR NCLEX

Activity E

Answer the following questions.

1. A patient has been prescribed cholinesterase inhibitors for the treatment of dementia. Which of the following adverse reactions should the nurse monitor for in the patient?

   a. Diarrhea

   b. High blood pressure

   c. Seizure disorders

   d. Renal dysfunction

2. Patients with Alzheimer's disease are prescribed tacrine to slow the progression of dementia. In which of the following cases should tacrine be used cautiously?

   a. Vaginitis

   b. Diabetes mellitus

   c. Cardiovascular problems

   d. Bladder obstruction

3. A patient is prescribed cholinesterase inhibitors for the treatment of dementia. The assigned nurse is required to perform a physical assessment of the patient before administering the drugs. Which of the following should the nurse monitor during physical assessment? Select all that apply.

   a. Pulse

   b. Respiratory rate

   c. Weight

   d. Brain waves

   e. Hepatic function

4. A nurse monitoring the ALT levels of a patient who received tacrine reports increased ALT levels to the primary health care provider. The provider decides to discontinue use of the drug because of the danger of hepatotoxicity. Which of the following could occur in the patient as a result of the abrupt discontinuation of tacrine?

   a. Loss of functional ability

   b. Decline in cognitive functioning

   c. Impulsive behavior

   d. Nervous breakdown

5. A nurse is caring for a patient with the dementia of Alzheimer's disease. Which of the following is an effect of the interaction of nonsteroidal anti-inflammatory drugs with cholinesterase inhibitors?

   a. Asthma

   b. Sick sinus syndrome

   c. Increased risk of gastrointestinal bleeding

   d. Increased risk of theophylline toxicity

6. A patient is administered tacrine to treat Alzheimer's disease. Which of the following conditions should the nurse monitor for when caring for the patient?

   a. Cardiovascular disease

   b. Pulmonary disease

   c. Liver damage

   d. Goiter

7. A nurse is caring for a patient receiving cholinesterase inhibitors. The drug is known to cause the adverse reactions of dizziness and syncope that can place the patient at risk for injury. Which of the following interventions should the nurse implement to reduce the risk of injury? Select all that apply.

   a. Use side rails

   b. Monitor the patient every 12 hours

   c. Keep bed in low position

   d. Use soft bedding

   e. Use night lights

8. A nurse is required to administer the prescribed tacrine to a patient for the treatment of moderate dementia of the Alzheimer type. How should the nurse administer this drug to the patient?

   a. 30 minutes before meals

   b. On an empty stomach

   c. 1 hour after meals

   d. Around the clock intravenously

9. Ginkgo, one of the oldest herbs in the world, is thought to improve memory and brain function and to enhance circulation to the brain, heart, limbs, and eyes. In which of the following patients is the use of ginkgo contraindicated?

   a. Patients receiving monoamine oxidase inhibitors

   b. Patients receiving sedatives and hypnotics

   c. Patients receiving opioid analgesics

   d. Patients receiving anticholinergic drugs

10. A nurse is caring for a patient receiving cholinesterase inhibitors for the treatment of Alzheimer's disease. Why is it important for the nurse to provide proper attention to the dosing of medication?

    a. Decreases the adverse gastrointestinal reactions

    b. Helps the patient to recover faster

    c. Helps the patient to maintain normal temperature

    d. Decreases variations in the pulse rate

Drugs Used to Treat Disorders of the Musculoskeletal System

SECTION I: ASSESSING YOUR UNDERSTANDING

Activity A MATCHING

1. Match the trade names of drugs used to treat musculoskeletal disorders in Column A with their uses in Column B.

Column A	Column B
___ 1. Rheumatrex	A. Management of symptoms of gout
___ 2. Azulfidine	B. Spasticity caused by multiple sclerosis
___ 3. Zyloprim	C. Cancer chemotherapy
___ 4. Lioresal	D. Ulcerative colitis

2. Match the musculoskeletal disorders in Column A with their descriptions in Column B.

Column A	Column B
___ 1. Synovitis	A. Inflammation of a joint involving pain or stiffness
___ 2. Arthritis	B. Inflammation of the synovial membrane of a joint
___ 3. Osteoarthritis	
___ 4. Paget's disease	

C. Chronic bone disorder characterized by abnormal bone remodeling

D. Noninflammatory degenerative joint disease marked by degeneration of the articular cartilage

Activity B FILL IN THE BLANKS

1. _____ are drugs used to treat musculoskeletal disorders such as osteoporosis and Paget's disease.

2. _____ reduces the production of uric acid, thereby decreasing serum uric acid levels and the deposit of urate crystals in joints.

3. Antirheumatic drugs have properties to produce _____, which in turn decreases the body's autoimmune response.

4. _____ is a condition in which uric acid accumulates in increased amounts in the blood and is often deposited in the joints.

5. _____ reduces the inflammation associated with the deposit of urate crystals in the joints.

SECTION II: APPLYING YOUR KNOWLEDGE

Activity C   SHORT ANSWERS

A nurse's role in managing a patient who is prescribed a drug for a musculoskeletal disorder involves assisting the patient with a preadministration assessment. The nurse helps in monitoring patients with drugs for musculoskeletal disorders. Answer the following questions, which involve the nurse's role in the management of patients who are on a drug therapy for a musculoskeletal disorder.

1. A patient with a musculoskeletal disorder is prescribed a drug. What preadministration assessments should the nurse conduct before administration of a musculoskeletal drug?

_____

_____

_____

2. After the preadministration assessment, the patient is administered a drug for the musculoskeletal disorder. What ongoing assessment should the nurse perform when caring for a patient who is administered a musculoskeletal drug?

_____

_____

_____

Activity D   DOSAGE CALCULATION

1. A physician prescribes 6 mg of the drug tizanidine daily to a patient. Tizanidine is available in 2-mg tablets. How many tablets should the nurse administer daily to the patient?

_____

2. A physician has prescribed 100 mg of orphenadrine daily to a patient. The orphenadrine therapy is to be continued for a period of 4 days. The drug is available in 100-mg tablets. How many tablets should the nurse administer to the patient?

_____

3. A patient has been prescribed 1.5 g of methocarbamol to be taken orally. The drug is available as 500-mg tablets. How many tablets should the nurse administer to the patient?

_____

4. A patient recovering from multiple sclerosis has been prescribed 60 mg of cyclobenzaprine. This drug is to be administered orally. On hand are 30-mg tablets. How many tablets should the nurse administer to the patient each time? _____

5. A physician prescribes 700 mg of carisoprodol per day to a patient recovering from painful musculoskeletal conditions. The drug is available in 350-mg tablets, and it has to be administered for a period of 3 days. How many tablets should the nurse administer to the patient? _____

SECTION III: PRACTICING FOR NCLEX

Activity E

Answer the following questions.

1. A patient with Paget's disease is receiving bisphosphonate drugs. What adverse reactions should the nurse monitor for in the patient?
   a. Dyspepsia
   b. Lethargy
   c. Sleepiness
   d. Constipation

2. A patient with Paget's disease is admitted to a local health care facility and is prescribed alendronate. In which of the following types of patients is the use of alendronate contraindicated?
   a. Hypertension patients
   b. Hypocalcemic patients
   c. Insomnia patients
   d. Diabetes patients

3. A patient with rheumatoid arthritis is receiving disease-modifying antirheumatic drugs (DMARDs) along with sulfa antibiotics. What possible interaction should the nurse monitor for in the patient?
   a. Rash
   b. Hepatotoxicity
   c. Methotrexate toxicity
   d. Theophylline toxicity

4. A patient is administered methotrexate for the treatment of rheumatoid arthritis. What should the nurse monitor for in patients receiving methotrexate?

a. Hematology

b. Liver function

c. Renal function

d. Pancreatic function

e. Cardiovascular function

5. A patient with rheumatoid arthritis is receiving DMARDs. What instructions should the nurse ask the patient to follow while administering DMARDs?

   a. Administer the drugs with food

   b. Drink 10 glasses of water a day

   c. Avoid hazardous tasks in case of drowsiness

   d. Notify the primary health care provider in the case of diarrhea

6. A patient is administered bisphosphonates for a musculoskeletal disorder. What ongoing assessments should a nurse perform for patients receiving bisphosphonates for musculoskeletal disorders?

   a. Obtain the patient's history of disorders

   b. Closely monitor the patient for adverse reactions

   c. Appraise the patient's physical condition and limitations

   d. Assess for pain in upper and lower back or hip

7. A patient is administered hydroxychloroquine for a musculoskeletal disorder. What nursing interventions are involved when a patient is administered hydroxychloroquine for a musculoskeletal disorder?

   a. Report adverse reactions, especially vision changes

b. Be alert to reactions such as skin rash, fever, cough, or easy bruising

c. Encourage liberal fluid intake and measure intake and output

d. Ask the patient to compensate for missed dosages

e. Be attentive to patient complaints such as tinnitus or hearing loss

8. A patient is prescribed sulfinpyrazone for the treatment of rheumatoid arthritis. In which of the following types of patients is the use of sulfinpyrazone contraindicated?

   a. Patients with peptic ulcer disease

   b. Patients with renal disorders

   c. Patients with hepatic disorders

   d. Patients with cardiac disease

9. A patient with rheumatic arthritis is administered the uric acid inhibitor sulfinpyrazone along with oral anticoagulants. What interactions should the nurse monitor for in the patient?

   a. Increased risk of bleeding

   b. Increased risk of hypoglycemia

   c. Increased effect of verapamil

   d. Decreased effectiveness of probenecid

10. A patient with gout is admitted to a local health care facility. What should the nurse examine in a patient with gout?

   a. Appearance of skin over joints

   b. Evidence of hearing loss

   c. Pain in upper and lower back or hip

   d. Mobility of affected joint

CHAPTER 35

Antitussives, Mucolytics, and Expectorants

SECTION I: ASSESSING YOUR UNDERSTANDING

Activity A MATCHING

1. Match the antitussive drugs in Column A with their uses in Column B.

Column A

C 1. Codeine sulfate

B 2. Guaifenesin

D 3. Diphenhy-
       dramine HCl

A 4. Acetylcysteine

Column B

A. Reduction of pul-
   monary complica-
   tion of cystic
   fibrosis

B. Relief of coughs
   associated with
   sinusitis

C. Relief of mild to
   moderate pain

D. Symptomatic relief
   of cough caused by
   bronchial irritation

2. Match the drugs Column A that are used to treat the discomfort associated with upper respiratory infection with their adverse reactions in Column B.

Column A

B 1. Codeine sulfate

D 2. Diphenhy-
       dramine

C 3. Potassium
       iodide

A 4. Acetylcysteine

Column B

A. Stomatitis, nausea,
   vomiting, fever,
   drowsiness, bron-
   chospasm, and
   irritation of the tra-
   chea and bronchi

B. Sedation, nausea,
   vomiting, dizziness,
   constipation, and
   central nervous
   system (CNS)
   depression

C. Iodine sensitivity or
   iodinism (sore
   mouth, metallic
   taste, increased sali-
   vation, nausea,
   vomiting, epigastric
   pain, parotid
   swelling, and pain)

D. Sedation, headache,
   mild dizziness, con-
   stipation, nausea,
   gastrointestinal (GI)
   upset, skin erup-
   tions, and postural
   hypotension

131

Activity B FILL IN THE BLANKS

1. An _Expectorant_ is a drug that aids in raising thick, tenacious mucus from the respiratory passages.

2. The ___opiod___ antitussives are contraindicated in premature infants or during labor, when delivery of a premature infant is anticipated.

3. When _dextromethorphan_ is administered with monoamine oxidase inhibitors, patients may experience jerking motions in the leg.

4. The mucolytic acetylcysteine is used to treat _atelectasis_ caused by mucus obstruction.

5. The patient should avoid drinking fluids for 30 minutes after the use of _lozenges_ to avoid losing effectiveness of the drug.

6. A mucolytic is a drug that loosens _respiratory_ secretions.

SECTION II: APPLYING YOUR KNOWLEDGE

Activity C SHORT ANSWERS

A nurse's role in managing a patient receiving an antitussive drug involves monitoring and managing the patient's needs after drug administration. The nurse also educates the patient about use of the drug. Answer the following questions, which involve the nurse's role in the management of such situations.

1. A patient with a cough has been prescribed an antitussive drug. What preadministration assessments should the nurse perform for the patient?
   document type of cough, and describe color + amount of any sputum. Record VS

2. What should be the nurse's role after he or she administers antitussives to the patient?
   Observe for therapeutic effect auscultate lung sounds,

Activity D DOSAGE CALCULATION

1. A patient with a cough has been prescribed 120 mg of the codeine sulfate drug to take daily. The drug is available as 30-mg capsules. How many capsules should a nurse administer to the patient every day? ___4___

2. A physician has prescribed 600 mg of Tessalon to take every 24 hours. The available drug is in 100-mg tablets. How many tablets should a nurse administer to the patient each day? ___6___

3. A 15-year-old patient has been prescribed 60 mg of DexAlone for the treatment of a cough. A nurse is required to administer the drug to the patient every 12 hours. It is available in 30-mg gelcaps. How many capsules should the nurse administer to the patient every 24 hours? ___4___

4. A patient has been prescribed 300 mg of Organidin, to be taken every 4 hours. The drug is available in 200-mg tablets. How many tablets should a nurse administer to the patient every 24 hours? ___6___

SECTION III: PRACTICING FOR NCLEX

Activity E

Answer the following questions.

1. A patient with a cough visits a health care facility and is prescribed an expectorant. What preadministration assessments should the nurse perform for this patient? Select all that apply.
   a. Ask the patient about throat infection
   b. Assess the respiratory status of the patient
   c. Document the lung sounds of the patient
   d. Examine the pulse rate every 30 minutes
   e. Document the consistency of sputum

2. A nurse at a health care center is assigned to prepare a teaching plan for a patient undergoing antitussive drug therapy. Which of the following instructions should the nurse include in the teaching plan? Select all that apply.

a. Take the medicine 1 hour before meals

b. Avoid irritants such as cigarette smoke, dust, or fumes

c. Avoid drinking fluids for 30 minutes after taking the drug

d. Take the medicine with milk to enhance absorption

e. Avoid chewing or breaking open the oral capsules

3. A patient with a cough visits a health care facility and is prescribed an antitussive. Which of the following reactions associated with antitussive administration should the nurse monitor for in the patient?

a. Diarrhea

b. Sedation

c. Somnolence

d. Dehydration

4. A nurse is assigned to care for a patient who has been prescribed an antitussive. The nurse knows that which of the following conditions contraindicate the use of antitussives?

a. Asthma

b. Liver dysfunction

c. Cardiac problems

d. Hypersensitivity

5. A nurse is caring for a patient who has been prescribed a medication containing potassium. The patient informs the nurse that he is taking a drug containing iodine products. What possible effect should the nurse be aware of concerning the interaction of potassium-containing medication with iodine products?

a. Hypokalemia

b. Hypoglycemia

c. Hypertension

d. Hemorrhage

6. A nurse is caring for a patient at a health care facility with ineffective airway clearance. Which of the following is an appropriate nurse's role to promote effective airway clearance?

a. Suggest avoiding consumption of milk products

b. Encourage fluid intake of up to 2000 mL per day

c. Monitor fluid intake of the patient every 8 hr

d. Encourage taking mucolytics after each coughing episode

7. A nurse is caring for a patient who has been prescribed a eucalyptus product for the treatment of nasal congestion. What instruction should the nurse provide while educating the patient about the use of this herbal medicine?

a. Take the medicine on an empty stomach

b. Dilute the medicine before use

c. Take the drug with warm milk

d. Warm the medicine before use

8. A patient experiencing a cough takes a non-prescription cough medicine. Under what conditions should the nurse instruct the patient to consult the primary health care provider?

a. Cough lasts more than 10 days

b. Cough is accompanied by dizziness

c. Frequency of coughing is 20 minutes

d. Cough is accompanied by vomiting

9. A nurse is caring for a patient with a severe cough at a health care facility. The physician has prescribed acetylcysteine for the patient, which is to be inserted into the patient's tracheostomy. What is the nurse's role in this case?

a. Ensure that the patient is not receiving any other drug therapy

b. Ensure that suction equipment is at the patient's bedside

c. Ensure that the patient gets continuous oxygen supply

d. Ensure that the patient keeps drinking warm water

10. A nurse is caring for a patient undergoing dextromethorphan therapy. The patient also needs monoamine oxidase inhibitors for the treatment of depression. What risk associated with the interaction of the two drugs should the nurse monitor for in the patient?

a. Hypotension

b. Dyspepsia

c. Bronchitis

d. Opisthotonos

Antihistamines and Decongestants

SECTION I: ASSESSING YOUR UNDERSTANDING

Activity A MATCHING

1. Match the medications that interact with antihistaminic drugs in Column A with the effect of the interaction in Column B.

Column A

C 1. Rifampin

E 2. Monoamine oxidase inhibitors

B 3. Beta-blockers

A 4. Opioid analgesics

D 5. Aluminum-based antacids

Column B

A. Causes additive central nervous system (CNS) depressant effect

B. Increases risk of cardiovascular effects

C. Reduces absorption of certain antihistamines

D. Decreases concentration of the antihistamine in the blood

E. Increases anticholinergic and sedative effects of antihistamines

2. Match the trade names of the medications in Column A with their generic names in Column B.

Column A

D 1. Clarinex

E 2. Aller-Chlor

A 3. Tavist

B 4. Benadryl

C 5. Phenergan

Column B

A. Clemastine fumarate

B. Diphenhydramine hydrochloride

C. Promethazine hydrochloride

D. Desloratadine

E. Chlorpheniramine maleate

Activity B FILL IN THE BLANKS

1. In allergic or hypersensitivity reactions, histamine is released from the ___mast___ cells.

2. A ___decongestant___ is a drug that reduces the swelling of the nasal passages, which, in turn, opens clogged nasal passages and enhances drainage of the sinuses.

3. Nasal decongestants produce localized ___vasoconstriction___ of the small blood vessels of the nasal membranes.

4. ___Histamine___ is produced from the amino acid histidine.

5. Antihistamines that penetrate the blood–brain barrier minimally exhibit fewer ___sedating___ effects.

SECTION II: APPLYING YOUR KNOWLEDGE

Activity C SHORT ANSWERS

A nurse's role in managing patients who are being administered antihistamines and decongestants involves monitoring and implementing interventions that aid in their recovery. Answer the following questions, which involve the nurse's role in the management of such situations.

1. A patient with mild angioneurotic edema is prescribed an antihistamine to relieve his symptoms. What teaching should the nurse provide to the patient and his family?

   Ⓧ hazardous tasks, frequent sips H2O,
   ⊖ Alcohol, Take w/food

2. A patient with sinusitis is on a decongestant medication. He wants to know about the possible side effects of the medication. What should the nurse tell him?

   Nasal burning or stinging, dryness
   of nasal mucosa

Activity D DOSAGE CALCULATION

1. A child, aged 10 years, is prescribed 30 mg of pseudoephedrine to relieve nasal congestion. The syrup contains 15 mg/5 mL (1 teaspoon) of pseudoephedrine. How many teaspoonfuls of the syrup should the nurse administer?

   _____

2. A 30-year-old patient has been prescribed 12 mg of brompheniramine for a runny nose caused by hay fever. Each tablet contains 4 mg of brompheniramine. How many such tablets per dose does the nurse need to give him? _____

3. A 17-year-old patient has been prescribed 4 mg of chlorpheniramine maleate every 6 hours. Chlorpheniramine maleate is available as 4-mg tablets. How many such tablets does the nurse need to give the patient in a single day? _____

4. An 8-year-old girl is prescribed 1.25 mg of clemastine fumarate twice daily for an allergic

rhinitis. The syrup contains 0.5 mg/5 mL of the medication. Each teaspoonful is 5 mL. How many teaspoonfuls of the medication should the nurse give her as a single dose?

_____

5. A patient has been prescribed 100 mg of hydroxyzine as a sedative. How many 25-mg tablets should the nurse give her?

_____

6. A patient is prescribed 25 mg of promethazine hydrochloride to relieve the symptoms of nausea. Each tablet contains 12.5 mg of promethazine hydrochloride. How many tablets does the nurse need to give to the patient? _____

SECTION III: PRACTICING FOR NCLEX

Activity E

Answer the following questions.

1. A patient has been prescribed an antihistamine for urticaria. He wants to know about the possible side effects of the drug. Which of the following are the possible side effects with this medication? Select all that apply.
   a. Thickening of bronchial secretions
   b. Disturbed coordination
   c. Increased frequency of micturition
   d. Anaphylactic shock or urticaria
   e. Excessive sweating and salivation

2. A nurse is required to care for a patient who has been prescribed an antihistamine to treat parkinsonism. In which of the following conditions should the nurse administer the drug with caution?
   a. Acute conjunctivitis
   b. Allergic rhinitis
   c. Angle-closure glaucoma
   d. Hypotension

3. A 70-year-old patient with acute sinusitis has been prescribed decongestant medication. At this age, he is at a greater risk of developing side effects caused by overdosage. Which of the following symptoms of overdosage should the nurse monitor for when caring for the patient? Select all that apply.

a. Hallucination

b. Dyspnea

c. Convulsion

d. Depression

e. Fatigue

4. A patient has been prescribed a nasal decongestant to relieve the symptoms of nasal congestion. The nurse needs to educate the patient about the method of drug administration. Which of the following procedures should the patient follow when administering the drug?

    a. Administer nasal spray by reclining on the bed with the head hanging

    b. Administer nasal drops by sitting upright and sniffing hard

    c. Administer nasal spray by touching the tip to the nasal mucosa

    d. Administer the inhaler by warming it in one's hand before use

5. Promethazine is prescribed to a patient who is also receiving an opioid analgesic. Which of the following factors should the nurse assess in the patient before administering promethazine?

    a. Bone density

    b. Urine output

    c. Blood pressure

    d. Skin turgidity

6. A patient has been prescribed an antihistamine drug to be given parenterally. Which of the following parenteral routes of drug administration should the nurse prefer?

    a. Intravenous

    b. Intramuscular

    c. Subcutaneous

    d. Intradermal

7. Given below, in a random order, are the steps of an inflammatory response to injury. Arrange the inflammatory responses in the order they occur in most situations.

2 a. Dilatation of arterioles

4 b. Increased capillary permeability

1 c. Release of histamine

5 d. Escape of fluid from blood vessels

3 e. Localized redness

6 f. Localized swelling

8. A 40-year-old patient is prescribed an antihistamine medication. The nurse needs to educate the patient about other drugs that he takes concomitantly that can interact with the antihistamine to either enhance or reduce its effects. Which of the following drugs reduces the effect of antihistamines?

    a. Beta-blocking agents

    b. Opioid analgesics

    c. Magnesium-based antacids

    d. Monoamine oxidase inhibitors

9. A patient is prescribed a decongestant for allergic rhinitis. In which of the following conditions should the nurse administer the drug cautiously? Select all that apply.

    a. Hypertension

    b. Hyperthyroidism

    c. Conjunctivitis

    d. Nephropathy

    e. Glaucoma

10. Which of the following instructions should the nurse provide to a patient who has been prescribed an antihistamine for hay fever? Select all that apply.

    a. Take an antacid 1 hour before the drug

    b. Avoid the use of alcohol and other sedatives

    c. Crush the sustained-release tablet before use

    d. Take the drug with food to avoid gastric upset

    e. Take frequent sips of water or suck on hard candy

Bronchodilators and Antiasthma Drugs

SECTION I: ASSESSING YOUR UNDERSTANDING

Activity A MATCHING

1. Match the bronchodilator and antiasthmatic drugs given in Column A with their class given in Column B.

Column A

D 1. Albuterol

C 2. Theophylline

E 3. Flunisolide

A 4. Zafirlukast

B 5. Zileuton

Column B

A. Leukotriene receptor antagonist

B. Leukotriene formation inhibitor

C. Xanthine derivative

D. Sympathomimetic bronchodilator

E. Corticosteroid

2. Match the interactant drugs given in Column A with their interactions with sympathomimetic agents in Column B.

Column A

B 1. Adrenergic drugs

E 2. Monoamine oxidase inhibitors

A 3. Methyldopa

C 4. Uterine stimulants

D 5. Theophylline

Column B

A. Increased pressor response

B. Possible additive effects

C. Possible severe hypotension

D. Increased risk of cardiotoxicity

E. Risk of severe headache and hypertensive crisis

Activity B FILL IN THE BLANKS

1. Methylxanthines stimulate the central nervous system to promote dilation of the bronchi.

2. In asthma, the airways become narrow, and extra mucous clogs the smaller airways.

3. The three most common symptoms of asthma are cough, dyspnea, and wheezing.

4. Cromolyn sodium acts by preventing calcium ions from entering mast cells, thus preventing the release of inflammatory mediators.

5. Terbutaline is a bronchodilator with beta-2 receptor agonist activity.

SECTION II: APPLYING YOUR KNOWLEDGE

Activity C SHORT ANSWERS

A nurse's role in managing patients who are receiving bronchodilators and antiasthma drugs involves monitoring and implementing interventions that aid in their recovery. Answer the following questions, which involve the nurse's role in the management of such situations.

1. A patient has been prescribed theophylline for the symptomatic relief of bronchial asthma.

   a. What should the nurse inform the patient about possible adverse effects of the drug?

_____

_____

_____

b. What points should the nurse include in the patient teaching plan in such a case?

_____

_____

_____

2. A patient with chronic bronchitis has been prescribed a bronchodilator agent. What preadministration assessments should the nurse implement when caring for the patient?

_____

_____

_____

Activity D   DOSAGE CALCULATION

1. A patient has been advised to take 4 mg of albuterol three times a day for the prevention of bronchospasm. The oral syrup available contains 2 mg/5 mL of albuterol. How many teaspoonfuls of the syrup should the nurse administer in a single dose? _____

2. A child weighing 25 kg has been prescribed 0.5 mg/kg of ephedrine sulfate as a subcutaneous injection for bronchial asthma. The strength of the injection is 50 mg/mL. What volume of the injection should the nurse administer? _____

3. A 35-year-old patient has bronchospasm during anesthesia. He is prescribed 0.01 mg of isoproterenol as a bolus intravenous (IV) injection. The 1-mL ampoule contains 0.2 mg of the drug. The nurse dilutes the contents of the ampoule with 10 mL of sodium chloride injection USP. How much of the diluted solution should be injected? _____

4. A 13-year-old patient is prescribed 0.25 mg of terbutaline to be injected subcutaneously (SC) for the reversal of bronchospasm. Each ampoule contains 1 mg of the drug in 1 mL of solution. What volume of the solution should the nurse administer? _____

5. A patient weighing 30 kg is prescribed 10 mg/kg of dyphylline for the symptomatic relief of bronchial asthma. How much of the drug should the nurse administer in a single dose? _____

6. A patient is prescribed 0.5 mg of epinephrine solution SC for respiratory distress. The solution contains 5 mg/mL of epinephrine. How much of the solution should the nurse administer? _____

SECTION III: PRACTICING FOR NCLEX

Activity E

Answer the following questions.

1. A pregnant client is admitted to a health care facility with acute respiratory distress. Which of the following drugs should the nurse consider as relatively safe for such a patient?

    a. Albuterol

    b. Epinephrine

    c. Terbutaline

    d. Salmeterol

2. A patient is prescribed aminophylline for the symptomatic relief of bronchial asthma. The nurse is required to inform the patient about other drugs that may interact with aminophylline. Which of the following drugs increases the effects of aminophylline?

    a. Ketoconazole

    b. Rifampin

    c. Loop diuretics

    d. Beta-blockers

3. A patient is prescribed aminophylline for emphysema. Which of the following factors should the nurse assess to check for the occurrence of any adverse effects?

    a. Electrocardiographic changes

    b. Fluid intake and output

    c. Consistency of the stool

    d. Changes in blood hemoglobin

4. A patient is admitted to a health care facility with complaints of cough, difficulty in breathing, and a wheezing sound during respiration. The patient is diagnosed as having asthma. Which of the following additional symptoms will the nurse observe in the patient?

    a. Decreased blood pressure

    b. Increased sweating

c. Decreased pulse rate

d. Increased urination

5. A patient is prescribed the antiasthmatic drug zafirlukast. The patient's medical history indicates that the patient is on aspirin for the pain relief of arthritis. For which of the following possible drug interactions should the nurse monitor?

a. Increased thrombolytic effect of aspirin

b. Increased plasma levels of zafirlukast

c. Decreased absorption of zafirlukast

d. Decreased plasma levels of aspirin

6. Given below, in random order, are the steps involved in the progress of chronic inflammation seen in asthma. Arrange the steps in the correct order.

5 a. Decreased airflow to the lungs

3 b. Bronchospasm and inflammation

1 c. Release of histamine from the mast cells

2 d. Increased mucus production and edema of the airway

4 e. Narrowing and clogging of the airways

7. A patient has been prescribed a multidrug regimen for the treatment of asthma. Which of the following drugs may be given as adjuncts to bronchodilator therapy in such a case? Select all that apply.

a. Corticosteroids

b. Leukotriene formation inhibitors

c. Uricosuric agents

d. Mast cell stabilizers

e. Leukotriene receptor antagonists

8. A patient with asthma has been prescribed an inhalational corticosteroid agent for the reduction of inflammation in the airways. Which of the following drugs are corticosteroid agents? Select all that apply.

a. Cromolyn

b. Flunisolide

c. Beclomethasone

d. Ipratropium

e. Triamcinolone

9. A patient complains of nausea after receiving antiasthmatic medication. Which of the following instructions should the nurse provide to alleviate the patient's condition? Select all that apply.

a. Keep head end of bed elevated

b. Eat frequent small meals

c. Suck on sugarless candy

d. Limit fluids with meals

e. Rinse mouth properly after food

10. A patient with asthma has been prescribed the use of montelukast taken orally. How often should the patient take the drug?

a. Once a day

b. Twice a day

c. Three times a day

d. Four times a day

Cardiotonics and Miscellaneous Inotropic Drugs

SECTION I: ASSESSING YOUR UNDERSTANDING

Activity A MATCHING

1. Match the drugs that interact with cardiotonics in Column A with the effects of their interaction with digitalis in Column B.

Column A

_____ 1. Amiodarone

_____ 2. Antacids

_____ 3. Thyroid hormones

_____ 4. Loop diuretics

Column B

A. Decreases plasma digitalis levels

B. Results in electrolyte imbalance

C. Increases plasma digitalis levels

D. Decreases the effectiveness of digoxin

2. Match the terms associated with congestive heart failure in Column A with their descriptions in Column B.

Column A

_____ 1. Ejection fraction

_____ 2. Nocturia

_____ 3. Congestive heart failure

Column B

A. Inability of the heart to pump sufficient quantities of blood to meet with the tissue demands

_____ 4. Cardiotonics

_____ 5. Cardiac hypertrophy

_____ 6. Orthopnea

B. Enlargement of cardiac musculature

C. Agents that increase contraction of the heart

D. Amount of blood ejected by the ventricles per beat in relation to the amount of blood available to eject

E. Difficulty in breathing when lying flat

F. Need to urinate frequently at night

Activity B FILL IN THE BLANKS

1. When cardiotonics are given by the _____ method, the site should be inspected for redness and infiltration.

2. _____ ventricular dysfunction results in pulmonary symptoms, which include dyspnea and moist cough.

3. Fetal toxicity and _____ death have been reported from maternal overdosage of digoxin.

4. During digoxin therapy, if severe _____ develops, atropine may be given.

5. Patients started on cardiotonic drug therapy are said to be _____.

143

SECTION II: APPLYING YOUR KNOWLEDGE

Activity C SHORT ANSWERS

A nurse's role in managing patients who are being treated with digoxin involves carefully monitoring and implementing interventions that aid in recovery. Answer the following questions, which involve the nurse's role in the management of such situations.

1. A patient is diagnosed with heart failure and requires digoxin therapy. What physical assessment should a nurse carry out before starting digoxin administration?

_____

_____

_____

2. A patient had rapid digitalization for his heart failure. He is required to continue taking digitalis for a prolonged period of time. What teaching plan should the nurse implement for patients taking digitalis?

_____

_____

_____

Activity D DOSAGE CALCULATION

1. A doctor prescribes 0.25 mg of digoxin to a patient with heart failure. The available digoxin tablet is 0.125 mg. How many tablets should a nurse administer to the patient?

_____

2. A doctor has prescribed 1.25 mg of digoxin as the loading dose for a patient with atrial fibrillation. Each ampoule contains 1 mL of digoxin in the strength of 0.25 mg/mL. How many ampoules of digoxin should the nurse administer? _____

3. A patient with heart failure has been prescribed 600 mg of digoxin immune fab to be given intravenously (IV) for digoxin toxicity. The patient's parents have brought 25 vials. Each vial contains 40 mg of the drug. How many of the vials need to be returned after the correct dose has been given? _____

4. A patient with severe heart failure has been prescribed 50 mg of milrinone lactate to be given IV. Each vial contains 100 mg/10 mL.

What volume of the injection should the nurse administer? _____

5. A doctor has prescribed 40 mg of inamrinone lactate to be given as an IV bolus for a patient with heart failure. Each vial contains 5 mg/mL. How many vials of inamrinone should the nurse administer? _____

6. A doctor has prescribed 0.75 mg of digoxin to be given IV for a patient with atrial flutter. Each ampoule contains 1 mL of digoxin in the strength of 0.25 mg/ampoule. How many ampoules of digoxin should a nurse administer? _____

SECTION III: PRACTICING FOR NCLEX

Activity E

Answer the following questions.

1. A patient arrives at a community health care center complaining of dyspnea and a hacking cough. The nurse assessing the patient notes that there are distended jugular veins, edema of the extremities, and reduced ejection fraction. Which of the following conditions do these symptoms indicate?
   a. Heart failure
   b. Glomerulonephritis
   c. Pulmonary disease
   d. Hypothyroidism

2. A patient is diagnosed with heart failure and is started on digoxin. The patient informs the nurse that he is taking benzodiazepines for seizures. Which of the following interventions should the nurse implement?
   a. Increase the dosage of digoxin
   b. Monitor for signs of digoxin toxicity
   c. Increase the dosage of benzodiazepines
   d. Monitor for signs of reduced effectiveness of digoxin

3. A nurse is educating a group of nursing students on the uses of digitalis. For which of the following conditions may digitalis be used?
   a. Ventricular tachycardia
   b. Atrioventricular block
   c. Atrial fibrillation
   d. Ventricular failure

4. When caring for a patient on digoxin, the nurse observes that the patient's pulse rate is 56 beats per minute. The patient is also complaining of nausea and vomiting. Which of the following is the most appropriate intervention in this situation?

    a. Administer milrinone lactate

    b. Increase the rate of digoxin infusion

    c. Perform a gastrointestinal suction

    d. Withhold the drug and notify the practitioner

5. A nurse is caring for a patient who requires rapid administration of digitalis for his heart failure. What amount of the total dose should the nurse administer as the first dose?

    a. Quarter of the total dose

    b. Half of the total dose

    c. Three quarters of the total dose

    d. The complete dose

6. A patient has been admitted for heart failure and is on digoxin. The nurse monitoring the patient notes that the serum digoxin level is 2.5 mg/mL. Which of the following signs should a nurse assess for in the case of digoxin toxicity? Select all that apply.

    a. Anorexia

    b. Headache

    c. Weakness

    d. Blurred vision

    e. Vomiting

7. A patient is given digitalis for congestive heart failure. The practitioner assessing the patient orders an analysis of serum electrolytes. Which of the following electrolyte changes indicates toxicity and needs to be reported? Select all that apply.

    a. Hyponatremia

    b. Hypokalemia

    c. Hypomagnesemia

    d. Hypocalcemia

    e. Hypophosphatemia

8. A nurse is caring for a patient on digitalis. The patient complains of nausea and vomiting after 2 days of digitalis administration. Which of the following are appropriate nursing interventions in this situation? Select all that apply.

    a. Ensure that the patient takes double the drug dosage

    b. Ensure the patient consumes small frequent meals

    c. Ensure the patient intakes fluids 1 hour before meals

    d. Ensure that the patient rinses his or her mouth after the consumption of meals

    e. Restrict fluid consumption at mealtimes

9. A patient is admitted to a health care center with atrial flutter. The patient complains of headache after the first dose of digitalis is administered. Which of the following adverse effects of digitalis should a nurse assess for in such a situation? Select all that apply.

    a. Hepatotoxicity

    b. Angina

    c. Drowsiness

    d. Vomiting

    e. Arrhythmia

10. A patient with heart failure has been advised to maintain digoxin therapy. Prior to discharge, the nurse teaches the steps of calculating the pulse. Arrange the steps involved in calculating the pulse in their correct order.

    a. Record the number of times the pulse beats in a minute

    b. Place the nondominant arm on a table or armchair

    c. Place the index and third fingers of the other hand on the wrist bone

    d. Feel for the beating or pulsing sensation, which is the pulse

    e. If the pulse rate is more than 100 beats per minute, notify the practitioner

CHAPTER 39

Antiarrhythmic Drugs

SECTION I: ASSESSING YOUR UNDERSTANDING

Activity A MATCHING

1. Match the terms associated with cardiac arrhythmias in Column A with their brief descriptions in Column B.

Column A

_____ 1. Arrhythmia

_____ 2. Cinchonism

_____ 3. Polarization

_____ 4. Depolarization

_____ 5. Repolarization

Column B

A. Hearing loss and ringing sensation in the ears caused by quinidine toxicity

B. Movement of positive ions into the nerve cell and negative ions to the outside of the cell

C. Movement of positive ions to the outside and negative ions to the inside of the nerve cell

D. Disturbance or irregularity in the heart rate, rhythm, or both

E. Positive ions on the outside and negative ions on the inside of the cell membrane when they are at rest

2. Match the interactant drugs in Column A with the effects of their interactions with antiarrhythmic agents in Column B.

Column A

_____ 1. Fluoro-quinolones

_____ 2. Anticholiner-gics

_____ 3. Local anes-thetics

_____ 4. Warfarin

_____ 5. Rifampin

Column B

A. Additive antivagal effects on atrioventricular (AV) conduction

B. Decreased levels of antiarrhythmic agent

C. Risk of life-threatening arrhythmias

D. Possible increased risk of central nervous system (CNS) side effects

E. Increased prothrombin time

Activity B FILL IN THE BLANKS

1. _____ is a term applied to any stimulus of the lowest intensity that will give rise to a response in a nerve fiber.

2. Beta-adrenergic blocking agents reduce the influence of the _____ nervous system in the heart and the kidney.

3. All antiarrhythmic drugs may cause new arrhythmias or worsen existing arrhythmias, even though they are administered to resolve an existing arrhythmia. This phenomenon is called the _____ effect.

4. Flecainide depresses fast _____ channels, decreases the height and rate of rise of action potentials, and slows conduction of all areas of the heart.

5. A transient increase in arrhythmias and _____ may occur within 1 hour after initial therapy with bretylium has begun.

SECTION II: APPLYING YOUR KNOWLEDGE

Activity C SHORT ANSWERS

A nurse's role in managing patients who are being administered antiarrhythmic drugs involves monitoring and implementing interventions that aid in recovery. Answer the following questions, which involve the nurse's role in the management of such situations.

1. A patient with paroxysmal atrial tachycardia is admitted to a health care facility. The patient is prescribed disopyramide.

   a. The nurse should inform the patient about which side effects of the drug?

   _____

   _____

   _____

   b. What conditions, if present, necessitate a cautious use of disopyramide?

   _____

   _____

   _____

2. A nurse is caring for a patient who has been prescribed an antiarrhythmic agent for atrial tachycardia. What assessments should the nurse perform before administering the drug to the patient?

   _____

   _____

   _____

Activity D DOSAGE CALCULATION

1. A patient with paroxysmal atrial tachycardia is prescribed 150 mg of disopyramide orally every 6 hours. The Norpace (disopyramide) tablets from the pharmacy are 100 mg each.

How many tablets should the nurse instruct the patient to take per dose? _____

2. A patient was prescribed mexiletine for the treatment of life-threatening ventricular tachycardia. By observing the patient's response, the health care provider has transferred to the 12-hour dosage schedule to improve compliance and convenience and has prescribed 300 mg of mexiletine every 12 hours. How many 150-mg tablets of mexiletine should the nurse administer in a single dose? _____

3. A patient weighing 55 kg has been prescribed 0.1 mL/kg of ibutilide fumarate for atrial fibrillation. How much of the drug should the nurse administer to the patient? _____

4. A patient with angina pectoris is prescribed 240 mg of propranolol hydrochloride daily in three divided oral doses. How much of the drug should the nurse instruct the patient to take in each dose? _____

5. A patient weighing 70 kg has supraventricular arrhythmia. He receives a loading dose of IV esmolol hydrochloride, which is to be followed by an intravenous (IV) infusion of 50 mg/kg/min for 4 minutes. How much of the drug should the nurse infuse during these 4 minutes? _____

6. A patient with hypertension has been prescribed 390 mg of acebutolol hydrochloride daily in two divided oral doses. How much of the drug should the nurse instruct him to take in each dose? _____

SECTION III: PRACTICING FOR NCLEX

Activity E

Answer the following questions.

1. When educating a group of nursing students on the Class IA antiarrhythmic drugs, the nurse cites which of the following drugs as an example of a Class IA antiarrhythmic drug?

   a. Lidocaine

   b. Disopyramide

   c. Propafenone

   d. Amiodarone

2. A patient is prescribed flecainide for the treatment of cardiac arrhythmia. Which of

the following channels in the heart does the drug depress?

a. Calcium

b. Chloride

c. Oxygen

d. Sodium

3. A patient has been prescribed an antiarrhythmic drug for cardiac arrhythmia. The nurse should inform the patient about which of the following possible adverse effects of the drug?

a. Hypertension

b. Insomnia

c. Light-headedness

d. Urinary frequency

4. A patient on amiodarone reports that she is pregnant. The primary health care provider informs her to stop use of the drug as it might cause fetal harm. To which of the following U.S. Food and Drug Administration (FDA) pregnancy categories does amiodarone belong?

a. Category B

b. Category C

c. Category D

d. Category X

5. A nurse is required to assess the vital signs of a patient with paroxysmal atrial tachycardia who is on an antiarrhythmic agent. Which of the following pulse rates alerts the nurse to immediately inform the primary health care provider?

a. 82 beats per minute

b. 92 beats per minute

c. 102 beats per minute

d. 122 beats per minute

6. A patient who is on antiarrhythmic drug therapy complains of nausea after taking the drug. Which of the following instructions should the nurse provide to the patient to help alleviate nausea?

a. Take the drug 2 hours before taking food

b. Lie down flat for at least 1 hour after taking the drug

c. Eat, small frequent meals rather than large meals

d. Drink lots of water after taking the medicine

7. A nurse caring for a patient who has been prescribed disopyramide to treat arrhythmia is required to obtain the patient's drug history. Which of the following drugs, if taken concurrently, can decrease the serum levels of disopyramide?

a. Erythromycin

b. Quinidine

c. Thioridazine

d. Rifampin

8. A nurse is required to closely monitor a patient with arrhythmia receiving IV lidocaine. Which of the following blood levels of lidocaine should the nurse report to the health care provider?

a. 1.5 mcg/mL

b. 3.0 mcg/mL

c. 4.5 mcg/mL

d. 6.0 mcg/mL

9. A patient has been admitted to a health care facility with the symptoms of cardiac arrhythmia. The patient is prescribed an antiarrhythmic agent. Which of the following adverse effects are possible with the use of an antiarrhythmic agent? Select all that apply.

a. Weakness

b. Hypertension

c. Insomnia

d. Arrhythmias

e. Light-headedness

10. A nurse is caring for an 86-year-old patient on antiarrhythmic drugs. Which of the following signs, if present, indicates the development of heart failure in the patient?

a. Decreased weight

b. Shortness of breath

c. Increased urine volume

d. Chills and fever

CHAPTER **40**

Antianginal and Peripheral Vasodilating Drugs

SECTION I: ASSESSING YOUR UNDERSTANDING

Activity A MATCHING

1. Match the antianginal and vasodilator drugs in Column A with their appropriate uses in Column B.

Column A

____ 1. Verapamil

____ 2. Amyl nitrite

____ 3. Cilostazol

____ 4. Nitroglycerin, intravenous (IV)

____ 5. Nifedipine

____ 6. Isoxsuprine hydrochloride

____ 7. Papaverine hydrochloride

Column B

A. Provides symptomatic relief in intermittent claudication

B. Treats cardiac arrhythmias

C. Controls blood pressure in perioperative hypertension associated with surgical procedures

D. Relieves angina pectoris

E. Treats myocardial ischemia complicated with arrhythmias

F. Treats Prinzmetal's variant angina

G. Treats peripheral vascular disease (PVD)

2. Match the terms associated with angina in Column A with their descriptions in Column B.

Column A

____ 1. Atherosclerosis

____ 2. Angina

____ 3. Ischemia

Column B

A. Condition where there is reduced blood supply to an area

B. Characterized by the presence of fatty plaque deposits on the inner wall of the arteries

C. Characterized by chest pain occurring as a result of decreased oxygen supply to the heart muscles

Activity B FILL IN THE BLANKS

1. Antianginal drugs relieve chest pain by dilating _____ arteries and thereby increasing the blood supply to the cardiac musculature.

2. The contractions of cardiac and vascular smooth muscles depend on the movement of extracellular _____ ions through specific ion channels.

3. Nitrates act by relaxing the _____ muscle layer of the blood vessels.

4. Contact _____ may occur with the use of transdermal nitrates.

5. Intermittent _____ is a group of symptoms characterized by pain in the calf muscle brought on by walking and relieved by rest.

SECTION II: APPLYING YOUR KNOWLEDGE

Activity C SHORT ANSWERS

A nurse's role in managing patients who are being administered antianginal drugs involves monitoring and implementing interventions that aid in the patient's recovery. Answer the following questions, which involve the nurse's role in the management of such situations.

1. A patient has been admitted to a health care facility with severe anginal attacks. What instructions should the nurse provide the patient on discharge?

_____

_____

_____

2. A nurse is monitoring a patient admitted to the primary health care facility for treatment of Raynaud's disease. What assessments should the nurse undertake during the therapy with peripheral vasodilators?

_____

_____

_____

Activity D DOSAGE CALCULATION

1. A patient is prescribed 20 mg of isoxsuprine hydrochloride daily for Raynaud's disease. The tablet is available in 10-mg strength. How many tablets should the nurse administer to give the correct dosage? _____

2. A nurse has to administer 40 mg of isosorbide dinitrate orally to a patient for the treatment of angina. The tablet is available in 20-mg strength. How many tablets should the nurse administer to the patient? _____

3. A patient is prescribed 10 mg of amlodipine for Prinzmetal's angina. The tablet is available

in 5-mg strength. How many tablets should the patient take to relieve his angina? _____

4. A patient has been prescribed 12.5 mg of IV diltiazem for atrial fibrillation. Each ampoule contains 5 mL of solution in the strength of 5 mg/mL. What amount of the solution should the nurse draw from the ampoule to give the correct dosage? _____

5. A patient requires 50 mg of nifedipine daily for the treatment of chronic stable angina. The drug is available in the strength of 25 mg per tablet. How many tablets should the patient consume daily? _____

6. The physician has prescribed 100 mg of cilostazol daily to a patient with PVD. The drug is available in 100-mg tablets. How many tablets should the patient buy for a week? _____

SECTION III: PRACTICING FOR NCLEX

Activity E

Answer the following questions.

1. A patient has been admitted to a health care facility for the treatment of severe acute angina. A nurse is administering sublingual nitroglycerin to the patient every 5 minutes. How many doses of nitroglycerin should the nurse administer before reporting no improvement to the practitioner?

   a. 3 doses in a 15-minute period
   b. 5 doses in a 30-minute period
   c. 7 doses in a 30-minute period
   d. 9 doses in a 60-minute period

2. A nurse is caring for a patient who has been prescribed cilostazol for treating intermittent claudication. Which of the following interventions should the nurse implement when administering cilostazol?

   a. Crush and mix cilostazol with food
   b. Administer cilostazol with grape juice
   c. Administer cilostazol with patient in supine position
   d. Administer cilostazol 30 minutes before food

3. A nurse is required to care for a patient receiving L-arginine for PVD. Which of the following functions should the nurse identify as the mode of action of L-arginine?

   a. Promotes sodium retention
   b. Increases nitric oxide levels
   c. Blocks calcium ion channels
   d. Blocks alpha-adrenergic receptors

4. A nurse is caring for a patient with PVD who delivered a baby 2 hours earlier. The patient complains of severe cramping pain in the calf muscles. Which of the following drugs should not be given in the immediate post-partum period?

   a. Isosorbide dinitrate
   b. Nitroglycerin
   c. Isoxsuprine
   d. Nifedipine

5. A patient has been admitted for the management of PVD. Which of the following drugs can be given in PVD?

   a. Papaverine
   b. Nitroglycerin
   c. Isosorbide mononitrate
   d. Amyl nitrite

6. A nurse is educating a group of nursing students on the various effects of calcium channel blockers on the heart. Which of the following are effects of calcium channel blockers on the heart? Select all that apply.

   a. Increase heart rate
   b. Retard conduction velocity
   c. Depress myocardial contractility
   d. Cause rapid atrial muscle contraction
   e. Dilate the coronary arteries

7. A patient is admitted to a health care center for angina management and is started on IV diltiazem. Which of the following adverse effects should the nurse monitor for in the patient? Select all that apply.

   a. Hypertension
   b. Tachycardia

   c. Arrhythmia
   d. Asthenia
   e. Flushing

8. A nurse is caring for a patient with Raynaud's disease who is receiving cilostazol. Which of the following indicates improvement following treatment with cilostazol? Select all that apply.

   a. Increased coldness of the affected limb
   b. Increase in painless walking distance
   c. Decreased pain and cramping in the legs
   d. Decreased amplitude of the peripheral pulse
   e. Decreased scaling of the affected area

9. A patient has been admitted for the treatment of arteriosclerosis obliterans and is started on isoxsuprine. Which of the following adverse effects should the nurse monitor for in patients on isoxsuprine? Select all that apply.

   a. Hypertension
   b. Sedation
   c. Flushing
   d. Bradycardia
   e. Headache

10. A patient is prescribed translingual nitrates for the management of angina. What instructions should the nurse give for a patient taking translingual nitrates? Arrange them in the correct sequence.

    a. If pain is not relieved after taking three metered doses in a 15-minute period, report to the health care provider immediately.
    b. Read the instructions supplied with the product for the use of translingual nitrates.
    c. At the occurrence of chest pain, spray one or two metered doses onto or under the tongue.
    d. Use the drug prophylactically 5–10 minutes before engaging in strenuous activities.

Study Guide to Accompany Introductory Clinical Pharmacology, 8th edition, by Sally S. Roach and Susan M. Ford.

Antihypertensive Drugs

SECTION I: ASSESSING YOUR UNDERSTANDING

Activity A MATCHING

1. Match the terms associated with hypertension in Column A with their correct descriptions in Column B.

Column A

___ 1. Hypertension

___ 2. Essential hypertension

___ 3. Hypertensive emergency

___ 4. Secondary hypertension

___ 5. Prehypertension

Column B

A. Blood pressure rise with no cause discernible; associated with risk factors such as diet and lifestyle.

B. Rise in blood pressure in which the cause is discernible.

C. Blood pressure that remains elevated over time.

D. Rise in blood pressure: systolic pressure between 120 and 139 mm Hg or diastolic pressure between 80 and 89 mm Hg.

E. Rise in blood pressure to extremely high levels, which can lead to damage of target organs such as kidneys, eyes, and the heart.

2. Match the antihypertensive drugs in Column A with their modes of action in Column B.

Column A

___ 1. Propranolol

___ 2. Prazosin

___ 3. Amlodipine

___ 4. Captopril

___ 5. Losartan

Column B

A. An angiotensin-converting enzyme (ACE) inhibitor

B. A beta-adrenergic blocking drug

C. An angiotensin II receptor antagonist

D. An alpha-adrenergic blocking drug

E. A calcium channel blocker

Activity B FILL IN THE BLANKS

1. Angiotensin I is converted to angiotensin II, which is a powerful _____.

2. Furosemide and hydrochlorothiazide are examples of _____ agents used in the treatment of hypertension.

3. Diazoxide and nitroprusside are drugs used in the management of _____ emergencies.

4. Aldosterone promotes the retention of _____ and water, which contributes to the rise in blood pressure.

5. Electrolyte imbalance such as _____, which is a low blood sodium level, occurs with diuretic usage.

SECTION II: APPLYING YOUR KNOWLEDGE

Activity C   SHORT ANSWERS

A nurse's role in managing patients who are being administered antihypertensive drugs involves monitoring and implementing interventions that aid in the recovery of the patients. Answer the following questions, which involve the nurse's role in the management of such situations.

1. A patient has been prescribed antihypertensive therapy with captopril. During the course of the therapy, what assessments should the nurse conduct?

   _____

   _____

   _____

2. A patient is prescribed amlodipine for hypertension. What points should the nurse include in the patient teaching plan?

   _____

   _____

   _____

Activity D   DOSAGE CALCULATION

1. A patient is advised to take 200 mg of captopril daily, in two divided doses, for hypertension. It is available as 25-mg tablets. How many tablets should the patient take in a day?

   _____

2. A patient is prescribed 40 mg of hydralazine to be given intravenously (IV) for hypertensive emergency management. Each ampoule contains 20 mg of hydralazine. How many ampoules should the nurse break to give the required dosage? _____

3. A patient is prescribed 100 mg of losartan daily for hypertension. The tablets are available in 50-mg strength. How many tablets should the patient take daily? _____

4. A nurse should give 150 mg of atenolol to a patient with hypertension. The tablets are available in 50-mg strength. How many tablets should the nurse administer?

   _____

5. A patient requires 1.2 mg of clonidine for hypertension management. The strength available is 0.3 mg per tablet. How many tablets should the nurse administer daily? _____

6. A doctor prescribes 2 mg of doxazosin daily for hypertension. The drug is available in 4-mg tablets. What fraction of the tablet should the patient consume? _____

SECTION III: PRACTICING FOR NCLEX

Activity E

Answer the following questions.

1. When assessing a 40-year-old patient, the nurse observes an increase in the patient's blood pressure. Which of the following changes in blood pressure is indicative of prehypertension?
   a. Systolic pressure between 120 and 139 mm Hg
   b. Systolic pressure between 100 and 119 mm Hg
   c. Systolic pressure between 80 and 99 mm Hg
   d. Systolic pressure between 60 and 79 mm Hg

2. A patient is diagnosed with renal impairment and hypertension. Which of the following drugs is contraindicated in renal impairment?
   a. Doxazosin
   b. Captopril
   c. Hydralazine
   d. Minoxidil

3. A nurse is monitoring a patient admitted to the emergency department with hypertensive emergency. Which of the following drugs should be administered in such situations?
   a. Amlodipine
   b. Acebutolol
   c. Diltiazem
   d. Nitroprusside

4. A patient with diabetes mellitus and hypertension is on insulin and enalapril for hypertension. Which of the following risks would increase with the simultaneous administration of both drugs?
   a. Hypersensitivity reaction
   b. Electrolyte imbalance
   c. Hypoglycemia
   d. Hypotensive effect

5. A patient has developed a headache following the use of prazosin for hypertension. Which of the following instructions should the nurse provide the patient receiving prazosin? Select all that apply.
   a. Lie down and elevate the legs above head level
   b. Withhold the consumption of prazosin
   c. Apply a cool cloth over the forehead
   d. Engage in progressive body relaxation
   e. Take an analgesic drug for the pain

6. A nurse is monitoring a patient on minoxidil for hypertension. Which of the following changes should the nurse report to the practitioner concerning patients on minoxidil? Select all that apply.
   a. Swelling of the face
   b. Pulse rate of more than 10 beats per minute
   c. Rapid weight gain of 1 lb
   d. Difficulty in breathing
   e. Angina and severe indigestion

7. A nurse is caring for a patient receiving captopril for hypertension. Which of the following precautions should the nurse take when administering captopril?
   a. Administer captopril 1 hour before or 2 hours after food
   b. Rub the patient's back before administering captopril
   c. Ensure that the patient exercises before administering captopril
   d. Take captopril along with antacids

8. A patient receiving terazosin for orthostatic hypertension complains of dizziness. Which of the following instructions should the nurse give the patient? Select all that apply.
   a. Rise slowly from a sitting or lying position
   b. Increase fluid intake
   c. Apply a cool cloth over the forehead
   d. Rest on the bed for 1 or 2 minutes before rising
   e. Stand still for a few minutes after rising

9. A nurse is required to educate patients on the consequences of hypertension. Which of the following will develop as a consequence of hypertension? Select all that apply.
   a. Adrenal tumor
   b. Blindness
   c. Stroke
   d. Heart diseases
   e. Obesity

10. A nurse is educating a patient with hypertension about the adverse effects associated with hawthorn use. Which of the following should the nurse include as the adverse effects of hawthorn? Select all that apply.
    a. Hypotension
    b. Arrhythmia
    c. Pruritus
    d. Neutropenia
    e. Sedation

Study Guide to Accompany Introductory Clinical Pharmacology, 8th edition, by Sally S. Roach and Susan M. Ford.

CHAPTER 42

Antihyperlipidemic Drugs

SECTION I: ASSESSING YOUR UNDERSTANDING

Activity A   MATCHING

1. Match the antihyperlipidemic drugs in Column A with their adverse reactions in Column B.

Column A	Column B
_D_ 1. Rosuvastatin	A. Coughing
_A_ 2. Ezetimibe	B. Tingling
_B_ 3. Niacin	C. Vertigo
_C_ 4. Gemfibrozil	D. Pharyngitis

2. Match the antihyperlipidemic drugs in Column A with their uses in Column B.

Column A	Column B
_C_ 1. Cholestyramine	A. Reduces elevated serum triglyceride levels
_A_ 2. Atorvastatin	
_D_ 3. Fluvastatin	B. Provides secondary prevention of cardiovascular events
_B_ 4. Lovastatin	
	C. Provides relief from partial biliary obstruction
	D. Slows progression of coronary artery disease

Activity B   FILL IN THE BLANKS

1. Hyperlipidemia is an increase in the lipids, which are a group of fats or fatlike substances in the blood.

2. Atherosclerosis is a disorder in which lipid deposits accumulate on the lining of blood vessels.

3. High-density lipoproteins take cholesterol from the peripheral cells and transport it to the liver.

4. A substance that accelerates a chemical reaction without undergoing a change itself is called a catalyst.

5. Rhabdomyolysis is a condition in which muscle damage results in the release of muscle cell contents into the bloodstream.

SECTION II: APPLYING YOUR KNOWLEDGE

Activity C   SHORT ANSWERS

A nurse's role in managing a patient who has been prescribed an antihyperlipidemic drug involves performing preadministration and ongoing assessments during the course of the drug therapy. The nurse also monitors the patients for any occurrence of adverse reactions. Answer the following questions, which involve the nurse's role in the management of patients on antihyperlipidemic drug therapy.

1. A nurse is caring for a patient with hyperlipidemia. What preadministration assessments should the nurse perform before administering a prescribed antihyperlipidemic drug?

_____

_____

_____

2. What is the nurse's role after an antihyperlipidemic drug is administered to a patient?

_____

_____

_____

Activity D   DOSAGE CALCULATION

1. A patient with partial biliary obstruction has been prescribed 16 g of cholestyramine to be taken four times a day in equal doses. The drug is available in packets of 4 g. How many packets would be required for 1 day? _____

2. A patient with hyperlipidemia has been prescribed 5 g of colestipol to be taken every day. Colestipol is available as tablets of 1 g each. How many tablets should be administered to the patient in a day? _____

3. A patient with hyperlipidemia has been prescribed 80 g of atorvastatin per day. The drug is available in 40-mg tablets. How many tablets should the nurse administer to the patient every day? _____

4. A patient with mixed dyslipidemia has been prescribed 60 mg of fluvastatin to be taken per day. The drug is available as 20-mg capsules. How many capsules should the nurse administer to the patient in a day? _____

5. An adolescent patient with hypercholesterolemia has been prescribed 40 mg of lovastatin per day. The drug is available in 10-mg tablets. How many tablets should the nurse administer to the patient daily? _____

SECTION III: PRACTICING FOR NCLEX

Activity E

Answer the following questions.

1. A nurse is caring for a patient undergoing ezetimibe drug therapy at a health care facility. What instruction should the nurse provide to the patient if the drug is to be taken with cholestyramine, a bile acid sequestrant?

a. Take the drug 2 hours before a bile acid sequestrant

b. Ensure a time gap of 1 hour between the intake of these drugs

c. Take both the drugs 30 minutes before the meals

d. Take the bile acid sequestrant with warm water

2. The nurse is required to initiate an atorvastatin drug therapy for a patient. For which of the following conditions of the patient is atorvastatin contraindicated?

a. Visual disturbances

b. Biliary obstruction

c. Serious liver disorders

d. Renal dysfunction

3. A nurse is caring for a patient with primary hypercholesterolemia who is undergoing ezetimibe drug therapy. What adverse reaction to the drug should the nurse monitor for in the patient?

a. Vertigo

b. Headache

c. Cholelithiasis

d. Arthralgia

4. A patient is undergoing gemfibrozil drug therapy for high serum triglyceride levels. The patient is also receiving an anticoagulant as a blood thinner. What effect should the nurse observe for in the patient resulting from the interaction of these two drugs?

a. Increased hypoglycemic effects

b. Increased risk of severe myopathy

c. Enhanced effect of the anticoagulant

d. Increased risk of hypertension

5. A nurse at a health care facility is caring for a patient who has been prescribed hydroxymethylglutaryl-coenzyme A (HMG-CoA) inhibitors. For which of the following conditions of the patient should the nurse use the prescribed drug cautiously? Select all that apply.

a. Peptic ulcer

b. Acute infection

c. Visual disturbances

d. Unstable angina

e. Endocrine disorders

6. A nurse is caring for a patient receiving garlic therapy for lowering serum cholesterol and triglyceride levels. The patient is also taking warfarin as an anticoagulant. What should the nurse monitor for in this patient?

a. Bleeding

b. Peptic ulcers

c. Irritation

d. Skin rashes

7. A nurse is caring for an elderly patient undergoing therapy with bile acid sequestrants. What should the nurse monitor for in the patient? Select all that apply.

a. Difficulty in passing stools

b. Hard dry stools

c. Constipation

d. Mouth dryness

e. Urinary hesitancy

8. A nurse is caring for a patient receiving an antihyperlipidemic drug. The nurse observes a paradoxical elevation of blood lipid levels in the patient. What should be the nurse's intervention in such a situation?

a. Notify the primary health care provider for a different antihyperlipidemic drug

b. Collect blood samples for further examination

c. Administer the next dose of the drug with milk

d. Record the fluid intake and output every hour

9. A patient informs the nurse that he has been taking flax powder for improving the blood lipid profile. Which toxic reaction is associated with the consumption of flax?

a. Abdominal pain

b. Dyspnea

c. Cramps

d. Dyspepsia

10. A nurse is caring for a patient who has been prescribed colestipol for the treatment of hyperlipidemia. This drug is known to cause constipation. What instructions should the nurse provide to the patient to help prevent constipation? Select all that apply.

a. Perform exercises daily

b. Consume foods high in dietary fiber

c. Take the drug 1 hour after meals

d. Increase the fluid intake

e. Take oral vitamin K supplements

CHAPTER 43

Anticoagulant and Thrombolytic Drugs

SECTION I: ASSESSING YOUR UNDERSTANDING

Activity A MATCHING

1. Match the drugs in Column A with their adverse reactions in Column B.

Column A	Column B
D 1. Heparin	A. Dyspepsia
C 2. Cilostazol	B. Pallor
A 3. Ticlopidine	C. Heart palpitations
B 4. Treprostinil	D. Chills

2. Match the antiplatelet drugs in Column A with their uses in Column B.

Column A	Column B
B 1. Clopidogrel	A. Intermittent claudication
D 2. Ticlopidine	B. Recent myocardial infarction
A 3. Cilostazol	C. Pulmonary arterial hypertension
C 4. Treprostinil	D. Thrombotic stroke

Activity B FILL IN THE BLANKS

1. _Prothrombin_ is essential for the clotting of blood.

2. Venous _Thrombus_ can develop as the result of venous stasis, injury to the vessel wall, or altered blood coagulation.

3. _Arterial_ thrombosis can occur because of atherosclerosis or arrhythmias.

4. Drugs that help to eliminate clots are known as _Thrombolytics_

5. Glycoprotein receptor blockers work to prevent _enzyme_ production.

6. The use of an adapter and tubing to stay in the vein for intermittent intravenous (IV) administration is called a _heparin_ lock.

SECTION II: APPLYING YOUR KNOWLEDGE

Activity C SHORT ANSWERS

A nurse's role in managing patients who are being administered anticoagulant and thrombolytic drugs involves monitoring the patients and implementing interventions that aid in their recovery. Answer the following questions, which involve the nurse's role in the management of such situations.

1. A nurse has been caring for a client with deep venous thrombosis (DVT). After treatment, the nurse has to evaluate the effectiveness of the treatment plan. What factors should the nurse consider to determine the success of the treatment plan?

_____

_____

_____

2. A nurse is caring for a patient who has been prescribed enoxaparin sodium for the treatment of pulmonary emboli (PE). What instructions should the nurse provide to help the patient cooperate with the prescribed therapy?

_____

_____

_____

Activity D DOSAGE CALCULATION

1. A patient undergoing treatment for venous thrombosis has been prescribed 250 mg of anisindione per day to take orally. The drug is available in 50-mg compressed tablets. How many tablets should the nurse administer to the patient in a day? _____

2. A patient has been prescribed 7.5 mg of warfarin per day for the prophylaxis of venous thrombosis. The drug is available in 2.5-mg tablets. How many tablets should the nurse administer to the patient every day?

_____

3. A patient with intermittent claudication has been prescribed 100 mg of cilostazol to be administered orally twice in a day. The drug is available in 50-mg tablets. How many tablets should be administered to the patient in a day? _____

4. A patient has been prescribed a single loading dose containing 300 mg of clopidogrel per day for the treatment of acute coronary syndrome. The drug is available in 75-mg tablets. How many tablets should the nurse administer to the patient in the course of 1 day? _____

5. A patient undergoing treatment for thrombotic stroke is prescribed ticlopidine drug therapy. The physician has instructed the nurse to administer 250 mg of ticlopidine twice a day to the patient. The drug is available in 250-mg tablets. How many tablets should the nurse get for the course of 3 days? _____

SECTION III: PRACTICING FOR NCLEX

Activity E

Answer the following questions.

1. Alteplase has been prescribed to a patient with acute ischemic stroke. Which of the following adverse reactions associated with drug administration should the nurse monitor for in the patient? Select all that apply.
   a. Gingival bleeding
   b. Erythema
   c. Epistaxis
   d. Ecchymosis
   e. Anemia

2. A nurse is caring for a patient who has been prescribed abciximab for coronary angioplasty. The patient is also taking aspirin for pain relief. What effects of the interaction between these two drugs should the nurse observe for in the patient?
   a. Decreased effectiveness of aspirin
   b. Increased effectiveness of abciximab
   c. Increased risk of bleeding
   d. Decreased absorption of abciximab

3. A nurse is required to start anticoagulant drug therapy for a patient. In which of the following conditions is an anticoagulant contraindicated? Select all that apply.
   a. Diabetic retinopathy
   b. Tuberculosis
   c. Gastrointestinal (GI) bleeding
   d. Leukemia
   e. Hemorrhagic disease

4. A nurse is caring for a patient who is undergoing anisindione drug therapy for the treatment of venous thrombosis. What assessment should the nurse perform during the course of the therapy?
   a. Draw blood for a complete blood count
   b. Determine the international normalized ratio (INR)
   c. Draw blood for a baseline prothrombin time (PT)/INR test
   d. Continually assess for any signs of bleeding

5. A nurse is caring for a patient taking antiplatelet drugs. What instruction should the nurse include in the teaching plan for this patient?
   a. Use a soft toothbrush
   b. Eat foods high in vitamin K
   c. Take the medication with food
   d. Take the drug at a different time each day

6. A patient is undergoing warfarin drug therapy. After taking the drug, the patient develops signs of GI bleeding. Which of the following interventions should the nurse perform for this patient?
   a. Inspect urine for red-orange color
   b. Monitor vital signs every 4 hours
   c. Inspect for bright red to black stools
   d. Monitor patient's fluid intake and output

7. A nurse is caring for a patient who has been administered heparin after the administration of a thrombolytic drug to prevent another thrombus from forming. What should the nurse monitor for in the patient after the administration of heparin?
   a. Internal bleeding
   b. Difficulty in breathing
   c. Excessive perspiration
   d. Skin rash

8. A nurse is required to administer heparin to a patient. What should the nurse do to avoid the possibility of local irritation, pain, or hematoma?
   a. Avoid application of firm pressure after the injection
   b. Avoid administration sites such as the buttocks and lateral thighs
   c. Use an area within 2 inches of the umbilicus for drug administration
   d. Avoid intramuscular (IM) administration of the drug

9. A nurse is caring for a patient receiving parenteral anticoagulant drug therapy. The nurse notices symptoms of overdosage of the drug. What intervention should the nurse perform if administration of this drug is necessary?
   a. Measure the patient's body temperature every hour
   b. Monitor the patient's pulse rate every 2 hours
   c. Observe the patient for new evidence of bleeding
   d. Administer the drug to the patient via the IV route

10. A patient is administered a thrombolytic drug, which is known to cause bleeding. Which of the following symptoms of internal bleeding should the nurse observe in the patient? Select all that apply.
    a. Black tarry stools
    b. Hematuria
    c. Chest pain
    d. Petechiae
    e. Coffee-ground emesis

CHAPTER 44

Agents Used in the Treatment of Anemia

SECTION I: ASSESSING YOUR UNDERSTANDING

Activity A MATCHING

1. Match the types of anemia in Column A with their corresponding descriptions in Column B.

Column A

_D_ 1. Iron deficiency anemia

_C_ 2. Anemia in chronic renal failure

_B_ 3. Pernicious anemia

_A_ 4. Folic acid deficiency anemia

Column B

A. Anemia occurring because of a dietary lack of folic acid, a component necessary in the formation of red blood cells

B. Anemia resulting from lack of secretions by the gastric mucosa of the intrinsic factor essential to the formation of RBCs and the absorption of vitamin B$_{12}$

C. Anemia resulting from a reduced production of erythropoietin, a hormone secreted by the kidney that stimulates the production of red blood cells (RBCs)

D. Anemia characterized by an inadequate amount of iron in the body to produce hemoglobin

2. Match the drugs used for treating anemia in Column A with their corresponding adverse reactions in Column B.

Column A

_D_ 1. Ferrous fumarate

_C_ 2. Darbepoetin alfa

_B_ 3. Folic acid

_A_ 4. Sodium ferric gluconate complex

Column B

A. Conjunctivitis

B. Allergic sensitization

C. Cardiac arrhythmias

D. Gastrointestinal (GI) irritation

Activity B FILL IN THE BLANKS

1. _Erythropoeisis_ is the process of making RBCs in the body.

2. _anemia_ is a condition caused by an insufficient amount of hemoglobin delivering oxygen to the tissues.

3. The technique of administering _leucovorin_ after a large dose of methotrexate is called folinic acid rescue.

4. _Megaloblastic_ anemia is characterized by the presence of large, abnormal, immature erythrocytes circulating in the blood.

5. A deficiency of the intrinsic factor results in the abnormal formation of erythrocytes because of the body's failure to absorb vitamin B_{12}, leading to _maurxytic_ anemia.

SECTION II: APPLYING YOUR KNOWLEDGE

Activity C SHORT ANSWERS

A nurse's role in managing patients who are being administered drugs for the treatment of iron deficiency anemia involves monitoring them and implementing interventions that aid in their recovery. Answer the following questions, which involve the nurse's role in the management of such situations.

1. A patient with iron deficiency anemia has been prescribed ferrous gluconate. What should a nurse assess for in the patient before administering the first dose of ferrous gluconate?

_____

_____

_____

2. A patient is administered sodium ferric gluconate complex for the treatment of iron deficiency anemia. What adverse reactions should the nurse monitor for in this patient?

_____

_____

_____

Activity D DOSAGE CALCULATION

1. A patient has been prescribed 75 mg of elemental iron for the treatment of iron deficiency anemia. Elemental iron is administered intramuscularly with the help of an iron dextran injection. Each milliliter of the available iron dextran contains 50 mg of elemental iron. How many milliliters of iron dextran will the nurse have to administer to the patient? _____

2. A patient is prescribed 25 mg of folic acid over 5 days for the treatment of megaloblastic anemia. The folic acid is to be administered intravenously (IV). The drug is available in a 5-mg/mL folic acid solution. How many

milliliters of folic acid will the nurse have to administer to the patient per day?

_____

3. A patient is prescribed 90 mg of oral Feosol in two equally divided doses per day. Feosol is available as tablets of 45 mg. How many tablets would the patient require for a week?

_____

4. A physician prescribes 6000 units of epoetin alfa per day for a patient with chronic renal failure (CRF)-associated anemia. Each 1 mL of epoetin alfa solution contains 3000 units of epoetin alfa. How many milliliters of epoetin alfa solution will the nurse have to administer to the patient per day? _____

SECTION III: PRACTICING FOR NCLEX

Activity E

Answer the following questions.

1. A patient with folic acid deficiency anemia is administered a Folvite injection. What adverse reactions should the nurse monitor for in this patient?
   a. Anorexia
   b. Allergic hypersensitivity
   c. Arthralgia
   d. Adrenal hyperplasia

2. A patient is prescribed epoetin alfa to treat CRF-associated anemia. In which of the following patients is epoetin alfa contraindicated?
   a. Patients with hypersensitivity to human albumin
   b. Patients with an allergy to cyanocobalamin
   c. Patients undergoing treatment for pernicious anemia
   d. Patients with hemolytic anemia

3. A nurse administers oral doses of vitamin B_{12} to a patient with vitamin B_{12} deficiency. During assessment, the nurse observes a reduction in the absorption of vitamin B_{12} in the patient's body. Which of the following has contributed to this reduction? Select all that apply.

a. Alcohol

b. Caffeine

c. Neomycin

d. Nicotine

e. Colchicine

4. A patient with iron deficiency anemia is prescribed iron dextran. Which of the following is the most appropriate assessment that a nurse should perform when calculating the dosage of iron dextran?

a. Weight and hemoglobin level

b. Heart rate

c. Blood pressure

d. Body temperature

5. A nurse is caring for a patient who has to be administered iron supplements. The patient informs the nurse that he has been taking methyldopa. Which of the following conditions should the nurse monitor in the patient as a result of the interaction between the two drugs once the iron drug regimen begins?

a. Decreased blood pressure

b. Increased heart rate

c. Decreased effect of Parkinson's medication

d. Increased absorption of iron

6. A nurse is caring for a patient who is receiving cyanocobalamin for vitamin B_{12} deficiency. Which of the following food items should the nurse ask the patient to consume in order to fulfill the nutritional deficiency of vitamin B_{12} through a balanced diet? Select all that apply.

a. Seafood

b. Meat

c. Eggs

d. Leafy vegetables

e. Breads and cereals

7. A patient receiving ferrous fumarate for the treatment of anemia is to be shortly discharged. What should the nurse include in the patient teaching plan when providing care on an outpatient basis?

a. Take antacids in case of acidity

b. Take drugs with meals in case of gastrointestinal upset

c. Drink the liquid iron preparation directly from a glass

d. Avoid using multivitamin preparations

8. A nurse is caring for a patient receiving parenteral administration of iron for the treatment of anemia. Which of the following adverse reactions should the nurse monitor for when caring for the patient? Select all that apply.

a. Urticaria

b. Dyspnea

c. Insomnia

d. Diabetes

e. Rashes

9. What information should the nurse offer when performing ongoing assessments for a patient receiving oral iron supplements?

a. The color of the stools will be black

b. His or her palpitations will be high

c. The patient's weight will increase

d. A rash may develop

10. A nurse is caring for a patient receiving iron supplements. Which of the following instructions should the nurse provide to the patient to prevent interference with the absorption of iron?

a. Avoid milk

b. Avoid poultry

c. Avoid meat

d. Avoid fish

45

Diuretics

SECTION I: ASSESSING YOUR UNDERSTANDING

Activity A MATCHING

1. Match the diuretics in Column A with their uses in Column B.

Column A

_E_ 1. Ethacrynic acid

_A_ 2. Mannitol

_B_ 3. Urea

_C_ 4. Amiloride

_D_ 5. Metolazone

Column B

A. Treatment of cerebral edema

B. Reduction of intracranial pressure

C. Prevention of polyuria with lithium use

D. Hypertension, edema caused by congestive heart failure (CHF), and cirrhosis

E. Short-term management of ascites caused by lymphedema

2. Match the loop diuretic and its interactant drug in Column A with the interaction results in Column B.

Column A

_C_ 1. Loop diuretic + thrombolytic

_A_ 2. Loop diuretic + lithium

Column B

A. Increased risk of lithium toxicity

B. Increased risk of arrhythmias

_D_ 3. Loop diuretic + aminoglycoside

_B_ 4. Loop diuretic + digitalis

C. Increased risk of bleeding

D. Increased risk of ototoxicity

Activity B FILL IN THE BLANKS

1. Retention of excess fluid in the tissue or body is known as **edema**.

2. **Carbonic** anhydrase inhibition, which is the action of a diuretic drug, results in the excretion of sodium, potassium, bicarbonate, and water.

3. Increase in the **potassium** in the blood is known as hyperkalemia.

4. Extremity **parasthesis**, meaning numbness, tingling, or flaccid muscles, may indicate hypokalemia, which is an adverse reaction to diuretics.

5. **Dermatolic** reactions to diuretics involve rash and photosensitivity.

SECTION II: APPLYING YOUR KNOWLEDGE

Activity C SHORT ANSWERS

A nurse's role in managing patients who have been prescribed diuretics involves performing preadministrative and ongoing assessments during the course of the drug therapy. The nurse also monitors patients receiving diuretic drugs for any adverse reactions. Answer the following questions, which involve the nurse's role in the management of patients on diuretic drug therapy.

1. A patient with edema is prescribed a diuretic drug. What preadministration assessments should the nurse perform before administration of this diuretic drug?

_____

_____

_____

2. What is the nurse's role after the administration of a diuretic drug to a patient?

_____

_____

_____

Activity D DOSAGE CALCULATION

1. A patient with edema has been prescribed acetazolamide. The physician instructs the nurse to administer 250 mg of the drug every 4 hours. The drug is available in 500-mg tablets. How many tablets should the nurse administer to the patient daily? _____

2. A patient with glaucoma is undergoing methazolamide drug therapy. The physician has prescribed 100 mg of the drug to be taken twice in a day. How many tablets should the nurse administer if the drug is available in 50-mg tablets? _____

3. A patient with edema caused by cirrhosis of the liver has been prescribed 6 mg of bumetanide (Bumex) on a daily basis. The drug is available in 2-mg tablets. How many tablets should the nurse administer the client every day? _____

4. A physician has prescribed 500 mg of chlorothiazide (Diuril) for a patient to take twice a day. The physician has instructed the nurse to administer the drug through the intravenous (IV) route. The drug is available in the form of 250 mg of chlorothiazide per 5 mL of solution. How much solution should the nurse prepare for this patient per day?

_____

5. A physician has prescribed 200 mg of furosemide (Lasix) per day. The drug is available in 80-mg tablets. How many tablets should the nurse administer the patient every day? _____

SECTION III: PRACTICING FOR NCLEX

Activity E

Answer the following questions.

1. A nurse is caring for a patient with edema. What assessments should the nurse perform on this patient to promote optimal response to therapy? Select all that apply.
   a. Measure and record patient's weight daily
   b. Check the pupils every 2 hours for dilation
   c. Measure fluid intake and output every 8 hours
   d. Assess respiratory rate every 4 hours
   e. Check the patient's response to light

2. A nurse is caring for a patient receiving diuretics. During assessment, the nurse observes that the patient is experiencing a gastrointestinal (GI) upset after taking the prescribed drug. Which of the following interventions should the nurse perform when caring for this patient?
   a. Ensure that the drug is taken on an empty stomach
   b. Ensure that the drug is taken with food or milk
   c. Instruct the patient to reduce fluid intake
   d. Caution the patient to avoid any consumption of fibrous food

3. A nurse is caring for a patient with edema caused by CHF. The physician has prescribed spironolactone for the patient. Which of the following adverse reactions to the drug should the nurse monitor for in the patient?
   a. Vertigo
   b. Paresthesias
   c. Hyperkalemia
   d. Anorexia

4. A physician has prescribed a chlorothiazide drug to a patient with hypertension. The patient informs the nurse that he is also taking an antidiabetic drug for controlling diabetes. What effect of the interaction between these two drugs should the nurse monitor for in the patient?
   a. Increased risk of ototoxicity
   b. Increased risk of hyperglycemia

c. Increased hypersensitivity to the antidiabetic

d. Increased chlorothiazide effect

5. A primary health care provider has prescribed an antihypertensive drug along with a diuretic to a patient as a treatment for hypertension. The patient informs the nurse about his preference for herbal extracts over medical drugs. What should the nurse inform the patient regarding herbal extracts? Select all that apply.

a. No herbal diuretic should be taken unless approved by the primary health care provider

b. Some herbal extracts have been associated with renal damage

c. Herbal extracts are more effective than caffeine

d. Most plant and herbal extracts that are available as diuretics are nontoxic

e. After consulting the primary health care provider, the patient may consume diuretic teas such as those made from juniper berries

6. A nurse is caring for a patient showing signs of excess fluid retention. The nurse knows that which of the following has caused this condition in the patient?

a. Endocrine disturbances

b. Hyperkalemia

c. Hematologic changes

d. Gastric distress

7. A nurse is caring for a patient with renal dysfunction. The physician has prescribed metolazone for the patient. What should the nurse monitor in the patient before administering the drug? Select all that apply.

a. Serum potassium levels

b. Levels of serum electrolytes

c. Fluid loss every hour

d. Creatinine clearance levels

e. Blood urea nitrogen level

8. A nurse is caring for a patient who complains of cramps and muscle pains. Assessment reveals that the patient is also experiencing oliguria, hypotension, and GI disturbances. Which of the following conditions is the patient experiencing?

a. Hyperkalemia

b. Electrolyte imbalance

c. Hypercalcemia

d. Hyponatremia

9. A physician prescribes the potassium sparing diuretic amiloride (Midamor). In which of the following conditions should the nurse discontinue the drug?

a. Gout attacks

b. Urine tests positive for glucose

c. Serum potassium levels greater than 5.3 mEq/mL

d. Excess fluid removed from the patient's body

CHAPTER 46

Urinary Tract Anti-Infectives, Antispasmodics, and Other Urinary Drugs

SECTION I: ASSESSING YOUR UNDERSTANDING

Activity A MATCHING

1. Match the urinary drugs in Column A with their uses in Column B.

Column A

___ 1. Amoxicillin

___ 2. Nitrofurantoin

___ 3. Oxybutynin

___ 4. Phenazopyridine

Column B

A. Treats acute bacterial urinary tract infections (UTIs)

B. Treats acute UTIs and other bacterial infections

C. Relieves pain associated with irritation of the lower genitourinary tract

D. Treats overactive bladder and neurogenic bladder

2. Match the anti-infectives and their interactant drugs in Column A with the interaction effects on the anti-infective drugs in Column B.

Column A

___ 1. Anti-infectives + anticholinergics

___ 2. Anti-infectives + metoclopramide

___ 3. Anti-infectives + oral anticoagulants

___ 4. Anti-infectives + magnesium trisilicate or magaldrate

Column B

A. Lowers plasma concentration and urinary tract excretion of fosfomycin

B. Decreases absorption of anti-infective

C. Delays gastric emptying

D. Increases risk for bleeding

Activity B FILL IN THE BLANKS

1. Clinical manifestations of _____ include urgency, frequency, pressure, burning, and pain on urination.

2. _____ drugs counteract the smooth muscle spasm of the urinary tract by relaxing the detrusor and other muscles through action at the parasympathetic nerve receptors.

3. _____ bladder is an impaired bladder function caused by a nervous system abnormality, typically an injury to the spinal cord.

4. Excessive urination caused during the night is called _____.

5. _____ incontinence is characterized by involuntary urination after a sudden sensation to void.

SECTION II: APPLYING YOUR KNOWLEDGE

Activity C SHORT ANSWERS

A nurse's role in managing patients who are being administered urinary tract anti-infectives, antispasmodics, and other urinary drugs involves monitoring the patients and implementing interventions that aid in their recovery. Answer the following questions, which involve the nurse's role in the management of such situations.

1. A nurse has been caring for a patient with a UTI. After treatment, the nurse has to evaluate the effectiveness of the treatment plan. What factors should the nurse consider to determine the success of the treatment plan?

_____

_____

_____

2. A patient with a UTI is undergoing anti-infective drug therapy. What instructions should the nurse offer the patient and the patient's family to ensure compliance with the medication regimen?

_____

_____

_____

Activity D DOSAGE CALCULATION

1. A patient with acute bacterial UTIs has been prescribed 500 mg of amoxicillin to be administered every 8 hours. On hand are 500-mg tablets. How many tablets should the nurse administer to the patient daily? _____

2. A patient with acute cystitis has been prescribed 6 g of fosfomycin to be taken with food daily. The drug therapy has to continue for 5 days. The drug is available in 3-g tablets. How many tablets should the nurse administer to the patient in 5 days? _____

3. A patient has been prescribed 1 g of methenamine to be administered orally twice a day. The treatment has to continue for 4 days. The drug is available in 1-g tablets. How many tablets should the nurse administer in 4 days? _____

4. A patient has been prescribed nitrofurantoin for acute bacterial UTI. The physician has prescribed 200 mg of the drug to be taken 4 times a day. The drug is available in 100-mg capsules in the pharmacy. How many capsules should the nurse administer to the patient in a day? _____

SECTION III: PRACTICING FOR NCLEX

Activity E

Answer the following questions.

1. A nurse is caring for a patient with an overactive bladder who has been prescribed darifenacin HCl (Enablex) drug. The drug is known to cause dry mouth. What instructions should the nurse offer the patient to get relief from dry mouth?
   a. Suck on sugarless lozenges
   b. Refrain from consuming hard candy
   c. Consume foods rich in fiber
   d. Always take the drug with milk

2. A nurse is caring for a patient receiving solifenacin drug therapy for the treatment of an overactive bladder. What adverse reaction to the drug should the nurse monitor for in the patient?
   a. Headache
   b. Dry eyes
   c. Pruritus
   d. Rash

3. A patient with acute bacterial urinary tract infections is undergoing sulfamethoxazole drug therapy. The patient is also receiving an oral anticoagulant as a blood thinner. What

condition should the nurse monitor for in this patient as a result of the interaction of the two drugs?

a. Increased risk of bleeding

b. Urinary tract excretion of the anti-infective

c. Delay in gastric emptying

d. Decreased effect of sulfamethoxazole

4. A nurse is required to initiate antispasmodic drug therapy. For which of the following patients is the use of antispasmodics contraindicated?

a. A patient with convulsive disorders

b. A patient with cerebral arteriosclerosis

c. A patient with myasthenia gravis

d. A patient with a hepatic impairment

5. A nurse is caring for a patient who has been prescribed a urinary anti-infective. What interventions should the nurse perform when administering the drug to decrease the pain experienced by the patient on voiding?

a. Administer the drug strictly with milk

b. Administer the drug after meals

c. Administer the drug with prune juice

d. Ensure drug administration with warm water

6. A nurse is caring for a patient receiving phenazopyridine to treat irritation of the lower genitourinary tract. The patient is also receiving an antibacterial drug for a UTI. What intervention should the nurse perform when administering phenazopyridine in combination with an antibacterial drug?

a. Encourage patient to drink at least 2000 mL of fluid daily

b. Administer the drug with cranberry or prune juice

c. Avoid administering phenazopyridine for more than 2 days

d. Administer phenazopyridine 2 hours before giving the antibacterial drug

7. A nurse is caring for a patient receiving flavoxate for the treatment of urinary problems. During assessment, the patient complains of constipation. What intervention should the nurse perform when caring for this patient?

a. Increase the patient's intake of fluids

b. Increase the patient's intake of citrus fruits

c. Decrease the patient's consumption of milk products

d. Administer the drug to the patient with warm water

8. A nurse is caring for a patient receiving nitrofurantoin urinary tract anti-infective at a health care facility. What nursing intervention should the nurse perform to prevent irritation in the stomach?

a. Administer the drug with apple juice

b. Administer the drug with milk

c. Administer the drug at bedtime

d. Administer the drug 1 hour before meals

9. A nurse is caring for a patient who has been prescribed a urinary tract anti-infective for the treatment of UTIs. What preadministration assessments should the nurse perform when caring for the patient? Select all that apply.

a. Question the patient regarding symptoms of infection

b. Assess for urinary frequency and bladder distension

c. Take and record vital signs

d. Constantly monitor body temperature

e. Assist in performing periodic urinalysis and culture tests

10. A nurse at a health care facility is caring for a patient who has been prescribed anti-infective drug therapy for acute otitis media. For which of the following patients should the nurse use the prescribed drug cautiously?

a. A patient with gastrointestinal infections

b. A patient with urinary retention

c. A patient with renal impairment

d. A patient with hypertension

47

Drugs That Affect the Upper Gastrointestinal System

SECTION I: ASSESSING YOUR UNDERSTANDING

Activity A MATCHING

1. Match the drugs in Column A with the disorders for which they are used in Column B.

Column A

C 1. Aluminum carbonate gel

D 2. Calcium carbonate

A 3. Lansoprazol

B 4. Pantoprazole

E 5. Misoprostol

Column B

A. Cystic fibrosis

B. Hypersecretory conditions

C. Hyperphosphatemia

D. Gastric ulcers

E. Osteoporosis

2. Match the drugs in Column A with the effect of their interactions with antacids in Column B.

Column A

B 1. Chlorpromazine

C 2. Tetracycline

A 3. Corticosteroids

E 4. Salicylates

D 5. Amphetamines

Column B

A. Decreased effectiveness of anti-inflammatory properties

B. Decreased absorption of the interactant drug

C. Decreased effectiveness of the anti-infective

D. Slow excretion of interactant drug from urine

E. Rapid excretion of pain reliever from urine

Activity B FILL IN THE BLANKS

1. The ___GI___ system is a long tube within the body where ingested food and fluids are prepared for absorption and ultimate replenishment of nutrients to the cells.

2. The __esophaus__ connects the mouth to the stomach where food is mixed with acids and enzymes to become a solution for absorption.

3. A forceful expulsion of gastric contents through the mouth is known as __vomiting__.

4. __Dronabnol__ is the only medically available cannabinoid prescribed for antiemetic use.

5. Proton pump inhibitors are particularly important in the treatment of *Helicobacter pylori* in patients with active __duodenal__ ulcers.

SECTION II: APPLYING YOUR KNOWLEDGE

Activity C SHORT ANSWERS

A nurse's role in managing patients receiving a drug for an upper gastrointestinal (GI) disorder involves assisting the patient for preadministration assessment. The nurse also monitors the patient for the occurrence of any adverse reactions. Answer the following questions, which involve the nurse's role in the management of such situations.

1. A patient with severe nausea and vomiting has been prescribed an antiemetic drug. What preadministration assessments should the nurse perform for the patient?

_____

_____

_____

2. After the preadministration assessment, the patient is administered an antiemetic drug. What is the nurse's role after administration of the drug?

_____

_____

_____

Activity D DOSAGE CALCULATION

1. A physician has prescribed 2.5 mg of dronabinol to a patient as a human immunodeficiency virus (HIV) appetite stimulant to be taken twice a day. The drug is available in 2.5-mg capsules at the facility's pharmacy. How many capsules should the nurse administer to the patient during the treatment course of 3 days? _____

2. A physician has prescribed 40 mg of esomeprazole magnesium to a patient daily for the treatment of erosive esophagitis. The drug is available as 20-mg capsules at a pharmacy store. How many capsules should the nurse administer to the patient per day?

_____

3. A patient has been prescribed 1600 mg of cimetidine for the treatment of gastric ulcers, to be taken orally each day. The drug is available in 400-mg tablets. How many tablets should the nurse administer to the patient per day? _____

4. A patient has been prescribed 600 mg of ranitidine per day for the treatment of erosive esophagitis. The drug is available as 150-mg tablets. How many tablets should the nurse administer to the patient daily? _____

5. A patient has been prescribed 30 mg of the lansoprazole drug daily for the treatment of cystic fibrosis. The drug is available as 15-mg capsules. How many capsules should the nurse administer to the patient for the treatment course of 3 days? _____

SECTION III: PRACTICING FOR NCLEX

Activity E

Answer the following questions.

1. A patient has been administered dronabinol for the prevention of chemotherapy-induced nausea. Which of the following adverse reactions should the nurse monitor for in the patient?
   a. Sedation
   b. Hypoxia
   c. Euphoria
   d. Asthenia

2. A nurse is caring for a patient who has been administered antacids for the treatment of gastric ulcers. The patient informs the nurse that he is also taking opioid analgesics for pain relief. What effect of the interaction between the two drugs should the nurse assess for in the patient?
   a. Increased risk of respiratory depression
   b. Decreased white blood cell count
   c. Increased risk of bleeding
   d. Increased risk of dehydration

3. A physician has asked a nurse to start promethazine therapy for a patient with nausea. For which of the following conditions should the nurse administer the drug with caution? Select all that apply.
   a. Hypertension
   b. Sleep apnea
   c. Glaucoma

d. Epilepsy

e. Viral illness

4. A nurse has administered aluminum hydroxide gel to relieve stomach hyperacidity. What should the nurse monitor for in the patient after administration of the drug?

a. Headache

b. Coffee–ground-colored emesis

c. Signs of electrolyte imbalances

d. Amount of fluid lost

5. A patient undergoing antacid drug therapy is to be discharged from a health care facility. What should the nurse include in the teaching plan for the patient?

a. Increase frequency of dose if symptoms worsen

b. Avoid direct exposure to sunlight

c. Take other drugs 1 hour before taking the antacid

d. Avoid driving when taking the drug

6. A nurse is caring for a patient who has intentionally ingested a poison. The nurse is required to administer an emetic drug to the patient. What information should the nurse obtain from a family member or friend of the patient before administration of the drug? Select all that apply.

a. Substances that have been ingested

b. Cause for ingesting the poison

c. Time when the substances were ingested

d. Patient's mental status before taking poison

e. Symptoms noted before seeking medical treatment

7. A nurse is caring for a patient experiencing nausea and vomiting. The physician has prescribed an antiemetic drug therapy for the patient. What symptoms of dehydration, a serious concern associated with nausea and vomiting, should the nurse monitor for in the patient? Select all that apply.

a. White streaks in stool

b. Decreased urinary output

c. Concentrated urine

d. Decreased respiratory rate

e. Dry mucous membranes

8. A patient who has undergone surgery is prescribed acid-reducing drugs intravenously (IV). What should the nurse monitor during administration of the drugs to the patient?

a. Rate of infusion at frequent intervals

b. Body temperature every hour

c. Irritation caused by drug administration

d. Blood pressure every 2 hours

9. A nurse is caring for a patient undergoing antacid drug therapy. The patient complains of diarrhea after taking the drug. What nursing interventions should the nurse perform in this case?

a. Remove items with strong odor

b. Change to a different antacid

c. Record the patient's temperature every hour

d. Record the patient's fluid intake and output

10. A nurse is caring for a patient undergoing antiemetic drug therapy to prevent nausea. The patient reports loss of appetite because of nausea. What should the nurse do to enhance the patient's appetite?

a. Suggest consumption of milk products

b. Suggest physical exercises to the patient

c. Remove items with a strong smell and odor

d. Avoid giving frequent oral rinses to the patient

CHAPTER 48

Drugs That Affect the Lower Gastrointestinal System

SECTION I: ASSESSING YOUR UNDERSTANDING

Activity A MATCHING

1. Match the drugs in Column A with their uses in Column B.

Column A

C 1. Loperamide
A 2. Simethicone
D 3. Lactulose
B 4. Psyllium

Column B

A. Prevents the formation of gas pockets in the intestine

B. Treats irritable bowel syndrome

C. Treats chronic diarrhea associated with irritable bowel disease (IBD)

D. Reduces blood ammonia levels in hepatic encephalopathy

2. Match the drugs used in managing lower gastrointestinal (GI) disorders in Column A with their adverse reactions in Column B.

Column A

D 1. Infliximab
B 2. Difenoxin

Column B

A. Abdominal cramping

B. Constipation

A 3. Olsalazine
C 4. Sulfasalazine

C. Anorexia

D. Sore throat

Activity B FILL IN THE BLANKS

1. Transit of contents rapidly through the bowel is called _diarrhea_.

2. _Chamomile_ herb protects against the development of stomach ulcers.

3. For short-term relief or prevention of constipation, a _laxitive_ is prescribed.

4. Charcoal may be used in the prevention of nonspecific _pruritis_ associated with kidney dialysis treatment.

5. _Aminosalicylates_ are used to treat Crohn's disease and ulcerative colitis.

SECTION II: APPLYING YOUR KNOWLEDGE

Activity C SHORT ANSWERS

A nurse's role in managing patients who have been prescribed drugs for lower GI disorders involves performing preadministrative and ongoing assessments during the course of drug therapy. The nurse also monitors the patients for the occurrence of any adverse reactions after administration of the drug. Answer the following questions, which involve the nurse's role in the management of such situations.

1. A patient with dyspepsia has been prescribed simethicone. What preadministration assessments should the nurse perform before administration of the drug?

_____

_____

_____

2. What is the nurse's role after administration of the drug to the patient?

_____

_____

_____

Activity D   DOSAGE CALCULATION

1. A physician prescribes balsalazide for a patient with active ulcerative colitis. The nurse needs to administer 2250 g of balsalazide on a daily basis. The drug is available in 750-mg capsules. How many capsules should the nurse administer to the patient to complete a course of 8 weeks? _____

2. A patient with proctitis has been prescribed mesalamine. The physician has prescribed 200 mg of mesalamine to be taken 4 times a day. The drug is available in 400-mg tablets. How many tablets should the nurse administer to the patient every day? _____

3. A patient has been prescribed 1 g of olsalazine daily in two doses to maintain remission of ulcerative colitis. The drug is available as 250-mg capsules. How capsules should the nurse administer in each dose? _____

4. A nurse is caring for a patient with rheumatoid arthritis. The physician has prescribed the patient 4 g of sulfasalazine daily in divided doses. The drug is available in 500-mg tablets. How many tablets will the nurse require to complete the 3-day course? _____

5. A physician has prescribed 10 mg of bisacodyl on a daily basis to a patient for the relief of constipation. The drug is available as 5-mg tablets. How may tablets should the nurse administer to the patient every day?

_____

SECTION III: PRACTICING FOR NCLEX

Activity E

Answer the following questions.

1. A nurse is caring for a patient with proctosigmoiditis. The physician has prescribed mesalamine to the patient, who informs the nurse that he is also taking hypoglycemic drugs to manage diabetes mellitus. What condition should the nurse monitor in this patient as a result of the interaction of the two drugs?
   a. Decreased absorption of hypoglycemic drugs
   b. Increased risk of bleeding
   c. Increased blood glucose level
   d. Reduced effect of mesalamine

2. A nurse is caring for a patient with acute diarrhea who has been prescribed loperamide. Which of the following adverse reactions should the nurse monitor for in the patient?
   a. Cramping
   b. Constipation
   c. Anorexia
   d. Sore throat

3. A physician has prescribed bismuth subsalicylate to a patient with abdominal cramps. For which of the following conditions should the nurse administer the drug with caution?
   a. Hepatic impairment
   b. Intestinal obstruction
   c. Acute appendicitis
   d. Rectal bleeding

4. A patient undergoing simethicone drug therapy for a peptic ulcer is to be discharged from the health care facility. What instruction should the nurse offer the patient regarding self-administration of the drug at home?
   a. Take the drug early in the morning
   b. Chew the tablets thoroughly
   c. Drink a glass of water after taking the drug
   d. Take the drug with a glass of juice

5. A nurse is caring for a patient with chronic diarrhea. The physician has prescribed diphenoxylate to the patient. What intervention

should the nurse perform when caring for this patient?

a. Encourage the patient to drink extra fluids

b. Avoid the use of commercial electrolytes

c. Encourage the patient to eat food high in fiber

d. Encourage the patient to exercise

6. A nurse is caring for an outpatient undergoing antidiarrheal therapy. Which of the following instructions should the nurse include in the teaching plan for this patient? Select all that apply.

a. Get sufficient exercise

b. Observe caution when driving

c. Avoid the use of alcohol

d. Eat foods high in roughage

e. Avoid the use of nonprescription drugs

7. A nurse is to instruct an outpatient in the right method of administering mineral oil for constipation. Which of the following should the nurse instruct the patient for optimal response to therapy?

a. Take it half an hour after a meal

b. Take it before breakfast

c. Take it at bedtime after dinner

d. Take it on an empty stomach in the evening

8. A nurse is caring for a patient undergoing methylcellulose therapy for the treatment of irritable bowel syndrome. Overuse of the drug results in constipation of the patient. What instruction should the nurse offer the patient to avoid constipation?

a. Take commercial electrolytes

b. Take the drug with food

c. Eat foods high in roughage

d. Avoid milk products

9. A nurse is caring for an outpatient undergoing laxative therapy. Which of the following should the nurse tell the patient is an effect of the prolonged use of a laxative?

a. Obstruction of the small intestine

b. Serious electrolyte imbalances

c. Fecal impaction

d. Renal impairment

10. A nurse needs to start antidiarrheal drug therapy for a patient. For which of the following categories of patients is an antidiarrheal drug contraindicated?

a. Patients with constipation

b. Patients with nausea

c. Patients with obstructive jaundice

d. Patients with abdominal distention

49

Antidiabetic Drugs

SECTION I: ASSESSING YOUR UNDERSTANDING

Activity A MATCHING

1. Match the antidiabetic drugs in Column A with their uses in Column B.

Column A	Column B
___ 1. Rosiglitazone	A. Hypoglycemia
___ 2. Diazoxide	B. Type 2 diabetes
___ 3. Glucagon	C. Hypoglycemia caused by hyperinsulinism

2. Match the antidiabetic drugs in Column A with their adverse reactions in Column B.

Column A	Column B
___ 1. Acetohexamide	A. Aggravated diabetes
___ 2. Metformin	B. Fluid retention
___ 3. Pioglitazone HCl	C. Heartburn
___ 4. Diazoxide	D. Asthenia

Activity B FILL IN THE BLANKS

1. Diabetes mellitus is a chronic disorder characterized by insufficient _____ production by the beta cells of the pancreas.

2. Increased urination is termed _____.

3. Insulin stimulates the synthesis of _____ by the liver.

4. Insulin in combination with glucose are used to treat _____.

5. Elevated blood glucose or sugar level is termed _____.

6. When blood glucose levels are high, glucose molecules attach to _____ in the red blood cells.

7. Diabetic _____ is a potentially life-threatening deficiency of insulin.

SECTION II: APPLYING YOUR KNOWLEDGE

Activity C SHORT ANSWERS

A nurse's role in managing patients who are being administered oral antidiabetic drugs involves monitoring the patients and implementing interventions that aid in their recovery. Answer the following questions, which involve the nurse's role in the management of such situations.

1. A nurse is caring for a patient with type 2 diabetes. The nurse evaluates the effectiveness of the treatment plan. What factors should the nurse consider to determine the success of the treatment plan?

_____

_____

_____

2. A nurse has been caring for a patient with type 2 diabetes. The nurse has to ensure that the patient complies with the drug regimen. What instructions should the nurse offer to the patient and patient's family to decrease the chance of noncompliance by the patient?

_____

_____

_____

Activity D DOSAGE CALCULATION

1. A physician at a health care facility prescribed 30 mg of pioglitazone HCl (Actos) to a patient with type 2 diabetes. The physician has instructed the nurse to continue the drug therapy for 2 days. The drug is available in 15-mg tablets at a pharmacy store. How many tablets should the nurse administer to the patient during the entire therapy?

_____

2. A patient diagnosed with type 2 diabetes has been prescribed 10 mg of repaglinide to be taken once daily. On hand, the drug is available in 2-mg tablets. How many tablets should the nurse administer to the patient daily?

_____

3. A patient at a health care facility has been prescribed 120 mg of nateglinide (Starlix) to be given three times a day. The drug is available in 60-mg tablets. How many tablets should the nurse administer to the patient through the entire day? _____

4. A patient has been prescribed 2650 mg of metformin to be taken orally. On hand, the drug is available in 850-mg tablets. How many tablets should the nurse administer to the patient daily? _____

5. A patient with type 2 diabetes has been prescribed miglitol drug therapy. The physician has instructed the nurse to administer 100 mg of the drug three times a day. On hand, the drug is available in 50-mg tablets. How many tablets should the nurse administer to the patient daily? _____

SECTION III: PRACTICING FOR NCLEX

Activity E

Answer the following questions.

1. A patient at a health care facility has been prescribed pioglitazone HCl to treat type 2 diabetes. What adverse reaction to the drug should the nurse monitor for in the patient?
   a. Congestive heart failure
   b. Myalgia
   c. Sodium retention
   d. Glycosuria

2. A nurse refers to the medical history of a patient who is to be administered chlorpropamide, a sulfonylurea. In which of the following preexisting conditions is the use of the sulfonylurea chlorpropamide contraindicated?
   a. Coronary artery disease
   b. Chronic intestinal diseases
   c. Colonic ulceration
   d. Inflammatory bowel disease

3. A nurse is caring for a female patient with gestational diabetes. The patient asks the nurse which stage of pregnancy has the greatest need for insulin. Which of the following should the nurse reply?
   a. Immediately after conception
   b. First trimester of pregnancy
   c. Third trimester of pregnancy
   d. Immediately after delivery

4. A nurse is assigned to administer a regular insulin dosage to a patient with type 1 diabetes mellitus. When should the nurse administer the insulin?
   a. 15 minutes before a meal
   b. 30 to 60 minutes before a meal
   c. Once at bedtime via the subcutaneous (SC) route
   d. Within 5 to 10 minutes of a meal

5. A patient has been prescribed miglitol. The administration of miglitol causes hypoglycemia in the patient. What should be the nurse's intervention in such a situation?

   a. Discuss the disease and methods of control with the patient

   b. Administer acetohexamide with insulin to the patient

   c. Administer dextrose to the patient rather than sugar

   d. Obtain capillary blood specimens of the patient

6. A nurse is to administer an insulin mixture of insulin lispro and long-acting insulin. What care should the nurse take in preparing the solution?

   a. Confirm with the primary health care provider whether the solution should be mixed in the same syringe

   b. Draw up insulin lispro first in the syringe while preparing the solution

   c. Confirm if the ratio of insulin to be administered is 70:30 or 50:50

   d. Keep the mixture for 1 hour if the patient has difficulty controlling diabetes

7. A nurse is preparing a teaching plan for a patient who has been prescribed α-glucosidase inhibitors. What instruction should the nurse include in the teaching plan for this patient?

   a. Avoid drug administration in case of a skipped meal

   b. Report respiratory distress or muscular aches to the primary health care physician

   c. Keep a source of glucose ready for signs of low blood glucose

   d. Take the drug at different times each day

8. A nurse is required to administer insulin to a patient who has undergone a renal transplantation. Which method of insulin delivery should the nurse adopt for the patient?

   a. Needle and syringe method

   b. Jet injection system method

   c. Syringe with pre-filled cartridge

   d. Insulin pump method

9. A nurse at a health care facility is preparing an insulin solution to be administered to a diabetic patient. What precaution should the nurse take before withdrawing the syringe from the insulin vial?

   a. Eliminate air bubbles from the syringe barrel

   b. Shake the vial vigorously just before withdrawal

   c. Ensure the vial has been undisturbed for an hour

   d. Use a syringe labeled with a higher concentration

10. A pregnant diabetic patient with early long-term complications is administered insulin with an insulin pump. Which of the following should the nurse instruct the patient?

    a. Monitor blood glucose levels twice per day

    b. Ensure that the needle is changed every 1 to 3 days

    c. Inject the same amount of insulin each time

    d. Use a mixture of isophane and regular insulin

CHAPTER 50

Pituitary and Adrenocortical Hormones

SECTION I: ASSESSING YOUR UNDERSTANDING

Activity A MATCHING

1. Match the drugs in Column A with their uses in Column B.

Column A	Column B
___ 1. Desmopressin acetate	A. Treatment of Parkinson's disease
___ 2. Bromocriptine mesylate	B. Treatment of von Willebrand's disease
___ 3. Budesonide	C. Partial replacement therapy for Addison's disease
___ 4. Fludrocortisone acetate	D. Treatment of Crohn's disease

2. Match the drugs in Column A with their adverse reactions in Column B.

Column A	Column B
___ 1. Octreotide acetate	A. Ovarian enlargement
___ 2. Vasopressin	B. Arthralgia
___ 3. Somatropin	C. Sinus bradycardia
___ 4. Clomiphene citrate	D. Tremor

Activity B FILL IN THE BLANKS

1. Adrenocorticotropic hormone (ACTH) stimulates the adrenal cortex to secrete the _____.

2. Anterior pituitary hormone _____ is the only hormone that is not used medically.

3. Follicle-stimulating hormone and luteinizing hormone are called _____ because they influence the organs of reproduction.

4. The nasal tube delivery system comes with a flexible calibrated plastic tube called a _____.

5. _____ are used in an assisted reproductive technology (ART) programs to stimulate multiple follicles for in vitro fertilization.

SECTION II: APPLYING YOUR KNOWLEDGE

Activity C SHORT ANSWERS

A nurse's role in managing patients receiving growth hormones involves assisting them to promote an optimal response to growth hormone therapy. The nurse also helps patients in educating them and their families about the successful implementation of therapy. Answer the following questions, which involve the nurse's role in the management of such situations.

1. A 10-year-old patient has enrolled in a growth hormone program. What is the nurse's role in promoting an optimal response to the growth hormone therapy?

_____

_____

_____

2. What is the nurse's role in educating the patient and his family about growth hormone therapy?

_____

_____

_____

DOSAGE CALCULATION

1. A physician has prescribed 2 g of amino-glutethimide on a daily basis to a patient for suppressing adrenal function. The drug is available as 250-mg tablets. How many tablets should the nurse administer the patient every day? _____

2. A patient has been prescribed 1 mg of caber-goline twice weekly for the treatment of acromegaly. The drug is available as 0.5-mg tablets. How many tablets should the nurse administer to the patient to complete the 3-week course? _____

3. A nurse is caring for a patient with salt-losing adrenogenital syndrome. The physician has prescribed 0.2 mg of fludrocortisone acetate daily for 5 days. The drug is available as 0.1-mg tablets. How many tablets will the nurse require to complete the course of drug administration? _____

4. A physician has prescribed 50 mg of cortisone on a daily basis as a treatment for systemic dermatomyositis. The drug is available as 25-mg tablets. How many tablets will the nurse need to complete a 3-day treatment course?

_____

5. A nurse is caring for a patient with psoriatic arthritis. The physician has prescribed 20 mg of prednisone on a daily basis. The drug is available as 10-mg tablets. How many tablets

should the nurse administer to the patient in 2 days? _____

SECTION III: PRACTICING FOR NCLEX

Answer the following questions.

1. A nurse is caring for a patient who has been prescribed corticotropin for acute exacerbations of multiple sclerosis. In which of the following types of patients should the nurse administer the drug cautiously? Select all that apply.
   a. Patients with diverticulosis
   b. Patients with sinus bradycardia
   c. Patients with febrile infections
   d. Patients with arthralgia
   e. Patients with myasthenia gravis

2. A nurse is caring for a patient with abnormal urination and thirst. The physician has pre-scribed vasopressin to the patient, who informs the nurse that he is also taking oral anticoagulants for blood thinning. What should the nurse inform the patient about the effect of interaction between these two drugs?
   a. Increased risk of hypokalemia
   b. Increased need for antidiabetic medication
   c. Decreased muscle function
   d. Decreased antidiuretic effect

3. A patient with mycosis fungoides is pre-scribed dexamethasone. Which of the following adverse reactions to the drug should the nurse monitor for in the patient? Select all that apply.
   a. Nasal congestion
   b. Acneiform eruptions
   c. Increased sweating
   d. Perineal itch
   e. Abdominal cramps

4. A physician has prescribed ACTH to a patient with nonsuppurative thyroiditis. What intervention should the nurse perform as a part of the ongoing assessment during the course of treatment?

a. Record the patient's abdominal girth

b. Monitor for a rise in the blood glucose level

c. Measure the specific gravity of the urine

d. Periodically monitor bone age

5. A physician prescribes hydrocortisone to a patient with regional enteritis. The patient informs the nurse of gastric irritation after taking the drug. Which of the following interventions should the nurse perform while managing the needs of the patient?

a. Give drug with a full glass of water

b. Administer enema before first dose of drug

c. Supply with large amounts of drinking water

d. Auscultate the abdomen

6. A physician prescribes fludrocortisone acetate for a patient undergoing replacement therapy for primary adrenocortical deficiency. For which of the following adverse reactions should the nurse monitor in the patient?

a. Joint pain

b. Hypothyroidism

c. Hypertension

d. Insulin resistance

7. A physician has prescribed ganirelix acetate to an infertile patient. During the course of the treatment, the patient complains of visual disturbances. Which of the following precautionary measures should the nurse take?

a. Discontinue the drug therapy

b. Administer the drug with food

c. Perform a complete blood count test, as ordered by the primary health care provider

d. Assess the skin integrity

8. A patient in a health care facility is prescribed glucocorticoids for systemic lupus erythematosus. What should the nursing diagnoses checklist include for this patient?

a. Pain related to abdominal distension

b. Deficient Fluid Volume related to inability to replenish fluid intake

c. Disturbed Body Image related to adverse reactions

d. Risk for Infection related to masking of signs of infection

9. A physician prescribes vasopressin for a patient with diabetes insipidus, and he or she also instructs the patient to undergo abdominal roentgenography. Which of the following interventions should the nurse perform for implementing the process?

a. Give enema before first dose

b. Check stools for evidence of bleeding

c. Monitor patient for rash, urticaria, and hypotension

d. Provide daily oral drug doses before 9 a.m.

10. A nurse is caring for a patient with congenital adrenal hyperplasia. The physician has prescribed prednisone to the patient. During the course of the treatment, the patient undergoes an overdose of prednisone. Which of the following conditions is the nurse most likely to observe in the patient as a result of the overdose? Select all that apply.

a. Swelling

b. Buffalo hump

c. Muscle pain

d. Moon face

e. Weight gain

Thyroid and Antithyroid Drugs

SECTION I: ASSESSING YOUR UNDERSTANDING

Activity A MATCHING

1. Match the drugs in Column A with their adverse reactions in Column B.

Column A	Column B
___ 1. Levothyroxine sodium (T_4)	A. Hives
___ 2. Methimazole	B. Palpitations
___ 3. Sodium iodine (^{131}I)	C. Agranulocytosis

2. Match the interactant drugs in Column A with the effect of their interaction with thyroid hormones in Column B.

Column A	Column B
___ 1. Digoxin	A. Increased risk of hypoglycemia
___ 2. Insulin	B. Decreased effectiveness of thyroid drug
___ 3. Oral anticoagulants	C. Decreased effectiveness of cardiac drug
___ 4. Antidepressant	D. Prolonged bleeding

Activity B FILL IN THE BLANKS

1. _____ is an increase in the amount of thyroid hormones manufactured and secreted.

2. Thyroid hormones are used as replacement therapy when the patient is _____.

3. _____ is an essential element for the manufacture of the thyroxine (T_4) and tri-iodothyronine (T_3) hormones.

4. Enlargement of a normal thyroid gland is called the _____ goiters.

5. _____ drugs inhibit the manufacture of thyroid hormones.

SECTION II: APPLYING YOUR KNOWLEDGE

Activity C SHORT ANSWERS

A nurse's role in managing patients who are being administered thyroid hormones involves monitoring the patients and implementing interventions that aid in their recovery. Answer the following questions, which involve the nurse's role in the management of such situations.

1. A patient undergoing thyroid hormone replacement therapy is discharged. What information should the nurse provide to the patient and family emphasizing the importance of taking the replacement therapy?

_____

_____

_____

2. A nurse is caring for a patient undergoing thyroid hormone therapy. After therapy, the nurse needs to evaluate the effectiveness of the therapy. What factors should the nurse consider to determine the success of the therapy?

_____

_____

_____

Activity D DOSAGE CALCULATION

1. A primary health care provider has prescribed 75 mcg per day of levothyroxine sodium, to be administered orally in three doses. The drug is available as 25-mcg tablets. How many tablets should the nurse administer to the patient per day? _____

2. A patient is prescribed methimazole to treat hyperthyroidism. The primary health care provider instructs the nurse to administer 10 mg of the drug in 8-hour intervals daily. The drug is available in 5-mg tablets. How many tablets should the nurse administer to the patient in a day? _____

3. A patient is prescribed 900 mg of propylthiouracil daily for the treatment of hyperthyroidism. The drug is available in 100-mg tablets. The nurse needs to administer the divided doses at 8-hour intervals. How many tablets should the nurse administer to the patient in each dose? _____

4. A patient with hypothyroidism is prescribed thyroid USP. The primary health care provider has initially prescribed 30 mg of the drug to be taken daily. The drug is available in 15-mg tablets. How many tablets should the nurse administer to the patient per day? _____

should notify the primary health care provider about which of the following adverse reactions to the drug?

a. Tachycardia

b. Agranulocytosis

c. Weight loss

d. Fatigue

2. A nurse is caring for a patient receiving thyroid hormones. The patient informs the nurse that he is also taking digoxin for a cardiac problem. What effect of the interaction between the two drugs should the nurse observe for in the patient?

a. Decreased effectiveness of the cardiac drug

b. Increased risk of prolonged bleeding

c. Decreased effectiveness of the thyroid drug

d. Increased potential for bleeding

3. A nurse is caring for a patient undergoing thyroid hormone therapy. What signs of therapeutic response should the nurse monitor after the thyroid hormone is administered to the patient?

a. Agranulocytosis

b. Headache

c. Mild diuresis

d. Loss of hair

4. A nurse is assessing a patient with hypothyroidism. Which of the following symptoms should the nurse document during the preadministration assessment? Select all that apply.

a. Weight loss

b. Cold intolerance

c. Confusion

d. Sweating

e. Unsteady gait

SECTION III: PRACTICING FOR NCLEX

Activity E

Answer the following questions.

1. A patient is administered methimazole for the treatment of hyperthyroidism. The nurse

5. A patient undergoing propylthiouracil drug therapy is discharged from the health care facility. What instruction should the nurse include in the teaching plan?

   a. Take the drug at regular intervals.

   b. Take the drug before breakfast.

   c. Record weight twice a week.

   d. Notify the primary health care provider if palpitations occur

   e. Avoid taking the drug in larger doses

6. A patient with cardiovascular disease is administered thyroid hormones. What should the nurse observe for in the patient to notify the primary health care provider to reduce the dosage of the thyroid hormone?

   a. High fever

   b. Chest pain

   c. Sweating

   d. Headache

7. The primary health care provider administers an antithyroid drug to a patient. What signs of thyroid storm should the nurse monitor for in the patient during the ongoing assessment?

   a. Nervousness

   b. Increased pulse rate

   c. Anxiety

   d. Altered mental status

8. A patient is prescribed an iodine procedure for the treatment of hyperthyroidism. What interventions should the nurse perform before administering the iodine procedure to the patient?

   a. Take an allergy history of seafood

   b. Monitor for signs of agranulocytosis

   c. Assess the patient for mouth infection

   d. Monitor the patient's stool color

9. A patient is prescribed thyroid hormone therapy. In which of the following conditions is the drug contraindicated?

   a. Agranulocytosis

   b. Adrenal cortical insufficiency

   c. Granulocytopenia

   d. Hypoprothrombinemia

10. A health care provider administers thyroid hormone therapy to a patient. Which of the following signs of hyperthyroidism should the nurse report to the primary health care provider before the next dose is due? Select all that apply.

    a. Moist skin

    b. Easy bruising

    c. Moderate hypertension

    d. Increased appetite

    e. Sore throat

CHAPTER 52

Male and Female Hormones

SECTION I: ASSESSING YOUR UNDERSTANDING

Activity A MATCHING

1. Match the hormones and their related drugs in Column A with the conditions they are used for in Column B.

Column A	Column B
____ 1. Androgens	A. Anemia of renal insufficiency
____ 2. Anabolic steroids	B. Endometriosis
____ 3. Androgen hormone inhibitors	C. Male hypogonadism
____ 4. Progestins	D. Atrophic vaginitis
____ 5. Estrogens	E. Benign hypertrophy of the prostate

2. Match the drugs used in hormonal therapy for cancer in Column A with their common adverse effects in Column B.

Column A	Column B
____ 1. Mitotane	A. Electrocardiogram (ECG) changes
____ 2. Testolactone	B. Hematuria
____ 3. Goserelin acetate	C. Maculopapular erythema
____ 4. Leuprolide acetate	D. Breast atrophy
____ 5. Bicalutamide	E. Leukocytosis

Activity B FILL IN THE BLANKS

1. The age of onset of first menstruation is called _____.

2. Hormones produced by the body are called _____ hormones.

3. _____ is called reverse tissue-depleting processes of the body.

4. The development of the _____ gland is dependent on the potent androgen 5 alpha-dihydrotestosterone (DHT).

5. Testosterone and its derivatives are collectively called _____.

SECTION II: APPLYING YOUR KNOWLEDGE

Activity C SHORT ANSWERS

A nurse's role in managing patients who are receiving hormone therapy involves monitoring and implementing interventions that aid in recovery. Answer the following questions, which involve the nurse's role in the management of such situations.

1. A nurse is caring for a patient who is on androgen therapy. What assessments should the nurse implement when monitoring for excess fluid volume in the patient?

_____

_____

_____

2. A nurse is educating a patient who plans to take oral contraceptives as a method of birth control. What points should the nurse include in the teaching plan when educating the patient regarding oral contraceptives?

_____

_____

_____

Activity D **DOSAGE CALCULATION**

1. A female patient has been prescribed 20 mg of Halotestin (fluoxymesterone) per day as a palliative therapy for advanced inoperable breast cancer. How many of the 5-mg tablets does she need to take in a single dose? _____

2. A patient weighing 30 kg has been prescribed 5 mg/kg of Anadrol-50 (oxymetholone) to be taken orally per day for anemia. Anadrol-50 is available as 50-mg tablets. How many of such tablets need the patient take each day?

_____

3. A patient with primary ovarian failure has been prescribed 1.5 mg of estropipate as a daily dose. How many of the Ortho-Est tablets (0.75 mg of estropipate) should the nurse instruct the patient to take daily? _____

4. A patient with endometriosis has been prescribed Aygestin (norethindrone acetate) to be taken at a dose of 5 mg/day for the first 2 weeks and 7.5 mg/day for the next 2 weeks. How many of the 5-mg tablets should the nurse instruct the patient to take during the 3rd and the 4th week? _____

5. A patient has been prescribed 200 mg of oral progesterone daily for the prevention of endometrial hyperplasia. How many of the 100-mg progesterone capsules should the patient take daily? _____

6. A patient weighing 75 kg has been prescribed 14 mg/kg/day of estramustine phosphate sodium in divided doses for prostate cancer. How many of the 140-mg tablets does the patient need to take daily? _____

SECTION III: PRACTICING FOR NCLEX

Activity E

Answer the following questions.

1. A patient has been prescribed androgen therapy. Which of the following conditions should the nurse consider to be an indication for such a prescription?

  a. Adrenal cortical cancer

  b. Testosterone deficiency

  c. Benign prostatic hypertrophy

  d. Male pattern baldness

2. Following a major road accident and disability 2 years ago, a patient had profound weight loss. The patient tells the nurse that he had been prescribed a certain drug to promote weight gain during that time. To which of the following groups should the nurse consider that the drug might have belonged?

  a. Androgen hormones

  b. Progestins

  c. Conjugate estrogens

  d. Anabolic steroids

3. A patient with obesity is receiving anticoagulant therapy as a prophylaxis for thromboembolism following an appendectomy. Which of the following interactions may be seen when androgens or androgen hormone inhibitors are used concomitantly in this patient?

  a. Increased antidiuretic effect

  b. Decreased anticoagulant effect

  c. Increased risk of hypoglycemia

  d. Increased risk of paranoia

4. A nurse is caring for a male patient with hypogonadism who has been prescribed androgen therapy, and he is required to educate the patient about the use of the drug and its possible adverse effects. Which of the following is an adverse effect of androgen therapy?

  a. Enlargement of testes

  b. Gynecomastia

  c. Virilization

  d. Frequent urination

5. A 44-year-old female patient complains of severe vasomotor symptoms of menopause, such as hot flashes and excessive sweating. The patient is prescribed estrogen to treat menopausal symptoms, along with a concurrent use of progestins. Which of the following is the reason for the concurrent use of progestins?

a. Reduces gastrointestinal irritation caused by estrogen

b. Treats associated atrophic vaginitis

c. Reduces risk of endometrial carcinoma

d. Decreases risk of postmenopausal osteoporosis

6. A 46-year-old woman is experiencing symptoms of menopause and is taking black cohosh, an herb, to alleviate these symptoms. The nurse should caution the patient about which of the following possible adverse effects of the herb?

a. Low blood pressure

b. Ringing in the ears

c. Impaired vision

d. Weight loss

7. A 30-year-old female patient arrives at the health care center complaining of abnormal uterine bleeding. Diagnosis indicates endometrial hyperplasia, and the patient receives a prescription for De-Provera (medroxyprogesterone acetate). Which of the following should the nurse keep in mind when administering this drug?

a. The drug is implanted in the subdermal tissue

b. The drug is to be shaken vigorously before use

c. The first dose is given on the tenth day of a menstrual cycle

d. The drug provides contraception for 5 years

8. A woman taking oral contraceptives has heard about health benefits associated with oral contraceptive use, apart from contraception, and is eager to know more about it. Which of the following risks are reduced with oral contraceptive use? Select all that apply.

a. Iron deficiency anemia

b. Ovarian cancer

c. Cervical erosion

d. Osteoporosis

e. Vaginal candidiasis

9. A 20-year-old woman taking oral contraceptives is anxious that she has missed one day's dose. Which of the following instructions should the nurse offer the patient?

a. Discontinue the drug and use another form of birth control till the next cycle

b. Take two tablets for the next 2 days and continue with the normal schedule

c. Remember to take one tablet the next day and forget about the missed dose

d. Take the missed dose as soon as remembered or take two tablets the next day

10. When educating a group of nursing students regarding the various female hormones, the nurse identifies which of the following hormones as a synthetic estrogen that is available only as a drug?

a. Estradiol

b. Estrone

c. Estriol

d. Estropipate

CHAPTER 53

Drugs Acting on the Uterus

SECTION I: ASSESSING YOUR UNDERSTANDING

Activity A **MATCHING**

1. Match the drugs acting on the uterus in Column A with their adverse reactions in Column B.

Column A	Column B
___ 1. Indomethacin	A. Diplopia
___ 2. Oxytocin	B. Anaphylactic reactions
___ 3. Magnesium sulfate	C. Vertigo
___ 4. Ritodrine hydrochloride	D. Hypokalemia
___ 5. Terbutaline	E. Fluid in the lungs

2. Match the drugs acting on the uterus in Column A with their contraindications in Column B.

Column A	Column B
___ 1. Tocolytics	A. Before delivery of placenta
___ 2. Oxytocin	B. Eclampsia
___ 3. Ergonovine and methylergonovine	C. Cephalopelvic disproportion
___ 4. Magnesium sulfate	D. With nonsteroidal anti-inflammatory drugs (NSAIDs)
___ 5. Indomethacin	E. Myocardial damage

Activity B **FILL IN THE BLANKS**

1. Oxytocic drugs are used antepartum to induce uterine _____.

2. Oxytocin is an endogenous hormone produced by the _____ pituitary gland.

3. A complication of pregnancy characterized by convulsive seizures and coma is known as _____.

4. Overdosage of ergonovine is known as _____.

5. Oxytocin leads to water intoxication due to its _____ effect.

SECTION II: APPLYING YOUR KNOWLEDGE

Activity C **SHORT ANSWERS**

A nurse's role in managing patients who are being administered drugs acting on the uterus involves monitoring and implementing interventions that aid in recovery. Answer the following questions, which involve the nurse's role in the management of such situations.

1. A nurse is required to monitor the uterine contractions of a patient who is receiving an oxytocin infusion. What conditions would alert the nurse to discontinue the oxytocin infusion?

_____

_____

_____

2. What ongoing nursing assessment should the nurse engage in when caring for a patient receiving tocolytic drugs?

_____

_____

_____

Activity D DOSAGE CALCULATION

1. A doctor prescribes 40 units of oxytocin in a 1000-mL intravenous (IV) solution to induce labor. The available 1-mL ampoule contains 10 units of oxytocin. How many ampoules will the nurse need to administer to the patient in 1000 mL of IV solution?

_____

2. A patient in preterm labor has been prescribed 2 g of magnesium sulfate intramuscularly. Each milliliter of the 50% solution for injection contains 0.5 g of magnesium sulfate. What volume of the solution should be administered to the patient? _____

3. A patient with postpartum bleeding has been prescribed 0.4 mg of methylergonovine maleate. The available methylergonovine maleate tablet is 0.2 mg. How many such tablets should the nurse administer to the patient? _____

4. A doctor prescribes 50 mg of indomethacin oral suspension to a patient in preterm labor. The available solution contains 25 mg of indomethacin per 5 mL. What volume of the solution should the nurse administer to the patient? _____

5. A doctor prescribes 0.25 mg of Brethine (terbutaline) to a patient in preterm labor. Each ampoule contains 1 mg of Brethine per 1 mL of solution. What volume of the available solution should the nurse administer to the patient? _____

6. A patient with postpartum bleeding has been prescribed 5 units of oxytocin. The available 1-mL ampoule contains 10 units of oxytocin. What volume of the solution should the nurse administer to the patient? _____

SECTION III: PRACTICING FOR NCLEX

Activity E

Answer the following questions.

1. A 32-year-old woman has been prescribed oxytocin intranasally to stimulate the milk ejection reflex. In which of the following positions should the nurse place the patient when administering oxytocin intranasally?

   a. Upright position

   b. Supine position

   c. Lateral position

   d. Standing position

2. A patient is receiving oxytocin to induce labor and is concerned about the use of the drug. Which of the following interventions should the nurse implement to help alleviate the patient's anxiety? Select all that apply.

   a. Explain the purpose of the IV infusion

   b. Do not inform the patient of the expected outcome

   c. Administer an antianxiety drug to the patient

   d. Offer encouragement and reassurance

   e. Spend time with the patient

3. A patient has been administered ergonovine after expulsion of the placenta following childbirth. The nurse observes that the patient's uterus is not responding well to the drug. Which of the following interventions is most appropriate in this situation?

   a. Increase the drug dosage

   b. Administer magnesium sulfate by IV injection

   c. Administer calcium by IV injection

   d. Administer terbutaline subcutaneously

4. A pregnant woman in her 28th week of gestation is admitted to a health care center with preterm labor. In which of the following conditions is magnesium sulfate contraindicated?

   a. Cephalopelvic disproportion

   b. Hypertension

   c. Total placenta previa

   d. Eclampsia

5. A 31-year-old patient in her 28th week of gestation is experiencing preterm labor. The

patient has been administered IV magnesium sulfate to prolong the pregnancy. Which of the following factors has to be monitored by the nurse when administering tocolytics?

a. Urine output

b. Pedal edema

c. Cardiac function

d. Vaginal bleeding

6. A 32-year-old pregnant woman is admitted to a hospital with labor pains. The patient is prescribed ergonovine during the third stage of labor after the placenta has been delivered. In which of the following conditions is this drug strictly contraindicated?

a. Renal disease

b. During lactation

c. Heart disease

d. Hypertension

7. A nurse is advised to administer methylergonovine to a patient with postpartum hemorrhaging. Which of the following nursing interventions should the nurse implement when administering the drug? Select all that apply.

a. Monitor vital signs every 4 hours

b. Discontinue the drug if the patient develops severe cramping

c. Notify the health care provider if abdominal cramping is severe

d. Note character and amount of vaginal bleeding

e. Place patient in a lateral position

8. When caring for a pregnant patient, the nurse observes signs of excess fluid volume in the patient. Which of the following drugs leads to the danger of an excessive fluid volume (water intoxication)?

a. Oxytocin

b. Ergonovine

c. Magnesium sulfate

d. Methylergonovine

9. When caring for a pregnant woman receiving ergonovine to increase the uterine contractions during labor, the nurse is required to monitor for signs and symptoms of ergotism. Which of the following symptoms are manifestations of ergotism? Select all that apply.

a. Dyspnea

b. Diplopia

c. Hallucinations

d. Water intoxication

e. Tachycardia

10. A patient in her 28th week of gestation is experiencing preterm labor and is prescribed magnesium sulfate. Which of the following is the property of magnesium sulfate?

a. It is a calcium antagonist

b. It blocks the production of prostaglandins

c. It has an antidiuretic action

d. Acts as a uterine stimulant

CHAPTER 54

Immunologic Agents

SECTION I: ASSESSING YOUR UNDERSTANDING

Activity A MATCHING

1. Match the generic name of immune globulins in Column A with their trade names in Column B.

Column A

C 1. Botulism immune globulin

A 2. Cytomegalovirus immune globulin

D 3. Immune globulin–Intravenous (IV)

B 4. Lymphocyte immune globulin

E 5. Rabies immune globulin

Column B

A. CytoGam

B. Atgam

C. BabyBIG

D. Gamimune N

E. BayRab

2. Match the terms associated with immunity in Column A with their definitions in Column B.

Column A

E 1. Active immunity

A 2. Passive immunity

D 3. Toxin

Column B

A. Injection of ready-made antibodies

B. Attenuated or killed antigen

C. Protein present in blood serum or plasma

B 4. Vaccine

C 5. Globulins

D. Poisonous substance produced by some bacteria

E. Use of agents to stimulate antibody formation

Activity B FILL IN THE BLANKS

1. When salicylates are administered with varicella vaccine, there is an increased risk of developing *Reyes* syndrome.

2. *Artificially* acquired active immunity occurs when an individual is given a weakened antigen that stimulates the formation of antibodies.

3. A *booster* injection is administered as an additional dose of vaccine to enhance the production of antibodies so that the desired level of immunity is maintained.

4. *Immunity* refers to the ability of the body to identify and resist microorganisms that are potentially harmful.

5. _____-mediated immunity depends on the actions of the T lymphocytes.

SECTION II: APPLYING YOUR KNOWLEDGE

Activity C SHORT ANSWERS

A nurse's role in managing patients receiving an immunologic agent involves diagnosis, planning, and implementation. Answer the following questions that involve the nurse's role in the management of such cases.

1. What information should the nurse document when preparing the patient's chart or form provided by the institution?

_____

_____

_____

2. What information should the nurse include in the teaching plan when educating the parents of a child receiving a vaccination?

_____

_____

_____

Activity D DOSAGE CALCULATION

1. A doctor prescribes an immunizing dose of 0.5 mL of meningococcal vaccine to a patient as part of a routine immunization program. After reconstitution, the solution consists of 8 mL. What amount of reconstituted solution is left in the vial after injecting the prescribed dose to the patient? _____

2. A single vial of Pneumovax 23 contains 3 mL of the vaccine solution. The nurse administers 0.5 mL of the solution subcutaneously to each patient. How many patients can be vaccinated using a single vial? _____

3. The diluent for a single dose of *Haemophilus influenzae* vaccine is available as 0.6 mL per ampoule. How many milliliters of diluent are necessary to prepare five doses of *Haemophilus influenzae* vaccine? _____

4. A nurse has been advised to inject 0.5 mL of reconstituted hepatitis B vaccine solution. The diluent supplied is 0.6 mL, and the vaccine in the vial is 0.25 mL. How many milliliters of the reconstituted solution are left in the syringe after injecting the prescribed dose?

_____

5. A doctor prescribes 0.5 mL of a single-dose poliovirus vaccine for each patient to be given intramuscularly (IM). The available vaccine solution after reconstitution is 4 mL. The vial can be used for how many patients?

_____

6. A patient has been prescribed 250 units of tetanus immune globulin. The available 7.5-mL ampoule contains 3750 units of tetanus immune globulin. What volume of the solution should the nurse administer to the patient? _____

SECTION III: PRACTICING FOR NCLEX

Activity E

Answer the following questions.

1. In Japan, health care providers use lentinan, a derivative of the shiitake mushroom, for general health maintenance. Which of the following are possible health benefits of this herb? Select all that apply.
   a. Boosts the body's immune system
   b. Helps in lowering blood cholesterol levels
   c. Prolongs the survival time of patients with cancer
   d. Reduces the risk of heart disease
   e. Helps in lowering blood pressure

2. A nurse is educating a group of nursing students about the health benefits of the shiitake mushroom. Which of the following is the recommended dose of the shiitake mushroom?
   a. 1 to 5 capsules daily
   b. 10 fresh shiitake mushrooms
   c. 1 dropper eight times a day
   d. 12 cups of shiitake juice per day

3. When educating patients on immunologic agents, the nurse identifies which of the following white blood cells as playing a major role in maintaining humoral immunity?
   a. Neutrophils
   b. Eosinophils
   c. Lymphocytes
   d. Basophils

4. When educating nursing students about vaccines, the nurse explains that humans can be administered vaccines and toxoids in which of the following cases? Select all that apply.
   a. Routine immunization of infants and children
   b. Adults at high risk for certain diseases

c. Immunization of pregnant women against rubella

d. Immunization of adults against tetanus

e. Immunization of children and adults with leukemia

5. A patient was rushed to a hospital following a rattlesnake bite. The nurse was advised to inject antivenins, which should be administered within which of the following time periods to yield the most effective response?

    a. Within 7 hours

    b. Within 6 hours

    c. Within 5 hours

    d. Within 4 hours

6. A nurse is caring for a patient with chickenpox. Which of the following is a late complication of chickenpox about which a nurse should alert the patient?

    a. Reye's syndrome

    b. Acute renal failure

    c. Herpes zoster

    d. Hepatitis

7. A patient traveling to South Africa and India is concerned about endemic diseases and is eager to know about any vaccination to prevent such diseases. Which of the following diseases are preventable by vaccination before traveling to endemic areas? Select all that apply.

    a. Typhoid

    b. Cholera diphtheria

    c. Tetanus

d. Yellow fever

e. Rubella

8. A child complains of pain at the injection site following the administration of the measles vaccine. Which of the following interventions should a nurse implement for pain management following vaccine administration? Select all that apply.

    a. Administer acetaminophen

    b. Massage the injection site

    c. Decrease fluid intake

    d. Encourage adequate rest

    e. Apply warm or cool compresses

9. When educating a group of nursing students on vaccines, the nurse identifies which of the following conditions as requiring vaccines to be administered with caution?

    a. Lactation

    b. Lymphoma

    c. Nonlocalized cancer

    d. Leukemia

10. A patient is advised to stay in the clinic for observation for about 30 minutes after receiving an immunologic agent. Which of the following signs should a nurse observe to identify hypersensitivity reaction? Select all that apply.

    a. Pruritus

    b. Laryngeal edema

    c. Dyspnea

    d. Renal failure

    e. Convulsions

CHAPTER 55

Antineoplastic Drugs

SECTION I: ASSESSING YOUR UNDERSTANDING

Activity A MATCHING

1. Match the terms in Column A with their corresponding meanings in Column B.

Column A	Column B
B **1.** Alopecia	**A.** Relief of symptoms at the end of life
E **2.** Metastasis	**B.** Loss of hair
A **3.** Palliation	**C.** Capable of soft tissue necrosis
C **4.** Vesicant	**D.** Inflammation of the mouth
D **5.** Stomatitis	**E.** Spread of cancer to other sites

2. Match the phases of cell growth in Column A with their corresponding characteristics in Column B.

Column A	Column B
C **1.** G_1	**A.** DNA is prepared
A **2.** S	**B.** Mitotic cell division occurs
E **3.** G_2	**C.** RNA and proteins are built
B **4.** M	**D.** Dormant or resting phase occurs
D **5.** G_0	**E.** Preparing for cell division

Activity B FILL IN THE BLANKS

1. **Malignant** cells appear to be more susceptible to the effects of alkylating drugs than normal cells.

2. Interference with the bone marrow's ability to make new cells is called **myelosupresoia**

3. Patients with **neutropenia** have a decreased resistance to infection.

4. **Erythemia** consists of a red, warm, and sometimes painful area on the skin.

5. **Chemotherap** refers to therapy with antineoplastic drugs

SECTION II: APPLYING YOUR KNOWLEDGE

Activity C SHORT ANSWERS

A nurse's role in managing patients undergoing antineoplastic drug therapy involves not just the treatment or the cause for treatment, but also managing the effects produced by a particular adverse reaction caused by the treatment. Answer the following questions, which involve the nurse's role in caring for a patient undergoing antineoplastic drug therapy.

1. A nurse is caring for a patient who has been undergoing chemotherapy. What factors determine the nursing care in a patient receiving antineoplastic drugs?

_____

_____

_____

2. A nurse is assigned to care for patients who will receive chemotherapy in a health care facility. What guidelines should the nurse follow when caring for patients receiving chemotherapeutic drugs?

_____

_____

_____

Activity D DOSAGE CALCULATION

1. A patient has been prescribed vincristine sulfate, to be taken intravenously (IV) for treatment of acute leukemia. The dosage indicated is 4 mg. The drug is available as vincristine sulfate injection (Oncovin) in 2-mL vials, and each milliliter contains 1 mg of vincristine sulfate. How many vials should the nurse administer to the patient? _____

2. A patient is to receive 50 mg of vinorelbine tartrate IV for the treatment of non-small cell lung cancer (NSCLC). The drug is available as Navelbine in 1-mL vials containing 10 mg of vinorelbine tartrate in water for injection. How many vials should the nurse administer to the patient? _____

3. The nurse will administer 60 mg of docetaxel IV to a patient being treated for solid prostate tumor. The drug is available as Taxotere (docetaxel) injection concentrate in single-dose vials containing 20 mg (0.5 mL) of docetaxel (anhydrous). Each milliliter contains 40 mg of docetaxel (anhydrous). How many vials should the nurse administer to the patient?

_____

4. A patient has been prescribed etoposide for the treatment of small cell lung cancer (SCLC). The dosage indicated is 100 mg. The drug is available as VePesid in 50-mg pink capsules. How many capsules should the nurse administer to the patient? _____

5. A patient is to receive 80 mg of irinotecan hydrochloride IV for the treatment of a rectal tumor. The drug is available as Camptosar injection in 2-mL vials containing 40 mg of irinotecan. Each milliliter of solution contains 20 mg of irinotecan hydrochloride. How many vials should the nurse administer to the patient? _____

6. A patient being treated for severe psoriasis has been prescribed 30 mg of methotrexate. The

drug is available as Trexall (methotrexate) tablets for oral administration. Each tablet contains methotrexate sodium in an amount equivalent to 7.5-mg strength. How many tablets should the nurse administer to the patient? _____

SECTION III: PRACTICING FOR NCLEX

Activity E

Answer the following questions.

1. A nurse is caring for a patient who has been receiving chemotherapy for breast cancer. The patient wants to know why chemotherapy is administered in a series of cycles. Which of the following responses should the nurse give to the patient? Select all that apply.
   a. To allow for recovery of the normal cells
   b. To release antioxidants into the system
   c. To release polyphenols and flavonoids
   d. To destroy more of the malignant cells
   e. To affect cells that rapidly divide and reproduce

2. A nurse is caring for a patient with hypertension. The patient asks the nurse if drinking green tea will be beneficial to him. Which of the following reasons should the nurse state for drinking green tea with caution? Select all that apply.
   a. Nervousness
   b. Insomnia
   c. Mouth ulcers
   d. Gastrointestinal (GI) upset
   e. Stomatitis

3. A nurse is caring for a patient who is prescribed Velban for leukemia. The nurse explains to the patient that Velban is a cell–cycle-specific drug. Which of the following is a characteristic of a cell–cycle-specific drug?
   a. Targets the cells at any phase of the cycle
   b. Targets only the cells that are malignant
   c. Targets the cells in various stages of cell division
   d. Targets the cells in one of the phases of cell division

4. The nurse is caring for a patient with osteosarcoma. The patient is prescribed Trexall, which is an antimetabolite drug. The patient asks the nurse to explain the action of the drug. Which of the following is the action of an antimetabolite?

   a. Changes the cell to a more alkaline environment

   b. Incorporates itself into the cellular components

   c. Interferes with amino acid production

   d. Interferes with the formation of microtubules

5. A nurse is assigned to care for an elderly patient who is receiving an antineoplastic drug. Which of the following factors should the nurse consider when preparing a nursing care plan for the ongoing assessment of the patient? Select all that apply.

   a. Guidelines established by the health care facility

   b. The patient's appetite

   c. The patient's general condition

   d. The patient's individual response to the drug

   e. The adequacy of health insurance coverage

6. A nurse is caring for a patient who is to be administered an antineoplastic drug subcutaneously. Which of the following is applicable to the subcutaneous administration of an antineoplastic drug?

   a. The injection should contain no more than 1 mL

   b. An Angiocath should be used for administration

   c. The z-track method should be used for administration

   d. The injection should contain only 3 mL

7. A nurse is caring for a patient receiving antineoplastic drugs. The patient's dietary requirements are not being met because of loss of appetite. What is the nurse's role in caring for a patient with imbalanced nutrition?

   a. Provide three large meals

   b. Provide food with less salt

   c. Provide frequent, small meals

   d. Provide food rich in fats

8. A patient being treated with antineoplastic drugs is at a high risk for thrombocytopenia. Which of the following must the nurse consider with regard to injections and blood withdrawal for tests?

   a. Use the same site for all withdrawals and injections

   b. Apply pressure to the injection site for 3 to 5 minutes

   c. Use electric razors when shaving

   d. Use nail trimmers to keep the patient's nails short

9. A nurse is caring for a patient who is experiencing anxiety after being diagnosed with cancer. What is the nurse's role when caring for this patient?

   a. Assist in making critical decisions regarding treatment

   b. Emphasize safety requirements for chemotherapy

   c. Plan and institute therapy to control the disease

   d. Offer consistent and empathetic support to the patient and his or her family

10. A nurse is caring for a patient prescribed antineoplastic drugs for oral therapy. Which of the following should the nurse include in the teaching plan for the patient and family?

    a. Take the exact amount of the drug at any time of the day

    b. Take the drug as directed on the prescription container

    c. Do not inform the dentist of the therapy

    d. Decrease the dose as the symptoms of illness decrease

Topical Drugs Used in the Treatment of Skin Disorders

SECTION I: ASSESSING YOUR UNDERSTANDING

Activity A MATCHING

1. Match the antibiotic drugs in Column A with their uses in Column B.

Column A	Column B
B 1. Azelaic acid	A. Relieves primary and secondary skin infections
D 2. Bacitracin	
A 3. Gentamicin	B. Treats acne vulgaris and rosacea
C 4. Mupirocin	C. Treats impetigo infections caused by *Staphylococcus aureus*
	D. Helps prevent infections in minor cuts and burns

2. Match the drugs in Column A with their adverse reactions in Column B.

Column A	Column B
D 1. Butenafine HCl	A. Alopecia, eye pain, facial edema
A 2. Loprox gel	B. Burning, itching, erythema

B 3. Clotrimazole

C 4. Haloprogin

C. Vesicle formation, scaling, pruritus

D. Contact dermatitis, erythema, irritation

Activity B FILL IN THE BLANKS

1. Prolonged use of topical antibiotic preparations may result in a superficial **superinfection**

2. Acyclovir is used in treating herpes simplex virus infections in **immuno compromised** patients.

3. Adverse reactions to topical anti-infectives may include rash, itching, urticaria (hives), or dermatitis, which may indicate a **hypersensitivity** reaction to the drug.

4. A/An **antiseptic** is a drug that stops, slows, or prevents the growth of microorganisms.

5. A drug that kills bacteria is known as a/an **germicide**

6. Topical **antipsoriatics** are drugs used to treat psoriasis.

SECTION II: APPLYING YOUR KNOWLEDGE

Activity C SHORT ANSWERS

Answer the following questions concerning the nurse's role in the management of patients receiving a topical drug for a skin disorder.

1. During a preadministration assessment, what are the required nursing interventions?

_____

_____

_____

2. What are the interventions required as a part of the ongoing assessment?

_____

_____

_____

Activity D **DOSAGE CALCULATION**

1. A patient with a herpes simplex virus infection has been prescribed acyclovir ointment to be applied every 3 hours, 8 times per day, for 7 days. How many total applications would the nurse administer for the entire treatment? _____

2. A patient with tinea corporis has been prescribed tolnaftate to be applied twice daily for 3 weeks. How many total applications would the nurse administer for the entire treatment?

_____

SECTION III: PRACTICING FOR NCLEX

Activity E

Answer the following questions.

1. A nurse is caring for a patient who has been prescribed masoprocol. The nurse should know that the administration of masoprocol is contraindicated for which of the following uses?
   a. For use on moles, birthmarks, or warts
   b. As monotherapy for bacterial skin infections
   c. For use on the face, groin, or axilla
   d. As sole therapy in plaque psoriasis

2. A patient undergoing treatment has been prescribed alclometasone dipropionate. The nurse should know that the administration of alclometasone dipropionate is contraindicated for which of the following uses?
   a. For use on moles and birthmarks
   b. As sole therapy in plaque psoriasis

   c. For use on genital or facial warts
   d. For use on infected skin

3. The primary health care provider has prescribed benzocaine for a patient. In which of the following should the nurse use benzocaine cautiously?
   a. Patients who are pregnant or lactating
   b. Immunocompromised patients with herpes simplex virus infections
   c. Patients receiving Class I antiarrhythmic drugs such as tocainide
   d. Patients with cutaneous candidiasis or tinea pedis

4. A nurse is caring for a patient being treated for psoriasis. The primary health care provider has prescribed anthralin. Which of the following should the nurse monitor for in the patient as an adverse reaction to anthralin?
   a. Hypothalamic-pituitary-adrenal axis suppression
   b. Cushing's syndrome
   c. Hyperglycemia and glycosuria
   d. Temporary discoloration of the fingernails

5. The primary health care provider has prescribed alclometasone dipropionate for a patient being treated for eczema. The nurse caring for the patient should know that which of the following is a systemic adverse reaction to alclometasone dipropionate?
   a. Hyperglycemia and glycosuria
   b. Mild and transient pain
   c. Numbness and dermatitis
   d. Flu-like syndrome

6. A patient is undergoing treatment for debriding chronic dermal ulcers, and the primary health care provider has prescribed collagenase. Which of the following should the nurse monitor for as an adverse reaction to the application of collagenase?
   a. Flu-like syndrome
   b. Numbness and dermatitis
   c. Cushing's syndrome
   d. Hyperglycemia and glycosuria

7. A nurse is caring for a patient who has been prescribed salicylic acid for the treatment of

hyperkeratotic skin disorders. Which of the following should the nurse monitor as an adverse reaction to salicylic acid?

a. Mild and transient pains

b. Temporary discoloration of the hair

c. Flu-like syndrome

d. Hyperglycemia and glycosuria

8. A nurse is caring for a patient who has been prescribed Accuzyme for treatment by the primary health care provider. The nurse should know that Accuzyme is used to treat which of the following?

a. Psoriasis

b. Eczema

c. Insect bites

d. Chronic dermal ulcers

9. A patient has been admitted to the health care facility with inflamed skin resulting from severe insect bites. The primary health care provider has prescribed topical corticosteroid therapy. The nurse caring for this patient should know that which of the following is the action of a topical corticosteroid?

a. Reduces itching, redness, and swelling

b. Reduces the number of bacteria on the skin

c. Prevents infection in the bite wounds

d. Cleanses the skin thoroughly

10. A nurse is caring for a patient with a chronic skin disease diagnosed as psoriasis. To avoid infections, which of the following should the nurse use to wash her hands before and after caring for the patient?

a. Topical antipsoriatics

b. Topical antiseptics and germicides

c. Topical enzymes

d. Topical antifungals

CHAPTER 57

Otic and Ophthalmic Preparations

SECTION I: ASSESSING YOUR UNDERSTANDING

Activity A MATCHING

1. Match the drugs in Column A with their uses in Column B.

Column A

B ____ 1. Brimonidine tartrate

D ____ 2. Apraclonidine hydrochloride 1% solution

A ____ 3. Dapiprazole hydrochloride

C ____ 4. Metipranolol hydrochloride

Column B

A. Reverses the diagnostic mydriasis after ophthalmic examination

B. Lowers intraocular pressure (IOP) in patients with open-angle (chronic) glaucoma

C. Treats elevated IOP in patients with ocular hypertension or open-angle glaucoma

D. Controls or prevents postoperative elevations in IOP

2. Match the drugs in Column A with their adverse reactions in Column B.

Column A

C ____ 1. 1% hydrocortisone, 5 mg neomycin sul-

Column B

A. Local irritation, itching, burning, and earache

fate, 10,000 units polymyxin B

A ____ 2. Floxacin otic

B ____ 3. Brimonidine tartrate

B. Burning and stinging

C. Ear irritation, burning, or itching

Activity B FILL IN THE BLANKS

1. Prolonged use of otic preparations containing an antibiotic, such as ofloxacin, may result in a/an **Superinfection**

2. **Glaucoma** is a condition of the eye in which there is an increase in the IOP, causing progressive atrophy of the optic nerve with deterioration of vision.

3. Dapiprazole acts by blocking the α-adrenergic receptor in the smooth muscles and produces **miosis** through an effect on the dilator muscle of the iris.

4. Silver possesses **antibacterial** activity against gram-positive and gram-negative microorganisms.

5. **Natamycin** is the only ophthalmic antifungal in use.

6. **Cycloplegia** is the paralysis of the ciliary muscle, resulting in an inability to focus the eye.

SECTION II: APPLYING YOUR KNOWLEDGE

Activity C SHORT ANSWERS

Answer the following questions concerning the nurse's role in the management of patients receiving otic preparations.

1. Before administration of an otic preparation, the primary health care provider examines the ear and external structures surrounding the ear and prescribes the drug indicated to treat the disorder. As a preadministration assessment, the nurse may be responsible for examining which areas of the ear?

Outer structures such as the earlobe + skin. Document any drainage / impacted cerumen

2. How should the nurse assess the patient's response to otic therapy, and what further examinations should be carried out?

Has pain / inflammation? Examine for irritation such as redness or drug sensitivity

Activity D DOSAGE CALCULATION

1. A patient has been prescribed an otic preparation of 1% hydrocortisone, 5 mg of neomycin sulfate, and 10,000 units of polymyxin. The dosage instructed is 4 gtt instilled 4 times daily. How many drops would the nurse be administering in a day? _____

2. A patient with trachoma has been prescribed 2 gtt of sulfacetamide sodium q2h. How many drops would the nurse administer in a day? _____

SECTION III: PRACTICING FOR NCLEX

Activity E

Answer the following questions.

1. A nurse is caring for a patient who has been using ofloxacin for a prolonged time. Which of the following are the risks associated with the prolonged use of such otic antibiotics?

a. Danger of superinfection in the ear

b. Systemic effects of cholinesterase inhibitors

c. Exacerbation of existing hypertension

d. Additive central nervous system (CNS) depressant effects

2. The nurse should know that ofloxacin is used with caution in which of the following?

a. Patients taking monoamine oxidase inhibitors

b. Patients who are pregnant or lactating

c. Patients with activities requiring mental alertness

d. Patients performing activities in dimly lit areas

3. A nurse is caring for a patient who is to be administered an antibiotic ear solution. Before instilling the otic solution, what should the nurse inform the patient?

a. Local effects such as headache and visual blurring may be felt

b. Fatigue and drowsiness may be experienced

c. A feeling of fullness may be felt in the ear

d. Hearing in the treated ear may temporarily improve

4. Prior to instillation of otic preparations, the nurse should hold the container in his or her hand for a few minutes. What is the reason for doing this?

a. To observe the number of drops in the applicator

b. To confirm the drug was kept refrigerated

c. To observe if the drug is in suspension form

d. To warm the preparation to body temperature

5. A nurse needs to administer otic drops to a patient. Which of the following should the nurse do to ensure correct administration of the otic drops?

a. Have the patient lie on his or her side with the ear toward the ceiling

b. In upright position, have the head tilted straight down towards the floor

c. Gently pull the cartilaginous portion of the outer ear down and forward

d. Properly insert the applicator tip or the dropper tip into the ear canal

6. A nurse is caring for a patient who is being administered Cerumenex for softening the dried earwax inside the ear canal. When should the nurse discontinue the use of Cerumenex?

   a. After using the medication for 1 week

   b. When absolutely no cerumen remains

   c. When drainage or discharge occurs

   d. When dizziness or other sensations occur

7. A nurse is caring for a patient who is being administered dipivefrin hydrochloride for the treatment of open-angle glaucoma. Which of the following should the nurse monitor for in the patient as a transient local reaction to dipivefrin hydrochloride?

   a. Deposits in conjunctiva

   b. Brow ache or headache

   c. Ocular allergic reactions

   d. Foreign body sensation

8. A patient has undergone an ophthalmic examination and is being administered dapiprazole hydrochloride to reverse the diagnostic mydriasis. The nurse should know that which of the following is a local effect of dapiprazole hydrochloride?

   a. Abnormal corneal staining

   b. Decreased night vision

   c. Frequent urge to urinate

   d. Drooping of the upper eyelid

9. A patient has been administered echothiophate iodide to treat accommodative esotropia. Which of the following ophthalmic adverse reactions should the nurse monitor for in the patient?

   a. Eyelid muscle twitching

   b. Abdominal cramps

   c. Cardiac irregularities

   d. Urinary incontinence

10. A patient with glaucoma who does not respond to other drugs has been administered travoprost to reduce increased intraocular pressure. The nurse should know that the patient is likely to exhibit which of the following as a local adverse reaction?

    a. Unpleasant taste

    b. Eyelid discomfort

    c. Asthma

    d. Cold or flu symptoms

CHAPTER 58

Fluids and Electrolytes

SECTION I: ASSESSING YOUR UNDERSTANDING

Activity A MATCHING

1. Match the electrolytes in Column A with their common uses in Column B.

Column A

_____ 1. Potassium

_____ 2. Magnesium

_____ 3. Sodium

_____ 4. Calcium

Column B

A. Plays an important role in the transmission of nerve impulses and the activity of many enzyme reactions such as carbohydrate metabolism

B. Necessary for the functioning of nerves and muscles, clotting of blood, building of bones and teeth, and other physiologic processes

C. Necessary for transmission of impulses; contraction of smooth, cardiac, and skeletal muscles; and other important physiologic processes

D. Important in maintaining acid–base balance, normal heart action, and regulation of osmotic pressure in body cells

Activity B FILL IN THE BLANKS

1. An _____ is an electrically charged substance essential to the normal functioning of all cells.

2. A low pH in the blood means the body is in an acidic condition, and a high blood pH indicates an _____ condition.

3. The term fluid _____ describes a condition in which the body's fluid requirements are met, and fluid administration occurs at a rate that is greater than the rate at which the body can use or eliminate the fluid.

4. Sodium as an electrolyte is administered for _____, or low blood sodium.

5. Protein _____ are amino acid preparations that act to promote the production of proteins.

SECTION II: APPLYING YOUR KNOWLEDGE

Activity C SHORT ANSWERS

A nurse's role in managing patients who are receiving fluids and electrolytes involves monitoring and managing interventions that aid in their recovery. Answer the following questions, which involve the nurse's role in the management of such situations.

1. A nurse has been caring for a patient who has been administered intravenous (IV) replace-

ment solutions. What factors should the nurse consider when evaluating the therapy to determine its effectiveness?

_____

_____

_____

2. A nurse has been caring for a patient who has been administered potassium. What instructions should the nurse offer as part of the patient teaching plan related to the intake of this electrolyte after discharge?

_____

_____

_____

Activity D **DOSAGE CALCULATION**

1. A patient has been prescribed 2 g of bicarbonate per day to be taken orally in two equally divided doses every 12 hr. The drug is available in 0.5-g tablets. How many tablets should the patient take in a day? _____

2. A patient is prescribed 5 g of magnesium sulfate to be taken IV every 3 hours. The drug is available in the form of 1 g/2 mL. How much magnesium sulfate should the nurse prepare in solution for the patient to take in 2 days? _____

3. A patient is prescribed 60 mEq of potassium per day to be taken orally. The drug is available in 30 mEq. How many tablets should the patient take in a day? _____

4. A standard dose of tromethamine is 30 mg/ 50 kg. The patient weighs 120 kg. The dose is available in the form of 15 mg/mL. If the physician prescribes a standard dose, how much tromethamine would the nurse prepare? _____

SECTION III: PRACTICING FOR NCLEX

Activity E

Answer the following questions.

1. A nurse is assigned to care for a patient who needs to be administered magnesium. What should the nurse determine from the patient's health history before administering magnesium to know that the use of the electrolyte is not contraindicated for the patient?
   a. Patient does not experience fluid retention
   b. Patient does not have heart block
   c. Patient does not have untreated Addison's disease
   d. Patient is not taking digitalis

2. A nurse is caring for a patient who is being administered electrolytes orally. During assessment, the nurse observes that the patient is experiencing gastrointestinal (GI) disturbances. What nursing interventions should the nurse perform when caring for this patient? Select all that apply.
   a. Offer smaller meals more frequently
   b. Monitor for any signs and symptoms of nausea
   c. Encourage patient to increase intake of fruit juices
   d. Ensure that drug is taken only with meals
   e. Administer antacids to the patient as prescribed for nausea

3. A nurse is assigned to care for a patient whose protein intake is significantly less than the amount required by the body. Which of the following conditions is the patient likely to experience?
   a. Metabolic acidosis
   b. GI disturbances
   c. Negative nitrogen balance
   d. Hypotensive episodes

4. A nurse is caring for a patient who is being administered fat emulsions. What interventions should the nurse perform when conducting ongoing assessments for the patient?
   a. Ensure the solution is colder than room temperature
   b. Monitor the patient for signs of diarrhea
   c. Monitor the patient's ability to eliminate infused fat
   d. Monitor the patient for signs of hypernatremia

5. A nurse is caring for a patient who is being administered plasma proteins. Which of the following adverse reactions should the nurse monitor for in this patient?

a. Urticaria

b. Flushing of skin

c. Dyspnea

d. Wheezing

6. A nurse is caring for a patient who is being administered sodium electrolyte solution IV. What interventions should the nurse perform as part of the ongoing assessment when caring for this patient? Select all that apply.

a. Ensure that a microscopic filter is attached to the IV line

b. Observe the rate of IV infusion every 15 to 30 minutes

c. Measure the patient's intake and output every 8 hours

d. Inform the primary health care provider if the patient voids less than 100 mL of urine every 4 hours

e. Monitor the patient's condition for signs of pulmonary edema

7. A nurse is caring for a patient who needs to be administered bicarbonate. What information should the nurse obtain from the patient's health history to know that bicarbonate should be administered cautiously in this patient?

a. The patient has metabolic alkalosis

b. The patient has congestive heart failure

c. The patient has hypocalcemia

d. The patient is on a sodium-restricted diet

8. A nurse is caring for a patient who is being administered potassium IV. When assessing the patient's condition, the nurse observes that the patient's heart rate is irregular. What nursing intervention should the nurse perform when caring for this patient?

a. Check the patient's pulse rate every 4 hours

b. Discontinue the IV infusion immediately

c. Monitor the patient for signs of nausea and vomiting

d. Administer a direct IV injection of potassium for the next dose

9. A nurse is caring for a 65-year-old patient who needs to be administered plasma proteins. What interventions should the nurse perform when monitoring and managing this patient's needs?

a. Carefully monitor the patient for signs and symptoms of fluid overload

b. Carefully observe the patient for difficulty in breathing, headache, or flushing

c. Immediately report any signs of hypercalcemic syndrome to the primary health care provider

d. Test the patient's patellar reflex before administering each dose

10. A nurse is caring for a patient who is being administered ammonium chloride. The nurse knows that the patient has been taking spironolactone. Which of the following adverse reactions should the nurse monitor for in this patient caused by the interaction of ammonium chloride and spironolactone?

a. Systemic alkalosis

b. Respiratory depression

c. Heart block

d. Systemic acidosis

Answer Key

CHAPTER 1

SECTION I: ASSESSING YOUR UNDERSTANDING

Activity A MATCHING

1. 1-B, 2-C, 3-A
2. 1-C, 2-D, 3-A, 4-B

Activity B FILL IN THE BLANKS

1. Absorption
2. Intravenous
3. Antagonistic
4. Synergism
5. Pharmacogenetic

SECTION II: APPLYING YOUR KNOWLEDGE

Activity C SHORT ANSWERS

1. Physical and chemical changes occur because of changes in the cellular environment:
   - Physical changes in the cellular environment include changes in osmotic pressures, lubrication, absorption, or the condition of the surface of the cell membrane.
   - Chemical changes in the cellular environment include inactivation of cellular functions or the alteration of the chemical components of body fluid, such as a change in the pH.
2. The U.S. Food and Drug Administration (FDA) is responsible for approving new drugs and monitoring drugs currently in use for adverse or toxic reactions. The process of drug development takes about 7 to 12 years and sometimes even longer.

Activity D

1. a. The patient should be informed that many botanicals have strong pharmacological activity, and some may interact with prescription drugs that the patient is taking. Botanicals may also produce toxic substances in the body.
   b. The nurse should inquire if the patient is using any herbs, teas, vitamins, or other dietary supplements. The nurse should explain that herbal supplements are not necessarily safe or without side effects.
2. The development of a new drug is divided into the pre-FDA phase and the FDA phase. During the pre-FDA phase, a manufacturer discovers a drug that looks promising. *In vitro* testing is performed using animal and human cells, followed by studies in live animals. The manufacturer then applies to the FDA for an Investigational New Drug (IND) status.
3. The nurse informs the patient that smoking or consumption of any type of alcoholic beverage carries risks to the fetus, such as low birth weight, premature birth, and fetal alcohol syndrome. Children born to mothers using addictive drugs, such as cocaine or heroin, are often born with an addiction to the drug abused by the mother.

SECTION III: PRACTICING FOR NCLEX

Activity E

1. **Answer: d**
   RATIONALE: The nurse should refer to a drug by its generic name to avoid confusion. A generic name is the name given to a drug before it becomes official and can be used in many countries by all the manufacturers. The official name is the name listed in *The United States Pharmacopeia-National Formulary.* The scientific name, also called the chemical name, gives the molecular structure of that particular drug. The trade name is the name registered by the manufacturer and is followed by the trademark symbol. Only the manufacturer can use this name.
2. **Answer: b, c, d**
   RATIONALE: The purpose of the *Controlled Substances Act* of 1970 is to regulate the manufacture, distribution, and dispensing of drugs that have abuse potential. Adverse drug effects are reported by physicians through the FDA-established reporting program called MedWatch. The *Orphan Drug Act* of 1983 was passed to encourage drug development.
3. **Answer: b**
   RATIONALE: During the pharmaceutic phase of drug activity, the liquid drug is absorbed into the body system. Solid tablets or capsules break into small pieces and dissolve into body fluids in the

gastrointestinal tract. Enteric-coated tablets disintegrate in the small intestine.

4. Answer: c

RATIONALE: The nurse should administer the drug intravenously as the drug is rapidly absorbed by the system. Absorption occurs slowly when the drug is administered orally, intramuscularly, or subcutaneously. Because of the complex membranes of the gastrointestinal mucosal layers, muscle and skin delay the drug passage.

5. Answer: a, c, e

RATIONALE: The nurse should monitor physiologic functions such as blood pressure, urine output, and heart rate in altered cellular function. Impaired vision and slurred speech may be symptoms of altered cellular function in patients with drug allergies.

6. Answer: a, c, e

RATIONALE: Cancer drugs act on the cell membrane and cell processes, eventually causing starvation and death of the cancer cells. Antacids cause chemical changes in body fluids by changing the pH to neutralize the acidity.

7. Answer: a, d, e

RATIONALE: The patient is likely to exhibit drug toxicity. The diseased kidney will not be able to eliminate excess drug amounts, so the drug levels in the blood will increase, causing a longer duration of action. A person who is addicted to certain drugs could be drug dependent and exhibit drug tolerance, in which case higher doses of the drug would have to be administered.

8. Answer: a, b, c

RATIONALE: The patient's age and weight are important in determining the drug dosage to be administered for effective action of the drug. If the patient has a disease, it could interfere with the drug action; the dosage would have to be adjusted accordingly. The patient's appetite and height do not influence the drug response.

9. Answer: c

RATIONALE: Patients with impaired liver function need to be monitored frequently during drug administration because impaired liver function influences drug response. Impaired vision, speech, or hearing does not affect the drug response.

CHAPTER 2

SECTION I: ASSESSING YOUR UNDERSTANDING

Activity A MATCHING

1. 1-C, 2-D, 3-A, 4-B
2. 1-C, 2-D, 3-B, 4-A

Activity B FILL IN THE BLANKS

1. Controllers
2. Subcutaneous
3. Unit

4. Sublingual
5. Buccal
6. Extravasation

SECTION II: APPLYING YOUR KNOWLEDGE

Activity C SHORT ANSWERS

1. There are two methods to ensure that the right patient receives the medication:
   - Check the patient's wristband containing the patient's name. If there is no written identification verifying the patient's name, the nurse can obtain a wristband or other form of identification before administering the drug.
   - Ask the patient to identify himself or herself and state his or her date of birth prior to administering the drug.
2. It is important to report drug errors so that:
   - Any necessary steps to counteract the action of the drug can be taken
   - Any observations can be made as soon as possible

Activity D CASE STUDY

1. The nurse should compare the medication, container label, and medication record to ensure that he is administering the right drug to the right patient.
2. Immediate documentation is particularly important when drugs are given on an as-needed (PRN) basis. Immediate documentation prevents accidental administration of a drug by another individual. Proper documentation is essential to the process of administering drugs correctly.
3. The nurse's responsibilities when administering a transdermal drug include:
   - Applying transdermal patches to clean, dry, non-hairy areas of intact skin
   - Removing the old patch when the next dose is applied in a new site
   - Rotating sites for transdermal patches to prevent skin irritation
   - Removing paper and tape and cleaning skin before next dose of ointment
   - Writing the nurse's initials, date, and time of application on the patch

SECTION III: PRACTICING FOR NCLEX

Activity E

1. Answer: a

RATIONALE: After administering an as-needed (PRN) drug, the nurse should immediately record the fact. Evaluating the patient's response to the drug or recording the site used for parenteral administration should be done after documentation of the drug's administration. The nurse should inform the physician only if there are any adverse reactions.

2. Answer: d

RATIONALE: The nurse should remove the old patch when the next dose is applied to a new site. The nurse should rotate sites for transdermal patches to prevent skin irritation and not place the new patch in the same location as the old patch. The nurse should not shave the area to apply the patch; shaving may cause skin irritation. The area where the transdermal patch is applied should be dry, not moist.

3. **Answer: b**

   RATIONALE: The nurse should obtain special instructions from the primary health care provider concerning application of the drug. The instructions may include whether to apply the drug in a thin or even layer or whether to cover the area after application of the drug to the skin. It is not essential to obtain information about the cause of skin infection, reasons for selecting the drug, and composition of the drug before administering the prescribed drug.

4. **Answer: c**

   RATIONALE: The inner part of the forearm is ideal for administering an intradermal injection. The nurse should not administer the drug near moles, areas with hair cover, or pigmented skin. The thigh and the upper arm are ideal sites for intramuscular injections, but not for intradermal injections.

5. **Answer: b**

   RATIONALE: A venipuncture is a difficult procedure; after three unsuccessful attempts, the nurse should ask for assistance from a more skilled nurse. It is not advisable for the nurse to repeatedly attempt a venipuncture; this may cause the patient great discomfort. The nurse should not change the administration route even if it is getting difficult to administer a drug in a particular manner. Shifting the patient to a more conducive position is unlikely to help significantly.

6. **Answer: a**

   RATIONALE: If an intramuscular injection volume is more than 3 mL, the nurse should divide the drug and give it as two separate injections. Volumes larger than 3 mL will not be absorbed properly. The nurse should use a needle with a 1½-inch length for the injection, not ½ inch. The upper back is not an ideal site for intramuscular injections. When giving a drug by the intramuscular route, the nurse should insert the needle at a 90° angle.

7. **Answer: c**

   RATIONALE: In thin or cachectic patients, there usually is less subcutaneous tissue. For such patients, the upper abdomen is the most appropriate site for injection. The thigh or upper arm is an administration site for intramuscular injections, not subcutaneous injections. The upper back, and not the lower back, is a site for subcutaneous injections.

8. **Answer: a, c, e**

   RATIONALE: The nurse should crush the tablets and ensure that the tablets are completely dissolved before administering them to the patient. The nurse should check the tube for placement and flush the tube with water to clear the tubing. The nurse should not put the tablets in water without crushing

them, as the drug may not dissolve properly. The tube should be fixed after the drug has been mixed.

CHAPTER 3

SECTION I: ASSESSING YOUR UNDERSTANDING

Activity A MATCHING

1. 1-B, 2-D, 3-A, 4-C
2. 1-D, 2-A, 3-B, 4-C

Activity B FILL IN THE BLANKS

1. Denominators
2. Lowest
3. Fractions
4. Numerator
5. Larger
6. Mixed
7. Improper
8. Proper
9. Ratio
10. Equality

CHAPTER 4

SECTION I: ASSESSING YOUR UNDERSTANDING

Activity A MATCHING

1. 1-C, 2-E, 3-A, 4-B, 5-D
2. 1-E, 2-A, 3-C, 4-B, 5-D

Activity B FILL IN THE BLANKS

1. Objective
2. Ongoing
3. Diagnosis
4. Implementation
5. Individual

SECTION II: APPLYING YOUR KNOWLEDGE

Activity C SHORT ANSWERS

1. a. Nursing process is a framework for nursing action consisting of problem-solving steps that help members of the health care team provide effective patient care. It is both a specific and orderly plan used to gather data, identify patient problems from the data, develop and implement a plan of action, and then evaluate the results of nursing activities, including the administration of drugs.

   b. These are the five phases of the nursing process: Assessment; Nursing diagnosis (analysis); Planning; Implementation; Evaluation.

2. An initial assessment is made based on objective and subjective data collected when the patient is first seen in a hospital, outpatient clinic, health care provider's office, or other type of health care

facility. The initial assessment is usually more thorough and provides a database from which later data can be compared and decisions made. An ongoing assessment is one that is made at the time of each patient contact and may include the collection of objective data, subjective data, or both. The scope of an ongoing assessment depends on many factors, such as the patient's diagnosis, the severity of illness, the response to treatment, and the prescribed medical or surgical treatment.

SECTION III: PRACTICING FOR NCLEX

Activity D

1. Answer: a
RATIONALE: In order to obtain subjective data from the patient, the nurse should inquire about the number of cigarettes smoked in a day. Subjective data include facts that are supplied to the nurse and other health care professionals by the patient and patient's family. Monitoring the patient's body temperature, blood pressure, and pulse rate and rhythm are objective data that the nurse should obtain. Objective data include facts, which the nurse obtains through physical assessment or examination.

2. Answer: c
RATIONALE: When caring for a patient of childbearing age, the nurse needs to determine and assess the patient's pregnancy status before administering a drug because the drug may be contraindicated or may require cautious use during pregnancy. Determining and assessing the patient for her relationship with her spouse, her menstrual history, or her family history are not appropriate interventions before administering a drug because they will not help in determining if the administration of the drug to the patient would be safe.

3. Answer: d
RATIONALE: When developing an expected outcome, the nurse should focus on the patient's ability to recuperate. Expected outcome describes the maximum level of wellness that is reasonably attainable for the patient. The expected outcome defines the expected behavior of the patient or family that indicates the problem is being resolved or that progress toward resolution is occurring. When developing an expected outcome, the nurse need not focus on the type of drug administered, its dosage pattern, or the patient's ability to recuperate considering these will not determine if the patient has the ability to achieve the maximum level of wellness.

4. Answer: a
RATIONALE: In her nursing diagnosis, a nurse should include problems that can be solved by independent nursing actions—actions that do not require a physician's order and may be legally performed by a nurse. The nurse should not include problems that have a definite cure or problems that cannot

be prevented by nursing actions. Nursing diagnosis also does not include identification of the patient's condition or criticality.

5. Answer: a, c, e
RATIONALE: Planning for nursing actions specific for the drug to be administered promotes a greater accuracy in drug administration, patient understanding of the drug regimen, and improved patient compliance with the prescribed drug therapy after hospital discharge. Planning for nursing actions does not prevent a relapse. Planning and implementing nursing actions does promote an optimal response to drug therapy, but it does not always promote an optimal response in minimal time.

6. Answer: b
RATIONALE: To combat the patient's noncompliant attitude, the nurse should try and find out the exact reason for noncompliance, if possible, so that it can be addressed. Often the noncompliant attitude develops out of patient-based fear and anxiety related to the drug regimen. Preparing a fixed schedule for the patient to take the drug and teaching the patient the importance of the drug regimen are not appropriate interventions considering they will do little to deal with the problem creating the noncompliant attitude. If the attitude stems from anxiety, then these interventions will do little to reduce patient anxiety. Though the nurse should monitor for a relapse caused by noncompliance with the drug regimen, doing so will not promote the patient to strictly follow the regimen.

7. Answer: c, a, d, b, e
The nursing process is a framework for nursing action consisting of problem-solving steps that help members of the health care team to provide effective patient care. It is both a specific and orderly plan used to gather data, identify patient problems from the data, develop and implement a plan of action, and then evaluate the results of nursing activities.

CHAPTER 5

SECTION I: ASSESSING YOUR UNDERSTANDING

Activity A MATCHING

1. 1-B, 2-C, 3-A
2. 1-C, 2-A, 3-B

Activity B FILL IN THE BLANKS

1. Physical
2. Affective
3. Chew
4. Sunlight
5. Scheduling

SECTION II: APPLYING YOUR KNOWLEDGE

Activity C SHORT ANSWERS

1. To ensure that the patient perfectly remembers all the exercises taught to him or her, the nurse should supervise while the patient demonstrates the exercises.
2. To ensure that the patient's relative has understood the procedure of measuring the patient's temperature by using an electronic thermometer, the nurse should:
   - Ask the relative to demonstrate the procedure.
   - Avoid posing questions such as, "Do you understand?" or "Is there anything you don't understand?" because the relative may be uncomfortable in admitting a lack of understanding.

Activity D

1. a. Because the patient is deficient in cognitive knowledge and psychomotor skills, the nursing diagnosis called Deficient Knowledge must be used to teach the patient administration of antimalarial drugs.
2. a. Learning how to perform breathing exercises involves the psychomotor domain, which involves physical skills.
   b. Ineffective Therapeutic Regimen Management must be used to teach the client breathing exercises.
3. a. The affective domain of learning is accessed when the patient implements the weight-loss program.

SECTION III: PRACTICING FOR NCLEX

Activity E

1. **Answer: a, b, c**
   RATIONALE: Ineffective Therapeutic Regimen Management targets discharge teaching, management of complicated medication regimens, and provision of positive results to patients. It also describes patients who successfully manage drug regimens. Effective Individual Therapeutic Regimen Management gives information about drug reactions and teaches management of adverse reactions. Effective Individual Therapeutic Regimen Management generally describes a patient who is successfully managing the medication regimen.
2. **Answer: a, b, d**
   RATIONALE: The teaching plan should be implemented a day or two before the patient's discharge. Care should be taken to see that the patient is alone, alert, and not sedated. Dividing the teaching material into sessions will make it easy for the patient to learn. The implementation of the teaching plan should not begin as soon as the patient is admitted to the hospital. Also, teaching everything all at once may make learning difficult for the patient.

3. **Answer: a, d, e**
   RATIONALE: Carrying out a patient assessment before formulating a teaching plan helps a nurse to determine obstacles that the patient could face in the learning process, to choose the best teaching methods, and to develop an effective teaching plan. An effective teaching plan can help improve patient motivation or participation.
4. **Answer: a**
   RATIONALE: The psychomotor domain involves the learning of physical skills. The cognitive domain involves the patient's or the caregiver's attitudes, feelings, beliefs, and opinions. The cognitive domain involves intellectual activities or intellectual domain such as thought, recall, decision making, and drawing conclusions.
5. **Answer: a**
   RATIONALE: Implementation of the teaching plan means actually performing the interventions identified in teaching plan. Determining the effectiveness of patient teaching comes under evaluation. Planning involves beginning with expected outcomes. Using patient experiences is an aspect of adult learning.
6. **Answer: c, d, e**
   RATIONALE: The three domains of learning are psychomotor domain, which involves the learning of physical skills; cognitive domain, which involves the patient's or the caregiver's attitudes, feelings, beliefs, and opinions; and the affective domain, which involves making decisions and drawing conclusions. The "intellectual" and "intuitive" domains are not defined domains of learning.
7. **Answer: c**
   RATIONALE: Different literacy levels can pose a major obstacle in the process of learning. Low grasping power, patient's nervousness in using the inhaler, and lack of awareness can be overcome if the literacy levels are matched.
8. **Answer: a**
   RATIONALE: The affective domain includes the patient's or the caregiver's attitudes, feelings, beliefs, and opinions. Here, the affective domain is involved in teaching the patient. The cognitive domain involves intellectual domain such as thought, recall, decision making, and ability to draw conclusions. The psychomotor domain involves learning physical skills.

CHAPTER 6

SECTION I: ASSESSING YOUR UNDERSTANDING

Activity A MATCHING

1. 1-C, 2-D, 3-A, 4-B
2. 1-D, 2-A, 3-B, 4-C

Activity B FILL IN THE BLANKS

1. 2
2. Bacteriostatic
3. Photosensitivity
4. Cranberry
5. Thrombocytopenia

SECTION II: APPLYING YOUR KNOWLEDGE

Activity C SHORT ANSWERS

1. A nurse is required to perform the following as part of the preadministration assessment:
   - Assess the patient's general appearance, general health history (surgeries, medical conditions, and medications), and allergies.
   - Take and record vital signs.
   - Obtain description of signs and symptoms of infection from the patient or family.
   - Review results of tests.
2. A nurse's teaching plan should include the following instructions:
   - Take the drug as prescribed.
   - Keep all follow-up appointments to ensure the infection is controlled.
   - Complete the full course of therapy.
   - Drink at least eight to ten 8-oz glasses of fluid every day.
   - Take the drug on an empty stomach either 1 hour before or 2 hours after a meal.
   - Avoid prolonged exposure to sunlight, which may result in skin reactions similar to severe sunburn.

Activity D DOSAGE CALCULATION

1. 6 tablets
2. 1 tablet
3. 20 mL
4. 3 tablets
5. 5 tablets

SECTION III: PRACTICING FOR NCLEX

Activity E

1. **Answer: a**
   RATIONALE: The nurse should clean and remove the debris present on the surface of the patient's burnt skin before the application of cream. The nurse should not apply a thick layer of cream on the burned area. The drug is normally applied 1/16-inch thick; thicker application is not recommended. Applying drugs with an open hand involves a risk of passing infection. It is advisable to use sterilized gloves while applying cream. The nurse should remove debris present on the surface of the skin before each application of the drug.
2. **Answer: d**
   RATIONALE: The nurse should inspect the patient's skin daily to assess the extent of bruising and evidence of exacerbation of existing ecchymotic areas. The patient can be shifted if required, but care should be taken to prevent bruising. There is no need to avoid brushing teeth as long as a soft-bristled toothbrush is used. While it is necessary to examine the patient's skin for trauma, palpating the patient's body can create unnecessary pain and may trigger bleeding.
3. **Answer: d**
   RATIONALE: The nurse should instruct the patient to wear protective clothing while outdoors. Applying sunscreen on exposed body parts is not enough to protect from photosensitivity, and the patient should wear protective clothing even after applying sunscreen. Sulfasalazine, not sulfadiazine, causes a yellow stain on contact lenses. There is no need to avoid indoor lights as the effects of photosensitivity are caused by sunlight.
4. **Answer: a, c, e**
   RATIONALE: The nurse should inform the patient that the chief reasons for increasing fluid intake during sulfonamide therapy is to remove microorganisms from the urinary tract, and prevent crystalluria and stone formation in the genitourinary tract. Sulfonamides are easily absorbed by the gastrointestinal system and also easily excreted by the kidneys. Increasing the fluid intake will not have any significant impact on the absorption and excretion of sulfonamides.
5. **Answer: c**
   RATIONALE: Edema is one of the possible allergic reactions that may be caused by mafenide, so the nurse should monitor the patient for edema. Urine turning an orange-yellow color is one of the symptoms of sulfasalazine, not mafenide. Crystalluria does not occur during mafenide therapy. A burning sensation while applying the drug to the skin is a normal reaction.
6. **Answer: c**
   RATIONALE: The nurse should inform the patient that using soft contact lenses during the sulfasalazine therapy might result in a permanent yellow stain on the lenses. Wearing lenses will not, however, cause a burning sensation in eyes, headache and dizziness, or impaired vision.
7. **Answer: a, b, d**
   RATIONALE: While caring for patients with ulcerative colitis, the nurse should inspect the stool samples, record their appearance, and monitor the patient for evidence of relief or intensification of the symptoms. The nurse should also ensure that sulfasalazine is administered during meals or immediately afterwards. There is no need to measure urine output, as the patient does not have impaired urinary elimination. Loss of appetite is a mild adverse effect of sulfonamides.
8. **Answer: a**
   RATIONALE: The nurse should inform the patient that using cranberries with antibiotics prevents bacteria from attaching to the walls of the urinary tract. Crystalluria, or the formation of crystals in

urine, can be prevented by increasing the fluid intake. However, specifically consuming cranberry juice will not have any significant effect in preventing crystalluria. The effects of photosensitivity can be reduced by wearing protective clothing or sunscreen when traveling outside, and consumption of cranberry juice will not have any effect on this. Clots can be prevented by using oral anticoagulants with sulfonamides.

9. **Answer: a**

   RATIONALE: The nurse should inform the patient that sulfonamides are used in the treatment of urinary tract infection because the GI system easily absorbs them. Sulfonamides don't kill bacterial cells directly. They inhibit the activity of folic acid in bacterial cell metabolism; the bacteria are subsequently destroyed by the body's defense mechanisms. Decrease in the number of white blood cells is caused by leucopenia, which is also an adverse effect of sulfonamides. Sulfonamides may have life-threatening complications such as Stevens-Johnson syndrome.

10. **Answer: b**

    RATIONALE: The nurse should assess for lesions on the mucous membranes to determine whether the patient is showing signs of Stevens-Johnson syndrome. Inflammation of the mouth (stomatitis), crystals in the urine (crystalluria), and diarrhea are some of the common adverse reactions of sulfonamides and do not necessarily indicate that the patient has Stevens-Johnson syndrome.

CHAPTER 7

SECTION I: ASSESSING YOUR UNDERSTANDING

Activity A MATCHING

1. 1-C, 2-D, 3-A, 4-B
2. 1-C, 2-D, 3-B, 4-A

Activity B FILL IN THE BLANKS

1. Intravenous
2. Extended
3. Hematopoietic
4. Antihistamines
5. Penicillinase

SECTION II: APPLYING YOUR KNOWLEDGE

Activity C SHORT ANSWERS

1. Before administering penicillin for the first time, a nurse should perform the following assessments:
   - Obtain patient's general health history, including medical and surgical treatments, drug history, history of drug allergies to penicillin or cephalosporin, and present symptoms of infection.
   - Take and record vital signs.

- Obtain description of signs and symptoms of infection from the patient or family.
- Assess infected area and record findings on the patient's chart.
- Describe signs and symptoms relating to the patient's infection, such as color and type of drainage from a wound, pain, redness and inflammation, color of sputum, and presence of odor.
- Note patient's general appearance.
- Obtain results of the culture and sensitivity test before giving the first dose.

2. When caring for a patient receiving penicillin who has developed impaired oral mucous membranes, a nurse should perform the following interventions:
   - If diet permits, provide yogurt, buttermilk, or acidophilus capsules to reduce risk of fungal superinfection.
   - Give frequent mouth care with a nonirritating solution.
   - Use a soft bristled toothbrush.
   - Recommend a nonirritating soft diet.
   - Monitor dietary intake to ensure adequate nutrition.
   - If recommended, administer antifungal agents and/or local anesthetics to soothe the irritated membranes.

Activity D DOSAGE CALCULATION

1. 15 cc
2. 3 cc
3. 3 mL
4. 2 mL
5. 2 tablets
6. 2.5 mL

SECTION III: PRACTICING FOR NCLEX

Activity E

1. **Answer: d**

   RATIONALE: In mild hypersensitivity cases, the drug may be continued with the nurse administering frequent skin care to provide relief to the patient. Reducing the dosage from the prescribed limit should not be done unless specifically instructed by the primary health care provider because it would lead to a fall in the blood level. A patient can take baths as long as he or she avoids harsh soaps and perfumed lotions. Avoiding clothing contact with the affected areas is not necessary as long as the clothing is not rough or irritating.

2. **Answer: a**

   RATIONALE: The nurse should instruct the patient to take the drug at the prescribed times of day to maintain the drug level. Stopping antibiotic therapy before finishing the prescribed course, even if the patient feels better, may allow the infection to return. Women who are prescribed ampicillin, bacampicillin, and penicillin V and who take birth control pills containing estrogen should use additional contraception measures, but they need not stop using birth control pills. Intramuscular or intravenous drugs may be administered without considering the food-intake time of the patient.

3. **Answer: b**

RATIONALE: It is important to inform the primary health care provider if previously used areas for injection appear red or the patient reports pain in the area. Penicillin solutions are often thick or viscous, and it is natural for the patient to feel pain at the injection site. Mild nausea is a normal reaction to any antibiotic and is not a cause for concern. Decrease in temperature is a response to the therapy and does not need to be reported to the primary health care provider.

4. **Answer: 5, 2, 1, 4, 3**

RATIONALE: Before beginning the treatment, the nurse obtains or reviews the patient's general health history, inquiring especially about any allergies to penicillins. A culture and sensitivity test is ordered in most of the cases; these tests help identify the appropriate penicillin. The prescribed penicillin is then administered, and any improvements are recorded in the patient's charts.

5. **Answer: c, d, e**

RATIONALE: As part of the ongoing assessment, the nurse evaluates the patient's response to the therapy, such as a decrease in temperature, relief from pain or discomfort, increase in appetite, and a change in the appearance or in the amount of drainage. These evaluations are then recorded on the patient's chart to monitor the progress. Additional culture and sensitivity tests may be performed to check if the microorganisms have become penicillin resistant or if a superinfection has occurred. The patient's general health history is obtained before the appropriate penicillin therapy is determined, and the patient's stools are saved only if he or she shows signs of diarrhea and there are signs of blood and mucus in the stools.

6. **Answer: 3, 2, 4, 1**

RATIONALE: In situations where diarrhea is suspected, the nurse first inspects all stools. The primary health provider has to be notified immediately if diarrhea occurs, because it may be necessary to stop the drug. If there are signs of blood and mucus in the stool, it is important to save a sample to test it for occult blood to confirm presence of blood. If the stool tests positive for blood, the nurse saves another sample for possible further laboratory analysis.

7. **Answer: a, c, d**

RATIONALE: Some of the signs of anaphylactic shock are severe hypotension, loss of consciousness, and acute respiratory distress. Pain at the injection site is normal for penicillins administered intramuscularly. Nausea and vomiting are signs of gastrointestinal disturbances that may or may not be serious.

8. **Answer: b, c, e**

RATIONALE: In cases of impaired comfort or increased fever, the nurse should take vital signs every 4 hours or more. The nurse should report any rise in temperature to the primary health care provider, who may take additional treatment measures, such as administering an antipyretic drug or changing the drug or dosage to bring down the temperature. The nurse should not discontinue the dosage unless specifically instructed by the primary health provider. Changing the patient's diet to a soft, nonirritating diet is not necessary unless the patient shows signs of impaired oral mucous membranes.

9. **Answer: a, c, e**

RATIONALE: Symptoms of bacterial superinfection of the bowel include diarrhea or bloody diarrhea, rectal bleeding, and abdominal cramping. Vomiting is a common adverse reaction to penicillins, and lesions may occur caused by a hypersensitivity reaction.

10. **Answer: 2, 5, 4, 1, 3**

RATIONALE: The nurse should first read the manufacturer's directions on the label of the drug to find out details of reconstitution and the diluent to be used. The next step is to obtain the diluent mentioned in the manufacturer's directions. The nurse needs to reconstitute the drug in the vial before extracting. After reconstitution, the nurse extracts the penicillin from the vial and administers it to the patient.

CHAPTER 8

SECTION I: ASSESSING YOUR UNDERSTANDING

Activity A MATCHING

1. 1-D, 2-C, 3-B, 4-A
2. 1-C, 2-A, 3-D, 4-B

Activity B FILL IN THE BLANKS

1. Inflammation
2. Disulfiram
3. Thrombophlebitis
4. Penicillins
5. Extravasation

SECTION II: APPLYING YOUR KNOWLEDGE

Activity C SHORT ANSWERS

1. The nurse must follow these steps before administering the first dose of cephalosporin:
   - Obtain the patient's general health history, including medical and surgical treatments, drug history, history of drug allergies to penicillins or cephalosporins, and present symptoms of infection.

- Check for any culture and sensitivity tests done before the first dose of the drug is administered.
- Keep in mind that approximately 10% of the people allergic to a penicillin drug are also allergic to a cephalosporin drug.

2. a. When a patient is to be administered cephalosporin IV, the following interventions are important:
   - The nurse should inspect the needle insertion site for signs of extravasation or infiltration.
   - The needle insertion site and the area above the site should be inspected several times a day for phlebitis or thrombophlebitis.
   - If problems occur, the nurse should contact the primary health care provider, discontinue the IV, and restart it in another vein.
   b. When a patient is to be administered cephalosporin IM, the following interventions are important:
   - The nurse should inject the drug into a large muscle mass, such as the gluteus muscle or lateral aspect of the thigh.
   - If the patient has been nonambulatory for any length of time, the nurse should assess the muscle carefully because the large muscle may be atrophied.
   - The nurse should remember to rotate injection sites.
   - The nurse should warn the patient that at the time the drug is injected into the muscle, there may be a stinging or burning sensation, and the area may be sore for a short time.
   - The nurse should inform the primary health care provider if previously used areas for injection appear red or if the patient reports continued pain in the area.

Activity D DOSAGE CALCULATION

1. 2
2. 2 capsules at 8 p.m.
3. 1 tablet twice daily
4. 22.2 mL
5. 0.5
6. 600 mg
7. 6 tablets

SECTION III: PRACTICING FOR NCLEX

Activity E

1. **Answer: c**
   RATIONALE: The nurse should measure and record the fluid intake and output and notify the primary health care provider when caring for a patient with renal impairment. In case of diarrhea or loose stools containing blood or mucus, the nurse should inspect each bowel movement and immediately report to the primary health care provider. An antipyretic drug is administered when the body temperature increases in a patient receiving cephalosporins. Administration of cephalosporins to a patient with renal impairment does not maximize the risk of excessive perspiration.

2. **Answer: a**
   RATIONALE: When cephalosporin is given IV, the nurse should monitor the needle insertion site and the area above the site several times a day for signs of redness, which may indicate phlebitis or thrombophlebitis. The nurse should inspect the site for tenderness when the drug is administered to the patient intramuscularly. Administration of cephalosporin by IV does not cause fever or angina.

3. **Answer: a**
   RATIONALE: The nurse should identify an increased risk for bleeding in the patient as an effect of interaction of oral anticoagulants administered with cephalosporin. The patient is at an increased risk for nephrotoxicity when aminoglycosides are administered with cephalosporins. Administration of cephalosporins with oral anticoagulants does not maximize the risk of hypertension or cause an increase in the number of WBCs.

4. **Answer: d**
   RATIONALE: The nurse should instruct the patient to take the drug 1 hour before or 2 hours after the meal. The patient can take the medication with food or milk if gastrointestinal (GI) upset occurs after administration. The patient need not avoid sunlight or lie down; the drug does not cause photosensitivity or dizziness. The patient should be instructed to avoid alcohol completely during the course of therapy.

5. **Answer: c**
   RATIONALE: If the patient has been nonambulatory for any length of time or has paralysis, the nurse should assess the muscle carefully when administering cephalosporin intramuscularly because the large muscle may be atrophied. The patient does not face an increased risk for hypersensitivity reactions. There is increased risk of phlebitis or thrombophlebitis when the drug is given IV. A stinging or burning sensation will occur when the drug is administered intramuscularly; the patient needs to be warned, but the nurse need not monitor the patient for this.

6. **Answer: b, c, e**
   RATIONALE: The expected outcomes for a patient receiving cephalosporin are optimal responses to therapy and understanding and compliance with treatment. Complete recovery and improved dietary patterns are not typical expected outcomes of drug therapy.

7. **Answer: c**
   RATIONALE: The patient has aplastic anemia, which is an adverse effect of cephalosporin therapy. The tests do not indicate nephrotoxicity or toxic epidermal necrolysis, which are also adverse effects of cephalosporin. Nephrotoxicity is damage to the kidney by toxic substances; toxic epidermal necrolysis is the death of the epidermal layer of the skin; anorexia is an eating disorder.

8. Answer: c, d, e

RATIONALE: The nursing interventions for a patient who has developed diarrhea as a result of cephalosporin are discontinuing the drug, reporting to the primary health care provider, and instituting treatment for diarrhea. An antipyretic drug is administered when there is an increase in the body temperature of a patient receiving cephalosporin. The nurse saves a sample of the stool and tests for occult blood if blood and mucus appear to be in the stool.

CHAPTER 9

SECTION I: ASSESSING YOUR UNDERSTANDING

Activity A MATCHING

1. 1-C, 2-A, 3-D, 4-B
2. 1-B, 2-C, 3-A

Activity B FILL IN THE BLANKS

1. Macrolides
2. Myoneural
3. Lincosamides
4. Telithromycin
5. Tetracyclines

SECTION II: APPLYING YOUR KNOWLEDGE

Activity C SHORT ANSWERS

1. The nurse assumes the following role in monitoring and managing a patient's needs:
   - Observes the patient at frequent intervals, especially during the first 48 hours of therapy.
   - Reports to the primary health care provider the occurrence of any adverse reaction before the next dose of the drug is due.
   - Immediately reports serious adverse reactions, such as a severe hypersensitivity reaction, respiratory difficulty, severe diarrhea, or a decided drop in blood pressure, to the primary health care provider because a serious adverse reaction may require emergency intervention.
2. In the teaching plan, the nurse should include the following information:
   - Take the correct dose of the drug as prescribed.
   - Complete the entire course of treatment.
   - Take each dose on an empty stomach with a full glass of water.
   - Avoid dairy products, antacids, laxatives, or products containing iron during the course of treatment.
   - Notify the primary health care provider of any adverse reactions.
   - Avoid the use of alcoholic beverages during therapy unless the primary health care provider has approved it.

Activity D DOSAGE CALCULATION

1. 2
2. 3
3. 2
4. 2
5. 15 mL
6. 2 mL

SECTION III: PRACTICING FOR NCLEX

Activity E

1. **Answer: a**

   RATIONALE: Lincosamides are contraindicated for patients with minor bacterial or viral infections. Patients younger than 9 years of age are contraindicated for tetracyclines. Patients with liver disease are contraindicated for macrolides.

2. **Answer: b**

   RATIONALE: Increased action of a neuromuscular blocking drug may lead to severe and profound respiratory depression. Increased risk for bleeding is caused by the interaction of oral anticoagulants with tetracyclines. Decreased absorption of the lincosamide is caused by the interaction of kaolin or aluminum-based antacids with lincosamides. Increased risk for digitalis toxicity is caused by the interaction of digoxin with tetracyclines.

3. **Answer: a, d, e**

   RATIONALE: General malaise, chills, fever, and redness are signs and symptoms of an infection. Diabetes is not a cause of any infection. Blood dyscrasia is an abnormality of the blood cell structure or function, which is an adverse effect of lincosamides.

4. **Answer: b, d, e**

   RATIONALE: Tests that should be done before the first dose of a drug is administered are culture and sensitivity, renal function tests, and urinalysis. A stress test is done to monitor heart conditions. A glucose tolerance test is done to check for diabetes.

5. **Answer: a, c, e**

   RATIONALE: The nurse must notify the primary health care provider if there is a significant drop in blood pressure, an increase in the pulse or respiratory rate, or a sudden increase in temperature. Regular urine output and normal blood sugar levels need not be immediately reported to the primary health care provider.

6. **Answer: b**

   RATIONALE: The nurse should instruct the patient not to perform any hazardous activities, such as driving or operating machinery, because Ketek (telithromycin) can cause the patient difficulty focusing his eyes and accommodating to light. Esophagitis, photosensitivity, and skin rashes are adverse effects of clindamycin.

7. **Answer: a.**

   RATIONALE: The teaching plan should instruct the patient to take the drug on an empty stomach with a full glass of water. Tetracyclines are not absorbed effectively if taken just before a meal or with dairy products. The dosage has to be distributed around the clock—not just at bedtime—to increase effectiveness.

8. **Answer: a**

RATIONALE: Dirithromycin can cause anorexia, constipation, dry mouth, hypersensitivity reactions, photosensitivity reactions, pseudomembranous colitis, and electrolyte imbalance. Visual disturbance, headache, or dizziness is caused by telithromycin. Abdominal pain, esophagitis, skin rash, or blood dyscrasias are caused by clindamycin. Photosensitivity reactions, hematologic changes, or discoloration of teeth is caused by demeclocycline.

9. **Answer: d**

RATIONALE: An immediate nursing intervention should be to save a sample of the stool for an occult blood test. Obtaining urine samples, measuring and recording vital signs, and checking blood pressure are not the immediate priorities; these may follow at a later stage as required.

10. **Answer: b**

RATIONALE: The patient should take nothing by mouth (except water) for 1 to 2 hours before and after taking lincomycin because food impairs the absorption of lincomycin. The patient can have food 1 to 2 hours before the drug's administration; he or she should not receive the drug on an empty stomach, but it should be administered only with water.

CHAPTER 10

SECTION I: ASSESSING YOUR UNDERSTANDING

Activity A MATCHING

1. 1-C, 2-D, 3-A, 4-B
2. 1-B, 2-C, 3-A

Activity B FILL IN THE BLANKS

1. Enteric-coated
2. Theophylline
3. Bactericidal
4. Hepatic
5. Respiratory

SECTION II: APPLYING YOUR KNOWLEDGE

Activity C SHORT ANSWERS

1. A nurse should perform the following assessments for a patient who is being administered fluoroquinolones:
   • Inspect needle site and area around the needle every hour.
   • Perform the assessment frequently if the patient is found restless or uncooperative.

• Check the rate of infusion every 15 minutes.
• Inspect the vein used for intravenous (IV) infusion every 4 hr for signs of tenderness, pain, and redness.
• If necessary, restart IV in another vein and notify the primary health care provider.

2. A nurse should perform the following assessments when caring for the patient with high fever:
   • Monitor vital signs, particularly body temperature
   • Monitor the drug's effectiveness in eradicating the infection
   • Check vital signs every 4 hr or more frequently if the temperature is elevated
   • Notify the primary health care provider if the temperature rises over 101°F

Activity D DOSAGE CALCULATION

1. 2 tablets every 12 hours
2. 4 tablets
3. 3 tablets
4. 2 injections of 10 mg/mL
5. 2 tablets each day
6. 3 mL

SECTION III: PRACTICING FOR NCLEX

Activity E

1. **Answer: a**

RATIONALE: Fluoroquinolones have to be administered cautiously in patients with a history of seizures. Aminoglycosides and not fluoroquinolones are administered cautiously to elderly patients, patients who have neuromuscular disorders, and patients who have renal failure.

2. **Answer: b**

RATIONALE: Using cephalosporins with aminoglycosides increases the risk of nephrotoxicity. There is an increased risk of ototoxicity when loop diuretics are administered with aminoglycosides. Neuromuscular blockage occurs when Pavulon interacts with aminoglycosides. Increased serum theophylline levels result from the interaction of theophylline with fluoroquinolones.

3. **Answer: a, d, e**

RATIONALE: As part of the preadministration assessment, the nurse should obtain the patient's urinalysis; the nurse should also ensure that patient's hepatic and renal function tests are conducted, and that the patient's complete blood count is obtained. Monitoring the patient's vital signs every 4 hr and recording observations in the patient's chart are interventions related to the patient's ongoing assessment, not preadministration assessment.

4. **Answer: d**

RATIONALE: The nurse should monitor the patient carefully for signs of dizziness when the patient is administered fluoroquinolones. The nurse should monitor the patient for anorexia, rash, and urticaria if the patient is administered aminoglycosides and not fluoroquinolones.

5. Answer: a

RATIONALE: The nurse is most likely to observe signs of lethargy in a patient who is administered kanamycin. Numbness and muscle twitching are seen as symptoms of neurotoxicity caused by amikacin. Abdominal pain is an adverse effect seen in patients who are taking fluoroquinolones.

6. Answer: a

RATIONALE: The nurse should know that the client has developed neuromuscular blockage, which is characterized by apnea and acute muscular paralysis. Ototoxicity is not marked by apnea and muscular paralysis. Nephrotoxicity is characterized by proteinuria and hematuria, not by muscular paralysis and apnea. Pseudomembranous colitis is an adverse reaction to fluoroquinolones.

7. Answer: b, d, e

RATIONALE: When caring for a patient receiving fluoroquinolones, the nurse should frequently inspect the vein used for infusion, inform the physician of any observations, and frequently perform assessments. The nurse should check the rate of infusion every 15 minutes and not every 2 hours. Also, the nurse should change the vein used for infusion only in case of thrombophlebitis or phlebitis.

8. Answer: a

RATIONALE: The nurse should ensure that the patient is not younger than 18 years of age to ensure that fluoroquinolone is not contraindicated in the patient. Preexisting hearing loss, myasthenia gravis, and parkinsonism are contraindications with aminoglycosides.

9. Answer: a, b, d

RATIONALE: The nurse should instruct the client to wear cover-up clothing, sunscreen, and brimmed hats to assist the patient in preventing photosensitivity reactions. Wearing light makeup will not help the patient avoid a skin reaction. Venturing out on hazy and cloudy days cannot be considered safe. The nurse should inform the patient that the glare during hazy or cloudy days could cause skin reactions as great as those on clear days.

10. Answer: c

RATIONALE: Pavulon is most commonly used as an anesthetic for surgery. Cephalosporins are used as anti-infective agents, loop diuretics are used to manage edema, and oral anticoagulants are used as blood thinners.

CHAPTER 11

SECTION I: ASSESSING YOUR UNDERSTANDING

Activity A MATCHING

1. 1-A, 2-C, 3-D, 4-B
2. 1-D, 2-C, 3-B, 4-A

Activity B FILL IN THE BLANKS

1. Oxazolidinone
2. Phenylketonuria
3. Ertapenem
4. Carbapenems
5. Vancomycin

SECTION II: APPLYING YOUR KNOWLEDGE

Activity C SHORT ANSWERS

1. To determine the effectiveness of the treatment plan, the nurse should ensure:
   • The therapeutic drug effect is achieved, and the infection is controlled.
   • Adverse reactions are identified, reported to the primary health care provider, and managed successfully.
   • Pain or discomfort following intramuscular (IM) or intravenous (IV) administration is relieved or eliminated.
   • Anxiety is reduced.
   • The patient and family demonstrate understanding of the drug regimen.

2. To decrease the chance of noncompliance, the nurse emphasizes the following points when any of the anti-infective drugs are prescribed on an outpatient basis:
   • Take the drug at the prescribed time intervals. These time intervals are important because a certain amount of the drug must be in the body at all times for the infection to be controlled.
   • Take the drug with food or on an empty stomach as directed on the prescription bottle.
   • Do not increase or omit the dose unless advised to do so by the primary health care provider.
   • Complete the entire course of treatment. Do not stop the drug, except on the advice of a primary health care provider, before the course of treatment is completed even if symptoms have improved or have disappeared. Failure to complete the prescribed course of treatment may result in a return of the infection.
   • Notify the primary health care provider if symptoms of the infection become worse or the original symptoms do not improve after about 5 to 7 days.
   • Contact the primary health care provider as soon as possible if a rash, fever, sore throat, diarrhea, chills, extreme fatigue, easy bruising, ringing in the ears, difficulty hearing, or other problems occur.
   • Avoid drinking alcoholic beverages unless they have been approved by the primary health care provider.

3. The nurse should focus on the following drug-specific diagnoses:
   • Anxiety related to feelings about seriousness of illness, route of administration, other factors

- Diarrhea related to adverse drug reaction, superinfection
- Acute Pain related to intramuscular injection or vein irritation
- Risk for Impaired Urinary Elimination related to adverse drug effects (nephrotoxicity)
- Risk for Disturbed Sensory Perception related to adverse drug effects (ototoxicity)

Activity D DOSAGE CALCULATION

1. 8 tablets
2. 5 tablets
3. 5.2 mL
4. 20 tablets
5. 6 tablets
6. 35 mL

SECTION III: PRACTICING FOR NCLEX

Activity E

1. **Answer: a**
   RATIONALE: The nurse should monitor for thrombocytopenia and pseudomembranous colitis as the most serious adverse reactions that could be caused by linezolid. Nephrotoxicity and ototoxicity are adverse reactions occurring due to the administration of vancomycin. Phlebitis occurs as a reaction when miscellaneous anti-infectives are administered through the IV route. It does not occur when anti-infectives are administered orally.

2. **Answer: a, c, d**
   RATIONALE: To maintain continuity of care, the nurse should instruct the patient and patient's family to complete the full course of treatment, avoid drinking alcoholic beverages, and understand potential adverse reactions. The nurse should instruct the patient to administer the drug with or without food in the stomach depending on the physician's instruction. All drugs need not be taken with food. The nurse should instruct the patient and patient's family to monitor for adverse symptoms for 5 to 7 days, after which if symptoms worsen, the physician should be contacted immediately.

3. **Answer: b**
   RATIONALE: The nurse should prepare and administer a dose of 10 mL of spectinomycin to the patient intravenously. The available strength of the drug dose is 5 mL/2 g. The prescribed dose is 4 g, so the nurse should prepare a dose of 10 mL. The nurse should not prepare a dose of 15 mL, 4 mL, or 2 mL.

4. **Answer: c**
   RATIONALE: When caring for a patient who has been administered spectinomycin, the nurse should monitor for urticaria as one of the adverse effects. Fever occurs as an adverse reaction of vancomycin when it is administered to patients. Throbbing neck pain occurs when vancomycin is

administered intravenously, and headache is an adverse effect of aztreonam.

5. **Answer: b**
   RATIONALE: When caring for a patient who has been administered quinupristin/dalfopristin, the nurse should monitor for secondary bacterial or fungal infections, which are caused by the disruption of the normal flora. The nurse has to monitor for cross-sensitivity with cephalosporins if the patient is receiving aztreonam and not quinupristin/dalfopristin. The nurse should monitor for bone marrow depression if the patient is administered linezolid and has had a history of bone marrow depression. Hearing and kidney problems can develop with vancomycin along with ototoxic or nephrotoxic drugs.

6. **Answer: c**
   RATIONALE: The nurse should be alert for a sudden decrease in the patient's blood pressure when vancomycin is administered through the parenteral route. Hypotension and shock occur only when the rate of infusion of drug through the IV route is rapid. She should remain alert for a ringing in the ears in the patient only if the patient has a disturbed sensory perception.

7. **Answer: b, c, d**
   RATIONALE: When conducting an ongoing assessment, the nurse should monitor vital signs of the patient every 4 hr, observe for a sudden increase in temperature, and observe the patient frequently during first 48 hours of therapy. Determining signs of infection in the patient is part of the nurse's preadministration assessment and not part of the ongoing assessment. The nurse should monitor for a sudden increase, not a decrease, in the pulse and respiratory rate.

8. **Answer: d**
   RATIONALE: Aztreonam has to be administered cautiously if the patient is taking penicillin. The interaction between aztreonam and penicillins could lead to cross-sensitivity. Linezolid has to be administered cautiously in case the patient takes antiplatelet drugs. Interaction between linezolid and antiplatelet drugs leads to increased risk of bleeding and thrombocytopenia. Vancomycin should be administered cautiously if the patient has been taking nephrotoxic drugs. Interaction between vancomycin and nephrotoxic drugs may not cause ototoxicity or nephrotoxicity, but the two drugs together increase risk of these adverse effects. Daptomycin has to be administered cautiously if the patient has been taking warfarin.

9. **Answer: b, c, d**
   RATIONALE: When caring for a patient receiving an anti-infective IM, the nurse should rotate the injection sites frequently and monitor them, inspect previous injection sites, and assess the vein used for infusion for any signs of irritation. It is important for the nurse to adjust the rate of infusion every 15 minutes, instead of 30 minutes. The nurse

should also check the infusion site once every 4 to 8 hours and not 12 hours.

10. **Answer: b**

RATIONALE: Quinupristin/dalfopristin will help reduce the infection caused by *Enterococcus faecium*. Quinupristin/dalfopristin is a bacteriostatic agent used in the treatment of vancomycin-resistant *Enterococcus faecium* (VREF). Daptomycin is a new category of antibacterial agents called cyclic lipopeptides. This drug binds to the cell membrane, depolarizing the cell wall and inhibiting protein DNA and RNA synthesis, which causes the bacteria cell to die. It does not help in the treatment of VREF. Fosfomycin tromethamine (Monurol) is an anti-infective used to treat urinary tract infections. Spectinomycin exerts its action by interfering with bacterial protein synthesis. It is used for treating gonorrhea in patients who are allergic to penicillin, cephalosporins, or probenecid, but it does not help in treating VREF.

CHAPTER 12

SECTION I: ASSESSING YOUR UNDERSTANDING

Activity A MATCHING

1. 1-D, 2-C, 3-A, 4-B

Activity B FILL IN THE BLANKS

1. Vancomycin
2. Immunodeficiency
3. Extrapulmonary
4. Tyramine
5. 2

SECTION II: APPLYING YOUR KNOWLEDGE

Activity C SHORT ANSWERS

1. When caring for a patient with tuberculosis, the nurse should perform the following interventions as part of the preadministration assessment:
   * Administer the prescribed drug that will best control the spread of the disease.
   * Assist the physician in helping to make the patient noninfectious to others.
   * Perform laboratory and diagnostic tests before starting antitubercular therapy.
   * Depending on the severity of the disease, patients may be treated initially in the hospital and then discharged for supervised follow-up care.
   * Obtain a family history and history of contacts if the patient has active TB.
2. To decrease the chance of noncompliance to the drug regimen, the nurse emphasizes the following points when any of these drugs are prescribed on an outpatient basis:

* Take the drug at the prescribed time intervals. These time intervals are important because a certain amount of the drug must be in the body at all times for the infection to be controlled.
* Take the drug with food or on an empty stomach as directed on the prescription bottle.
* Do not increase or omit the dose unless advised to do so by the primary health care provider.
* Complete the entire course of treatment. Do not stop taking the drug, except on the advice of a primary health care provider, before the course of treatment is completed—even if symptoms have improved or disappeared. Failure to complete the prescribed course of treatment may result in a return of the infection.
* Notify the primary health care provider if symptoms of the infection worsen or the original symptoms do not improve after about 5 to 7 days.
* Contact the primary health care provider as soon as possible if the following occur: rash, fever, sore throat, diarrhea, chills, extreme fatigue, easy bruising, ringing in the ears, difficulty hearing, or other problems.
* Avoid drinking alcoholic beverages unless the primary health care provider has approved them.

3. The nurse should keep the following goals in mind when evaluating the treatment plan:
   * The therapeutic drug effect is achieved and the infection is controlled.
   * Adverse reactions are identified, reported to the primary health care provider, and managed successfully.
   * Pain or discomfort is relieved or eliminated following intramuscular or intravenous administration.
   * Anxiety is reduced.
   * The patient and family demonstrate understanding of the drug regimen.

Activity D DOSAGE CALCULATION

1. 3 tablets
2. 2 tablets
3. 2 tablets

SECTION III: PRACTICING FOR NCLEX

Activity E

1. **Answer: c**

RATIONALE: When caring for a patient who has been administered rifampin, the nurse should monitor for reddish-orange discoloration of body fluids as one of the drug's generalized adverse reactions. Myalgia is the generalized adverse reaction of pyrazinamide, not rifampin. Jaundice is the generalized adverse reaction of isoniazid, and dermatitis and pruritus are generalized adverse reactions of ethambutol.

2. **Answer: a, b, c**

RATIONALE: The nurse should ensure that the patient is not under 13 years of age, the patient does not have cataracts, and the patient does not have a hypersensitivity to the drug. Any of these conditions contraindicate the use of ethambutol. The nurse should ensure that the patient does not have diabetes mellitus or acute gout only if the patient has to be administered pyrazinamide and not ethambutol.

3. Answer: a

RATIONALE: The nurse knows that following an alternative-dosing regimen of twice weekly promotes nutrition and decreases the incidence of gastric upset in the patient. It also promotes patient compliance to the drug regimen on an outpatient basis. An alternative-dosing regimen of twice weekly does not promote fluid balance in the body or reduce the incidence of liver dysfunction. Taking vitamin B_6 or pyridoxine prevents the occurrence of neuropathy.

4. Answer: b, c, e

RATIONALE: Liver, kidneys, and spleen can be affected by extrapulmonary tuberculosis. On the other hand, the heart and brain are not affected by extrapulmonary tuberculosis.

5. Answer: a, b, c

RATIONALE: The nurse should know if the patient is taking digoxin, oral anticoagulants, or oral contraceptives along with prescribed rifampin. Rifampin, taken along with digoxin, decreases the serum level of digoxin. When taken with oral anticoagulants, rifampin decreases anticoagulant effectiveness, and when taken with oral contraceptives, it decreases contraceptive effectiveness. Colchicine and allopurinol more commonly interact with pyrazinamide, leading to decreased effectiveness.

6. Answer: c

RATIONALE: The nurse should monitor for severe hepatitis as the manifestation of a severe toxic reaction to isoniazid. Severe, sometimes fatal hepatitis may occur after many months of treatment. Hepatotoxicity is the principal adverse reaction seen with pyrazinamide use, which is characterized by severe jaundice. Anaphylactoid reactions are more severe reactions seen in patients administered ethambutol. Epigastric distress is a generalized reaction and not a severe toxic reaction to isoniazid.

7. Answer: a

RATIONALE: The nurse should monitor for severe jaundice as a manifestation of a severe hepatotoxic reaction to pyrazinamide. Epigastric distress and hematologic changes are some of the generalized reactions of isoniazid. Severe hepatitis is a manifestation of a severe toxic reaction to isoniazid and not pyrazinamide.

8. Answer: d

RATIONALE: The nurse should instruct the patient to reduce alcohol consumption to prevent the risk of hepatitis. Administering pyridoxine promotes nutrition and prevents neuropathy, but it does not reduce the risk of hepatitis. Using the direct observation therapy (DOT) method to administer medication encourages patient compliance to the

medication regimen but does not prevent the risk of hepatitis. Administering antitubercular drugs in combination also promotes patient compliance to the drug regimen but does not prevent the risk of hepatitis.

9. Answer: b

RATIONALE: Rifampin is contraindicated in patients with hepatic or renal impairment. Pyrazinamide is contraindicated in patients with diabetes mellitus and those who have tested positive for HIV. Ethambutol is contraindicated in patients with diabetic retinopathy.

CHAPTER 13

SECTION I: ASSESSING YOUR UNDERSTANDING

Activity A MATCHING

1. 1-C, 2-D, 3-A, 4-B
2. 1-B, 2-C, 3-A

Activity B FILL IN THE BLANKS

1. Nodular
2. Gastric
3. Pigmentation
4. Hemolysis

SECTION II: APPLYING YOUR KNOWLEDGE

Activity C SHORT ANSWERS

1. The nurse should focus on the following when assessing a patient on leprostatic drug therapy:
   a. Preadministration assessment
      It is important to perform a complete physical examination and to obtain a complete medical history before initiation of therapy. The nurse should examine the involved areas and describe them in detail on the patient's record to provide a database, or baseline, for comparison during therapy.
   b. Ongoing assessment
      Each time the patient is seen in the clinic or primary health care provider's office, the nurse should perform a general physical examination, paying particular attention the affected areas.
2. The nurse must spend time with the patient, allowing her to verbalize her anxieties, anger, and fears. It is also important for the nurse to acknowledge these feelings as being both valid and important to the patient. The nurse should also refer the patient to a support group or encourage her to talk to other patients.

Activity D DOSAGE CALCULATION

1. 2 tablets
2. 2 capsules

SECTION III: PRACTICING FOR NCLEX

Activity E

1. **Answer: a**

   RATIONALE: Clofazimine is used cautiously in patients with gastrointestinal disorders; the patient should be carefully assessed before therapy is initiated. The nurse should assess for cardiopulmonary disease if the patient is to be administered dapsone. While the nurse should assess a patient for any disorder, including cardiopulmonary disease, liver dysfunction, and renal impairment, these do not affect clofazimine therapy.

2. **Answer: a, b, c**

   RATIONALE: The nurse should closely monitor a patient on dapsone therapy for jaundice, hemolysis, and toxic epidermal necrolysis (TEN); these are the adverse reactions associated with the drug. The nurse should monitor a patient on clofazimine for abdominal/epigastric pain and conjunctiva.

3. **Answer: d**

   RATIONALE: A nurse should administer leprostatic drugs orally with food as this practice minimizes gastric upset. Leprostatic drugs should not be given on an empty stomach or administered with aluminum salts or anticoagulants.

4. **Answer: b**

   RATIONALE: The nurse should inform the patient that substantial amounts of dapsone are excreted in breast milk, which causes hemolytic reactions in the neonates. The drug does not cause skin eruptions, and it is unlikely that the neonate will reject breast milk because of the drug's presence.

5. **Answer: c**

   RATIONALE: The nurse must spend time with the patient to allow him to verbalize his anxieties, anger, and fears. Noting signs of depression or indifference and being alert to the patient's compliance with drug therapy are important activities, but they will not help alleviate the patient's anxiety. The nurse should not trivialize the patient's feelings, act indifferent, or simply instruct him to "deal with it."

6. **Answer: b**

   RATIONALE: To ensure compliance with the treatment regimen, the nurse should explain the dosage schedule, possible adverse effects, and the importance of scheduled follow-up visits to the patient. The nurse should also emphasize the importance of adhering to the prescribed dosage schedule. During the ongoing assessment stage, the nurse should report necessary adjustments in the dosage schedule and adverse drug reactions; however, these interventions do not ensure compliance. Communication with family members does not help ensure that the patient complies with his or her treatment regimen either.

CHAPTER 14

SECTION I: ASSESSING YOUR UNDERSTANDING

Activity A   MATCHING

1. 1-C, 2-A, 3-D, 4-B
2. 1-A, 2-D, 3-B, 4-C

Activity B   FILL IN THE BLANKS

1. Lemon
2. Cidofovir
3. Ritonavir
4. Indinavir
5. Antiretroviral

SECTION II: APPLYING YOUR KNOWLEDGE

Activity C   SHORT ANSWERS

1. Before administering an antiviral drug, a nurse should perform a series of assessments. Preadministration assessment of the patient receiving an antiviral drug depends on the patient's symptoms or diagnosis. These patients may have a serious infection that decreases their natural defenses against disease. Before administering the antiviral drug, the nurse should determine the patient's general state of health and resistance to infection. The nurse then records the patient's symptoms and complaints. In addition, the nurse takes and records the patient's vital signs. Other assessments may be necessary in certain types of viral infections or in patients who are acutely ill. For example, before treatment of patients with HSV 1 or 2, the nurse inspects the areas of the body affected with the lesions (e.g., the mouth, face, eyes, or genitalia) as a baseline for comparison during therapy.

2. During administration of an antiviral drug, a nurse should perform the following assessments:
   The ongoing assessment depends on the reason for giving the antiviral drug. It is important to make a daily assessment for comparison to the signs and symptoms identified in the initial assessment. The nurse monitors for and reports any adverse reactions from the antiviral drug. Additionally, the nurse inspects the intravenous (IV) site several times a day for redness, inflammation, or pain and reports any signs of phlebitis.

Activity D   DOSAGE CALCULATION

1. 5 mL
2. 35 mL
3. 70 mL
4. 4 tablets
5. 4 mL
6. 120 mL

SECTION III: PRACTICING FOR NCLEX

Activity E

1. **Answer: a, b, d**
   RATIONALE: While administering ribavirin, the nurse should use a small particle aerosol generator and discard and replace the solution every 24 hours. Ribavirin can worsen the respiratory status, and the nurse should monitor the patient's respiratory system for any signs of deterioration. Ribavirin does not induce anorexia or nephrotoxicity in the patient.

2. **Answer: b**
   RATIONALE: When clarithromycin is taken along with an antiretroviral drug, it results in increased serum levels of both drugs. Interaction between antifungals and antiretroviral drugs increases the serum level of just the antiretroviral. No toxicity risk is associated with combining the two drugs. This combination also does not significantly decrease the effectiveness of either of the drugs.

3. **Answer: c**
   RATIONALE: Before beginning the treatment of the patient with HSV 1, the nurse should inspect the areas of the body affected with the lesions as a baseline for comparison during therapy. Recording a patient's temperature and blood pressure are routine interventions that the nurse should follow and are not specific to the treatment of HSV 1. There is no need to save a sample of the patient's urine unless specifically instructed to do so by the health care provider.

4. **Answer: b, c, e**
   RATIONALE: The nurse should include soft nonirritating foods in the client's diet, keep the atmosphere clean and free of odors, and provide good oral care before and after meals. The nurse should administer small, frequent meals to the client and not reduce the frequency of the meals. Frequent sips of carbonated beverages or hot tea may be helpful and should not be eliminated from the patient's diet.

5. **Answer: c**
   RATIONALE: Phlebitis refers to inflammation of the patient's veins. It commonly occurs when drugs are administered intravenously. Phlebitis does not occur in patients who are being administered drugs orally, intramuscularly, or transdermally.

6. **Answer: d**
   RATIONALE: The nurse should exercise caution while caring for patients who have been administered indinavir and have a history of bladder stone formation. Indinavir does not significantly exacerbate the condition of patients with cardiac disorders or renal impairment. The drugs fosamprenavir and amprenavir, not indinavir, should be used cautiously in patients with sulfonamide allergy.

7. **Answer: c**
   RATIONALE: The nurse should avoid generating dust while preparing to administer didanosine to the patient. Didanosine should be given on an empty stomach and not with meals. The drug should be dissolved in 4 oz of water and not 2 oz. The solution should be given immediately to the patient after preparation and not refrigerated.

8. **Answer: b**
   RATIONALE: 1 mL of solution contains 24 mg of the drug. Therefore, the required amount is 225 mL (5400/24).

9. **Answer: c**
   RATIONALE: Required dosage is 800 mg. Available drug is 200 mg. Number of tablets required is 4 (800/200) per dosage.

10. **Answer: c**
    RATIONALE: Required dosage is 200 mg. Available drug is 50 mg/5mL. Therefore, solution of drug in 1 mL is 10 mg (50/5). Required quantity is 20 mL (200/10) per dosage.

CHAPTER 15

SECTION I: ASSESSING YOUR UNDERSTANDING

Activity A MATCHING

1. 1-B, 2-D, 3-A, 4-E, 5-C

Activity B FILL IN THE BLANKS

1. Systemic
2. Superficial
3. Creatinine
4. Liver
5. Heart
6. Electrolyte
7. Lesions

SECTION II: APPLYING YOUR KNOWLEDGE

Activity C SHORT ANSWERS

1. The nurse should perform the following preadministration assessments before administering an antifungal drug:
   - Assess the patient for signs of infection before first dose of drug.
   - Inspect superficial fungal infections, such as skin or skin structures, and provide baseline data.
   - Document observations, such as skin lesions, rough itchy patches, cracks between the toes, and sore and reddened areas to obtain an accurate database.
   - Ask about pain; describe white plaques or sore areas on mucous membranes, oral or perineal areas; and inquire about any vaginal discharge.
   - Take and record vital signs.

- Weigh the patient scheduled to receive an amphotericin or flucytosine dose.
2. When caring for a patient on antifungal drug therapy, the nurse's role is to:
   - Inspect the application site for localized skin reactions
   - Ask patient about discomfort or other sensations experienced after insertion of the antifungal preparation, which is administered vaginally
   - Note in the chart any improvement or deterioration of skin lesions, mucous membranes, or vaginal secretions
   - Evaluate and chart daily the patient's response to therapy

Activity D DOSAGE CALCULATION

1. 2 tablets
2. 4 tablets
3. 8 tablets
4. 5 mL
5. 12 capsules
6. 2 capsules

SECTION III: PRACTICING FOR NCLEX

Activity E

1. **Answer: b**
   RATIONALE: The nurse should check the lungs for deep mycotic infections. Deep mycotic infections develop inside the body, in areas such as the lungs, brain, or gastrointestinal tract. The nurse need not check the liver, mouth, or heart because deep mycotic infections occur only in the lungs, brain, or gastrointestinal tract.

2. **Answer: c**
   RATIONALE: The nurse needs to observe for any redness or stinging in a patient who is treated with a topical antifungal drug. Topical administration is unlikely to cause nausea and diarrhea; these adverse reactions can be caused by systemic administration of an antifungal drug.

3. **Answer: c**
   RATIONALE: History of heart failure is a contraindication the nurse must consider when assessing a patient for itraconazole therapy. The drug is not contraindicated in patients with bone marrow suppression, severe liver disease, or history of asthma. Severe liver disease is a contraindication to be considered when assessing a patient for griseofulvin therapy.

4. **Answer: a**
   RATIONALE: When administering an IV solution of amphotericin B, the nurse should ensure that the IV solution is protected from light because it is light sensitive. The solution must be used within 8 hours after the drug is reconstituted, not 24, to prevent loss of drug activity. The nurse should not freeze the unused solution; it should be discarded. It should not be stored either.

5. **Answer: a**
   RATIONALE: The nurse needs to monitor the patient for vomiting as it is an adverse reaction to IV administration of amphotericin B. Abdominal pain, muscle pain, and anorexia are not adverse reactions of IV amphotericin B. Topical administration of an antifungal drug can cause abdominal pain, while systemic administration of an antifungal drug can result in anorexia and muscle pain.

6. **Answer: b**
   RATIONALE: The nurse should encourage the patient to verbalize his or her feelings because it will help reduce the patient's anxiety. The nurse need not check the patient's blood pressure, provide the client with a blanket, or keep the patient away from light because these efforts won't help reduce the patient's anxiety. The patient's blood pressure needs to be taken during the administration of an antifungal drug. Providing warm blankets will only comfort the patient and not reduce the anxiety.

7. **Answer: d**
   RATIONALE: In the teaching plan, the nurse should inform the patient about keeping towels and washcloths separate from those of other family members to avoid spreading the infection. It is important to keep the affected area clean and dry. Antifungal drugs neither cause photosensitivity nor do they affect mental status, so the patient does not need to avoid sunlight or activities. Sexual contact will not spread the infection unless it is in the vagina.

8. **Answer: c**
   RATIONALE: The nurse should instruct the patient taking ketoconazole to expect headache, dizziness, and drowsiness. The patient is unlikely to experience unusual fatigue, yellow skin, darkened urine, fever, sore throat, skin rash, nausea, vomiting, or diarrhea because these are not adverse reactions caused by ketoconazole. Unusual fatigue, yellow skin, and darkened urine are reactions caused by itraconazole, while fever, sore throat, and skin rash are caused by griseofulvin. Flucytosine causes nausea, vomiting, and diarrhea.

CHAPTER 16

SECTION I: ASSESSING YOUR UNDERSTANDING

Activity A MATCHING

1. 1-B, 2-C, 3-D, 4-A
2. 1-C, 2-A, 3-B

Activity B FILL IN THE BLANKS

1. Mebendazole
2. Chloroquine
3. Paromomycin
4. Iodoquinol
5. Retinal

SECTION II: APPLYING YOUR KNOWLEDGE

Activity C SHORT ANSWERS

1. Before administering anthelmintic drugs for the first time, a nurse should perform the following assessments:
   - Instruct the patient how to take a specimen from the perianal area with a cellophane tape-covered swab early in the morning before the patient gets out of bed.
   - Weigh the patient if the drug's dosage is determined by weight or if the patient is acutely ill.
2. If a patient develops nausea, vomiting, or abdominal pain during treatment for anthelmintic drugs, the nurse should perform the following interventions:
   - Give the drug with food to alleviate the nausea.
   - Provide small meals of easily digestible food.
   - Consider the patient's food preferences and encourage the patient to eat nutritious, well-balanced meals.
   - If vomiting is present, recommend an antiemetic or a different anthelmintic agent.

Activity D DOSAGE CALCULATION

1. 2 tablets
2. 3 tablets
3. 5 mL
4. 5 tablets
5. 5 mL

SECTION III: PRACTICING FOR NCLEX

Activity E

1. **Answer: d**
   RATIONALE: Because the patient is acutely ill, the nurse should carefully measure and record the fluid intake and output. The nurse should record the patient's vital signs every 4 hours, not 12 hours, and observe the patient every 2 hours, not 4 hours, for malaria symptoms. There is no need to collect urine samples of the patient for testing.
2. **Answer: a**
   RATIONALE: Quinine is contraindicated in patients with myasthenia gravis because the drug might cause respiratory distress and dysphagia. Quinine, however, is not contraindicated in patients with thyroid disease, blood dyscrasias, or diabetes.
3. **Answer: a, b, d**
   RATIONALE: Drowsiness, dizziness, nausea, vomiting, abdominal pain, and cramps are some of the adverse reactions associated with anthelmintic drugs. Visual disturbances and tinnitus, or a ringing sound in the ears, are not generally associated with anthelmintic drugs.
4. **Answer: b**
   RATIONALE: The nurse should follow hospital procedure for transporting the stool sample to the laboratory. Unless ordered otherwise, the nurse should save all stools that are passed after the drug is given. The nurse should visually inspect all stools, not just when the patient reports something unusual. Specimens should be taken by swabbing the perianal area with a cellophane tape-covered swab, not any container.
5. **Answer: a, d, e**
   RATIONALE: The primary health care provider should be notified immediately if the patient experiences unusual muscle weakness, ringing in the ears and visual changes after the chloroquine drug has been administered. Yellow or brownish discoloration of urine is a natural and harmless side effect of chloroquine and need not be reported. Peripheral neuropathy is an adverse effect of metronidazole and is not associated with chloroquine.
6. **Answer: a**
   RATIONALE: The nurse should caution the patient that albendazole can cause serious harm to a developing fetus. Albendazole does not, however, cause miscarriage, decrease the chances of conception, or reduce estrogen levels.
7. **Answer: c**
   RATIONALE: The nurse should educate the patient to use chlorine bleach to disinfect toilet facilities or the shower stall after bathing. The nurse should recommend the barrier method and not birth control pills for contraception. The dosage regimen should be adhered to even if the symptoms have disappeared, and chloroquine should be taken with water and not milk.
8. **Answer: b**
   RATIONALE: Nephrotoxicity and ototoxicity are adverse reactions associated with paromomycin. Peripheral neuropathy may occur with metronidazole use but not paromomycin. Thrombocytopenia is associated with anthelmintic medications, and vertigo and hypotension are the adverse effects of chloroquine.
9. **Answer: a**
   RATIONALE: The nurse should instruct the patient to take metronidazole with meals or immediately afterwards. Alcohol should be avoided for the duration of the treatment and not just for the first week. Cimetidine should not be taken as it decreases the metabolism of metronidazole. Also, metronidazole does not cause photosensitivity, so there is no need to wear clothing to protect the skin from the sun.
10. **Answer: a**
    RATIONALE: The nurse should caution the patient against exposure to sunlight as the skin becomes photosensitive during the administration of doxycycline. Skin eruptions, cinchonism, and thrombocytopenia are not adverse effects caused by doxycycline.

CHAPTER 17

SECTION I: ASSESSING YOUR UNDERSTANDING

Activity A MATCHING

1. 1-B, 2-D, 3-A, 4-C
2. 1-C, 2-A, 3-D, 4-B

Activity B FILL IN THE BLANKS

1. Prostaglandins
2. Platelets
3. Pancytopenia
4. Reye's
5. Tinnitus

SECTION II: APPLYING YOUR KNOWLEDGE

Activity C SHORT ANSWERS

1. The nurse can assess the patient's pain in the following ways:
   - The patient is taught to rate the pain on a scale of 0 to 10, with 0 being "no pain" and 10 being the "most severe pain imagined" by the patient.
   - Other methods to rate paint may be used, including scales of colors or facial expressions such as the Wong-Baker FACES Pain Rating Scale.
2. The nurse can monitor and manage the discomfort of the patient receiving a salicylate or a nonsalicylate in the following ways:
   - Notify the primary health care provider if there has been no relief from pain or discomfort.
   - Assess the patient for bleeding or inflammation.
   - To minimize gastrointestinal (GI) distress, administer the drug with food or milk or give antacids.
   - Check the color of the patient's stools, with bright red or black indicating bleeding, and report it.

Activity D DOSAGE CALCULATION

1. 12 tablets
2. 6 tablets
3. 6 tablets
4. Half a tablet
5. 4 tablets
6. 2 tablets

SECTION III: PRACTICING FOR NCLEX

Activity E

1. **Answer: b**
   RATIONALE: The nurse needs to monitor the patient for GI bleeding because it is an adverse reaction caused by the administration of salicylates. Skin eruptions, jaundice, and bleeding disorders are not adverse reactions to salicylates. Skin eruptions and jaundice are adverse reactions to administration of acetaminophen. Incidence of a bleeding disorder contraindicates the administration of salicylates, but they do not cause bleeding disorders.

2. **Answer: a, c, d**
   RATIONALE: For patients with influenza or viral illness and those with bleeding disorders, salicylate use is contraindicated. Salicylates are also contraindicated for patients with a known history of hypersensitivity to the drug. Salicylates are not contraindicated in patients with heart disease. The drugs are administered with caution in patients with hepatic or renal disorders, but incidence of these conditions does not contraindicate administration of salicylates.

3. **Answer: c**
   RATIONALE: Unlike aspirin, acetaminophen does not inhibit platelet aggregation; therefore, it is the analgesic of choice when bleeding tendencies are an issue. Acetaminophen and aspirin are both used to treat high fever or severe pain, and there is no reason why acetaminophen is preferred over aspirin for treating pain or fever. Acetaminophen is not used to treat inflammatory disorders.

4. **Answer: d**
   RATIONALE: The nurse should assess for a decrease in inflammation and greater mobility as part of the ongoing assessment. The nurse should reassess the patient's pain rating in 30 to 60 minutes, not 2 hours, following administration of the drug, and he or she should monitor vital signs every 4, not 8, hours. There is no need to immediately send a sample for testing if stools are dark as long as the nurse informs the primary care provider.

5. **Answer: a**
   RATIONALE: Nausea is one of the symptoms that can be observed in a patient with salicylate levels between 150-250 mcg/mL. Respiratory alkalosis, hemorrhage, and asterixis are associated with salicylate levels in excess of 400 mcg/mL.

6. **Answer: d**
   RATIONALE: Combining loop diuretics with acetaminophen may result in decreased effectiveness of the diuretic. Combining loop diuretics with acetaminophen does not increase the possibility of toxicity or bleeding, nor does it decrease the effectiveness of acetaminophen.

7. **Answer: a, d, e**
   RATIONALE: The nurse should instruct the patient to avoid over-the-counter drugs that may contain aspirin in the label. The patient should purchase the drug in small quantities when used on an occasional basis to prevent deterioration. If a surgery or a dental procedure is anticipated, the patient should notify the primary health care provider or dentist. The patient should avoid eating foods such as paprika, licorice, prunes, and raisins because they are rich in salicylates. Also, salicylates should be stored in tightly closed containers and not in ventilated locations.

8. **Answer: a**
   RATIONALE: One of the adverse reactions that the nurse should monitor for in a patient who has

been administered salicylates such as salsalate is GI bleeding. Hypoglycemia, pancytopenia, and hemolytic anemia are symptoms associated with acetaminophen and not salsalate.

9. **Answer: b**
   RATIONALE: Aspirin can be used to treat inflammatory conditions such as rheumatoid arthritis. Because aspirin increases bleeding tendencies, it is contraindicated in patients with hemophilia, patients who have just undergone surgical operations, or patients taking anticoagulants.

10. **Answer: a**
    RATIONALE: Malaise is one of the symptoms associated with acetaminophen toxicity. Increased anxiety, hyperglycemia, and bradycardia are not symptoms generally associated with acetaminophen toxicity.

CHAPTER 18

SECTION I: ASSESSING YOUR UNDERSTANDING

Activity A MATCHING

1. 1-C, 2-A, 3-B
2. 1-D, 2-C, 3-A, 4-B

Activity B FILL IN THE BLANKS

1. Cyclooxygenase
2. Celecoxib
3. Ibuprofen
4. Reye's
5. Inflammation

SECTION II: APPLYING YOUR KNOWLEDGE

Activity C SHORT ANSWERS

1. NSAIDs are used for the treatment of the following:
   - Pain associated with osteoarthritis, rheumatoid arthritis, and other musculoskeletal disorders
   - Mild to moderate pain
   - Primary dysmenorrhea (menstrual cramps)
   - Fever reduction
2. The nurse should monitor the patient for the following adverse reactions of NSAIDs on the sensory organs:
   - Visual disturbances, such as blurred or diminished vision, diplopia (double vision), swollen or irritated eyes, photophobia (sensitivity to light), and reversible loss of color vision
   - Tinnitus (ringing in the ears)
   - Taste change
   - Rhinitis (runny nose)

ACTIVITY D: DOSAGE CALCULATION

1. 3 tablets
2. 5 tablets
3. 1.5 tablets
4. 2 tablets
5. 4 tablets

SECTION III: PRACTICING FOR NCLEX

Activity E

1. **Answer: a, c, e**
   RATIONALE: The nurse should inform the patient that epigastric pain, abdominal distress, and intestinal ulceration are adverse reactions of NSAIDs on the gastrointestinal system. Appendicitis is the inflammation of the vermiform appendix. Appendicitis and indigestion are not adverse reactions of NSAIDs.

2. **Answer: c**
   RATIONALE: Celecoxib is not used to relieve postoperative pain for a patient who has undergone coronary artery bypass graft (CABG) surgery because it increases the risk of myocardial infarction in the patient. Duodenal ulcer, gastric bleeding, and diarrhea are adverse reactions of ketoprofen in the treatment of rheumatoid disorder.

3. **Answer: b**
   RATIONALE: The nurse should identify that patients with peptic ulceration are contraindicated for treatment with ibuprofen. Celecoxib is contraindicated in patients with an allergy to sulfonamides, history of cardiac disease, or stroke.

4. **Answer: d**
   RATIONALE: Before administering an NSAID to the patient, the nurse should assess the patient for bleeding disorders. Visual disturbances, skin allergies, and dizziness are monitored during ongoing assessments.

5. **Answer: a**
   RATIONALE: The nurse should document limitations in mobility before administration of the prescribed NSAID. Examining the level of consciousness, checking mental stability, and examining body temperature are not relevant assessments for a patient with osteoarthritis.

6. **Answer: c**
   RATIONALE: The nurse should suggest that the patient take the medication with food. This will promote an optimal response to therapy. Avoiding exercise, restricting intake to a liquid diet, or restricting mobility will not promote an optimal response to therapy. Exercise and mobility would be essential to maintain free movement of the joints. The patient undergoing therapy may be affected by acidity, hence the need to have a complete nutritious diet, not just a liquid diet.

7. **Answer: d**
   RATIONALE: The nurse should monitor the patient for gastrointestinal bleeding, which is an adverse reaction of indomethacin administration. Tinnitus, diarrhea, and rash are adverse reactions of etodolac administration.

8. Answer: d

RATIONALE: NSAID treatment for patients older than 65 years of age should begin with a reduced dosage, which is increased slowly because there is a risk of serious ulcer diseases. NSAIDs do not cause an increased risk for inflammation, erythema, or large numbers of red blood cells in the elderly.

9. Answer: a

RATIONALE: The nurse should administer 2 500-mg tablets of nabumetone for the recommended dose of 1 g per day.

10. Answer: b, d, e

RATIONALE: The nurse should advise the patient not to use the drugs on a regular basis unless the patient notifies the primary health care physician. The patient should also avoid the use of aspirin and take the drug with a full glass of water or with food. Avoiding physical activities during drug therapy and keeping towels separate from those of other family members are not points that the nurse should include in the patient's teaching plan.

CHAPTER 19

SECTION I: ASSESSING YOUR UNDERSTANDING

Activity A MATCHING

1. 1-B, 2-D, 3-A, 4-C
2. 1-C, 2-A, 3-D, 4-B

Activity B FILL IN THE BLANKS

1. Morphine
2. Hypersensitivity
3. Opium
4. Heroin
5. Cachectic

SECTION II: APPLYING YOUR KNOWLEDGE

Activity C SHORT ANSWERS

1. When a patient is receiving drugs through a patient-controlled analgesia (PCA) infusion pump, the nurse should educate him or her on the following points:
   - The location of the control button that activates the administration of the drug
   - The difference between the control button and the button to call the nurse (when both are similar in appearance and feel)
   - The machine-regulation of the drug dose and the time interval between doses
   - What happens if the control button is used too soon after the last dose (the machine will not deliver the drug until the correct time)
   - When pain relief should occur (shortly after pushing the button)

   - How to call the nurse if pain relief does not occur after two successive doses
2. The nurse should evaluate the following factors to confirm the success of an opioid treatment plan:
   - The therapeutic effect occurs and pain is relieved.
   - The patient demonstrates the ability to effectively use PCA.
   - Adverse reactions are identified, reported to the primary health care provider, and managed through appropriate nursing interventions.
   - No evidence of injury is seen.
   - Body weight is maintained.
   - Diet is adequate.
   - The patient and family demonstrate understanding of the drug regimen.

Activity D DOSAGE CALCULATION

1. 2 tablets
2. 1 tablet
3. Physician has prescribed 6.3 mg of butorphanol. 18.9 mg of the drug should be taken a day.
4. 1 mL
5. 12.5 mL
6. 2 tablets

SECTION III: PRACTICING FOR NCLEX

Activity E

1. **Answer: b**

   RATIONALE: The nurse should monitor for urticaria as one of the allergic reactions of opioid analgesics in the patient. Other allergic reactions include rashes and pruritus. Although constipation, palpitations, and facial flushing are all adverse reactions to opioid analgesics, they are not allergic reactions specifically. Constipation is an adverse gastrointestinal reaction to opioid analgesics. Palpitations and facial flushing are specific cardiovascular system reactions to the administration of opioid analgesics.

2. **Answer: b**

   RATIONALE: The preadministration assessment conducted by the nurse before the administration of an opioid analgesic involves assessing and documenting the type, onset, intensity, and location of the pain. Other preadministration assessments include reviewing the patient's health history, allergy history, and past and current drug therapies. The nurse obtains the blood pressure, pulse and respiratory rate, and pain rating in 5 to 10 minutes if the drug is given intravenously (IV), 20 to 30 minutes after the drug is taken intramuscularly or subcutaneously, and 30 or more minutes if the drug is given orally. However, these interventions are a part of the ongoing assessment conducted while the patient is on the drug therapy and not before administration of the drug.

3. **Answer: a**

   RATIONALE: The nurse should confirm that the patient is not taking monoamine oxidase inhibitors to ensure that the use of passion flower is not contraindicated in the patient. Use of passion flower is also contraindicated in patients who are pregnant. Administration of passion flower is not known to be contraindicated in patients taking opioid analgesics, patients with acute ulcerative colitis, or patients with a history of asthma, so the nurse need not ensure the absence of these conditions in patients.

4. **Answer: b**
RATIONALE: The nurse should assess the patient's food intake after each meal when caring for a patient with imbalanced nutrition as a result of anorexia. It is important for the nurse to notify the primary health care provider of continued weight loss and anorexia. The nurse need not complement the patient's meal with additional protein supplements. Patient's bowel movements would be recorded daily if the patient suffered from constipation, not nutritional imbalance. Ensuring an increase in the patient's fluid intake specifically is not a necessary intervention considering it will not help improve the patient's condition.

5. **Answer: a, b, c**
RATIONALE: The nurse should look for withdrawal symptoms such as excessive crying, vomiting, and yawning in the newborn of an opioid-dependent mother. Withdrawal symptoms in the newborn usually appear during the first few days of life. Other withdrawal symptoms in the infant include increased respiratory rate, tremors, fever, vomiting, and diarrhea. Coughing and sneezing are not known to occur as withdrawal symptoms in the newborn of an opioid-dependent mother.

6. **Answer: a**
RATIONALE: A nurse should administer naloxone with great caution to a patient who has been receiving an opioid. While naloxone will counteract a decrease in respiratory rate, it also removes all the pain-relieving effects of the opioid and leads to withdrawal symptoms or a return of intense pain. Naloxone is not known to cause vomiting, dizziness, or headache.

7. **Answer: a, b, c**
RATIONALE: The primary health care provider should be contacted immediately if the nurse observes a significant decrease in the respiratory rate or a respiratory rate of 10 breaths/min or below, a significant increase or decrease in the pulse rate or a change in the pulse quality, or a significant decrease in blood pressure (systolic or diastolic) or a systolic pressure below 100 mm Hg. Opioid analgesics do not lead to an increase in body weight or an increase in body temperature therefore the nurse is not likely to make these observations when caring for the patient.

8. **Answer: a, c, d**
RATIONALE: The nurse should know that opioid analgesics are administered with caution in patients with undiagnosed abdominal pain, hepatic or renal

impairment, and hypoxia. Other conditions that require cautious use of opioid analgesics include supraventricular tachycardia, prostatic hypertrophy, lactating patients, patients of an advanced age, opioid-naïve patients, and patients undergoing biliary surgery. The drug need not be used cautiously with patients who are 13 years or younger or in patients with fungal infections.

9. **Answer: c**
RATIONALE: Administration of barbiturates when the patient is on opioid therapy leads to respiratory depression, hypotension, and sedation. Barbiturates interacting with opioid analgesics are not known to cause bacterial infections, hypertension, or hypoxia.

10. **Answer: b**
RATIONALE: The nurse should instruct the patient to avoid alcohol after being treated with opioid analgesics. Alcohol may intensify the action of the drug and cause extreme drowsiness or dizziness. In some instances, the use of alcohol and an opioid can have extremely serious and even life-threatening consequences that may require emergency medical treatment. The nurse need not instruct the patient to avoid traveling, exercising, and eating starchy foods because they will not have a negative effect on the patient's health when using opioids.

CHAPTER 20

SECTION I: ASSESSING YOUR UNDERSTANDING

Activity A / FILL IN THE BLANKS

1. Antagonist
2. Opioid
3. Naloxone
4. Hypersensitivity
5. Postanesthesia
6. Respiratory
7. Narcan

SECTION II: APPLYING YOUR KNOWLEDGE

Activity B SHORT ANSWERS

1. The nurse should perform the following preadministration assessments when caring for a patient who is prescribed opioid antagonists:
   • Arouse the patient from somnolence and instruct the patient regarding the different breathing patterns.
   • Before the administration of the antagonist, the nurse should obtain the blood pressure, pulse, and respiratory rate.
   • The nurse should review the record for the drug suspected of causing the symptoms of respiratory depression.

- The nurse should review initial health history, allergy history, and current treatment modalities for the patient.
2. The nurse should know that opioid antagonists are used in the following circumstances:
   - Postoperative acute respiratory depression
   - Reversal of opioid adverse effects
   - Suspected acute opioid overdosage

Activity C DOSAGE CALCULATION

1. 5 tablets
2. 6 mL
3. 5 mL

SECTION III: PRACTICING FOR NCLEX

Activity D

1. **Answer: b**
   RATIONALE: The nurse should know that an opioid antagonist reverses pain relief. An antagonist is given to reverse a specific adverse reaction; therefore, the antagonist reverses all effects. A patient who receives an antagonist to reverse respiratory effects will also experience a reversal of pain relief (i.e., the pain will return). The opioid antagonist does not relieve or decrease pain, nor does it neutralize the effect of the opioid drug.

2. **Answer: a, c, d**
   RATIONALE: The critical factors that a nurse should evaluate in a patient receiving an opioid antagonist for respiratory depression are positive response to the therapeutic treatment, normal respiratory rate, and resumption of pain. The nurse need not evaluate normal blood pressure and normal heart rate in a patient who has received treatment for respiratory depression.

3. **Answer: c**
   RATIONALE: To promote an optimal response to naloxone in the patient, the nurse should balance the need for continued pain relief and the ability of the person to breathe independently. The nurse need not specifically monitor for an increase in the patient's body temperature because naloxone is not known to cause a rise in body temperature. Similarly, administration of naloxone is not known to cause dehydration or any other form of water loss, so the nurse need not monitor the patient for this condition. Naloxone is always given by slow intravenous (IV) push. The drug should not be administered through a rapid IV push because it is known to cause withdrawal and return of intense pain if administered with a rapid bolus.

4. **Answer: b, c, d**
   RATIONALE: In monitoring and managing the patient's needs during and after naloxone administration, the nurse should make suction equipment readily available for use because abrupt reversal of opioid respiratory depression causes vomiting. The nurse must maintain a patent airway and should turn and suction the patient as needed. Depending on the patient's condition, the nurse should use artificial ventilation and cardiac monitoring. Opioid antagonists are not known to cause hypotension or hematologic changes, so the nurse need not monitor the patient for these conditions.

5. **Answer: b**
   RATIONALE: The nurse should know that opioid antagonists are administered cautiously in patients who are lactating. Antagonists are also used cautiously in those who are pregnant (pregnancy category B), in infants of opioid-dependent mothers, and in patients with an opioid dependency and/or cardiovascular disease. Use of opioid antagonists is contraindicated in patients who are hypersensitive to the drug. Liver impairment or renal failure is not known to enforce a cautious use of opioid antagonists in patients.

6. **Answer: a**
   RATIONALE: The expected outcome for the patient with respiratory depression is an optimal response to therapy. This involves a return to normal respiratory rate, rhythm, and depth. The nurse meets the patient's needs by providing adequate ventilation of the body as well as continued pain relief. The nurse need not provide the patients with controlled analgesic pumps, administer prescribed IV sedatives, or provide an odor-free room, considering these interventions will not help bring about an optimal response to the drug therapy.

CHAPTER 21

SECTION I: ASSESSING YOUR UNDERSTANDING

Activity A MATCHING

1. 1-C, 2-D, 3-A, 4-B
2. 1-D, 2-C, 3-B, 4-A

Activity B FILL IN THE BLANKS

1. Conduction
2. General
3. Anesthesia
4. Anesthetist
5. Anesthesiologist
6. Volatile

SECTION II: APPLYING YOUR KNOWLEDGE

Activity C SHORT ANSWERS

1. The nurse must ensure that the surgeon and the anesthesiologist are made aware of the abnormality. The nurse must attach a note to the front of the chart and also try to contact the surgeon or anesthesiologist via telephone.
2. After surgery, the nurse has the following responsibilities, which vary according to where the nurse first sees the postoperative patient:

- Admit the patient to the unit according to hospital procedure or policy.
- Check the patient's airway for patency, assess the respiratory status, and give oxygen as needed.
- Position the patient to prevent aspiration of vomitus and secretions.
- Check the patient's blood pressure and pulse, intravenous (IV) lines, catheters, drainage tubes, surgical dressings, and casts.
- Review the patient's surgical and anesthesia records.
- Monitor the patient's blood pressure, pulse, and respiratory rate every 5 to 15 minutes until the patient is discharged from the area.
- Check the patient every 5 to 15 minutes for emergence from anesthesia. Provide suctioning as needed.
- Exercise caution in administering opioids. Check the patient's respiratory rate, blood pressure, and pulse before these drugs are given, and 20 to 30 minutes after administration. Contact the physician if the respiratory rate is below 10 before the drug is given or if it falls below 10 after the drug is given.
- Discharge the patient from the area to his or her room or another specified area. Record all drugs administered and nursing tasks performed before the patient leaves the PACU.

3. The administration of general anesthesia requires the use of one or more drugs. The choice of anesthetic drug depends on many factors, including:
- General physical condition of the patient
- Area, organ, or system being operated on
- Anticipated length of surgical procedure

Activity D DOSAGE CALCULATION

1. 3 mL
2. 2 tablets
3. 5 doses in 5 days; 1 dose each day
4. 3 tablets
5. 45 minutes

SECTION III: PRACTICING FOR NCLEX

Activity E

1. **Answer: c**
   RATIONALE: The nurse should know that methohexital is a barbiturate, and it depresses the CNS to produce hypnosis and anesthesia, but it does not produce analgesia. Recovery after a small dose is rapid. Enflurane, which is a volatile anesthetic liquid, produces mild stimulation of respiratory and bronchial secretions when used alone. Halothane, another volatile anesthetic liquid, causes moderate muscle relaxation. Cholinergic blocking drugs, such as glycopyrrolate, decrease secretions of the upper respiratory tract.

2. **Answer: a**
   RATIONALE: Stage 1 of anesthesia, known as the induction or the analgesic stage of general

anesthesia, begins with a loss of consciousness. Delirium along with excitement are part of the second stage of anesthesia. Surgical analgesia and respiratory paralysis are noted in the third and fourth stage, respectively.

3. **Answer: b**
   RATIONALE: Topical anesthesia leads to desensitization of the skin and the mucus membranes. Topical anesthesia does not decrease anxiety and apprehension, stimulate cardiovascular tissue, or create a loss of feeling in the lower extremities. Opioids, which are anesthetic drugs used for general anesthesia, bring about a decrease in anxiety and apprehension. Ketamine, a drug used for general anesthesia, causes cardiovascular and respiratory stimulation. Administration of spinal anesthesia causes a loss of feeling (anesthesia) and movement in the lower extremities.

4. **Answer: c**
   RATIONALE: As part of postoperative interventions after anesthesia administration, the nurse should position the patient to prevent aspiration of vomitus and secretions. The nurse should review the patient's laboratory test records before the administration of anesthesia and not after. As part of the postoperative interventions done after anesthesia administration, the nurse should review the patient's surgical and anesthesia records. The nurse should also monitor the blood pressure, pulse, and respiratory rate every 5 to 15 minutes until the patient is discharged from the area, and not every 12 hours. The nurse should know that a hypnotic agent is administered to the patient before anesthesia administration and not after.

5. **Answer: b**
   RATIONALE: If a patient shows an increase in respiratory secretions on administration of the preanesthetic drug, the nurse should understand that the preanesthetic drug was not given to the patient on time. Preanesthetic drugs must be administered on time to produce their intended effects. Failure to give the preanesthetic drug on time may result in such events as increased respiratory secretions caused by the irritating effect of anesthetic gases and the need for an increased dose of the induction drug because the preanesthetic drug has not had time to sedate the patient. Not assessing patient's IV lines well, not assessing patient's respiratory status, and not reviewing the patient's anesthesia records do not cause an increase in the patient's respiratory secretions.

6. **Answer: a, b, c**
   RATIONALE: When caring for a patient receiving local anesthesia, the nurse should apply a dressing to surgical areas and observe for bleeding and oozing, if any. Assessing the patient's pulse rate every 5 to 15 minutes and exercising caution when administering opioids to the patient are postoperative interventions that a nurse has to

perform. These interventions are not appropriate when caring for a patient about to undergo local anesthesia for the suturing of a wound.

7. **Answer: a**

   RATIONALE: The nurse should confirm that the patient is not older than 60 years of age. Preanesthetic drugs may be omitted in patients aged 60 or older because many of the medical disorders for which these drugs are contraindicated are seen in older individuals. Epinephrine used with local anesthesia is contraindicated in cases when local anesthesia is to be applied to the extremities, but preanesthetic drugs are not contraindicated in these cases. Preanesthetic drugs are also not contraindicated in patients who have a low body weight.

8. **Answer: a**

   RATIONALE: The nurse should administer a cholinergic blocking drug as it decreases the secretions of the upper respiratory tract. Scopolamine and glycopyrrolate are mild sedatives. Opioids are used to decrease the anxiety and apprehension of the patient before the surgery. Diazepam or Valium is used as an antianxiety drug for preoperative sedation.

9. **Answer: a**

   RATIONALE: The trans-sacral block is injected into the epidural space at the level of the sacrococcygeal notch when administering a trans-sacral block as anesthesia for a cesarean delivery. A trans-sacral block is often used in obstetrics. An epidural block is injected for anesthesia into the space surrounding the dura of the spinal cord. Spinal anesthesia is injected into the subarachnoid space of the spinal cord. A brachial plexus block involves the injection of a local anesthetic into the brachial plexus.

10. **Answer: d**

    RATIONALE: The nurse should confirm that the patient does not require anesthesia to be administered on the extremities to ensure that the use of epinephrine along with local anesthesia is not contraindicated in the patient. The anesthetic stays in the tissue longer when epinephrine is used. This is contraindicated, however, when the local anesthetic is used on an extremity. Epinephrine used with local anesthesia is not known to be contraindicated in patients who are anemic, have a low blood pressure, or are older than 60 years of age.

CHAPTER 22

SECTION I: ASSESSING YOUR UNDERSTANDING

Activity A MATCHING

1. 1-B, 2-C, 3-D, 4-A
2. 1-C, 2-A, 3-B

Activity B FILL IN THE BLANKS

1. Anxiolytics
2. Digoxin
3. Preanesthetic
4. Parenteral
5. Withdrawal

SECTION II: APPLYING YOUR KNOWLEDGE

Activity C SHORT ANSWERS

1. Before administering alprazolam for the first time, a nurse should perform the following assessments:
   - Obtain patient's complete medical history, including mental status and anxiety level.
   - Obtain portions of the patient's history from a family member or friend.
   - Observe the patient for behavioral signs indicating anxiety.
   - Assess the blood pressure, pulse, respiratory rate, and weight.
   - Obtain a history of any past drug or alcohol use.
2. When caring for a patient receiving alprazolam who has developed constipation, a nurse should perform the following interventions:
   - Offer frequent sips of water to relieve dry mouth and to provide adequate hydration.
   - Administer oral antianxiety drugs with food or meals to decrease the possibility of gastrointestinal upset.
   - Include fiber, fruits, and vegetables with meals to prevent constipation.

Activity D DOSAGE CALCULATION

1. 1.5 tablets
2. Every 6 hours
3. 3 tablets
4. 10 tablets
5. 1.5 mg
6. 6 tablets

SECTION III: PRACTICING FOR NCLEX

Activity E

1. **Answer: b**

   RATIONALE: Diarrhea is an adverse reaction to the antianxiety drug, which is a cause of concern and should be immediately reported by the nurse to the primary health care provider. Antianxiety drugs do not cause seizures. On the contrary, they are used to control seizures or convulsions in patients. Abdominal cramps and bradycardia are not known to be adverse reactions to antianxiety drugs either.

2. **Answer: c**

   RATIONALE: The nurse should assess for increased anxiety as the withdrawal symptom of benzodiazepines. Increased red blood cell (RBC) count and decreased pulse rate are not known to be observed in patients exhibiting benzodiazepine withdrawal symptoms. The withdrawal symptoms are marked by a decrease in appetite in patients, bordering on anorexia. An increased appetite is not observed in patients with benzodiazepine withdrawal symptoms.

3. **Answer: d**
RATIONALE: The nurse should monitor the patient for increased risk of digitalis toxicity caused by the interaction of digoxin with diazepam. Increased risk for central nervous system (CNS) depression is caused by the interaction of alcohol with diazepam. Increased risk for respiratory depression and sedation are caused by the interaction of tricyclic antidepressants or antipsychotics with diazepam.

4. **Answer: a, c, e**
RATIONALE: The nurse should take precautions when administering hydroxyzine drugs to patients with impaired liver function, impaired kidney function, and patients with debilitation. Impaired pancreas function or bone marrow depression is not known to be contraindicated with hydroxyzine.

5. **Answer: b**
RATIONALE: Acute panic is an alcohol withdrawal symptom. Diarrhea, dry mouth, and light-headedness are not known to be alcohol withdrawal symptoms. These are adverse reactions to chlordiazepoxide therapy, which is administered for acute alcohol withdrawal.

6. **Answer: b**
RATIONALE: The nurse should ensure that the patient is not hypersensitive. When administering fluoroquinolones, the nurse should ensure that the patient is not younger than 18 years of age. When administering aminoglycosides, the nurse should ensure that the patient does not have myasthenia gravis or parkinsonism.

7. **Answer: c**
RATIONALE: The nurse should provide the patient with a fiber-rich diet including plenty of fluids to prevent the occurrence of constipation. Providing vitamin supplements, a fluid-only diet, or vegetarian food are ineffective measures to prevent constipation caused by chlordiazepoxide.

8. **Answer: b**
RATIONALE: The nurse should inform the patient to avoid alcohol. The patient with photosensitivity should be instructed to avoid sunlight. Photosensitivity is an adverse reaction to tricyclic antidepressants. The patient who is being treated with monoamine oxidase inhibitors should be instructed to avoid sour cream and yogurt as these foods are rich in tyramine, which should be avoided when the patient is being treated with monoamine oxidase inhibitors.

9. **Answer: a**
RATIONALE: The nurse should administer the drug intramuscularly in the gluteus muscle, which is a large muscle mass, and not in the arm, which has less muscle mass. The nurse should monitor for hearing and kidney problems if the patient is to receive vancomycin, along with ototoxic or nephrotoxic drugs. The nurse should monitor for secondary bacterial or fungal infections if the patient is administered quinupristin/dalfopristin.

10. **Answer: c**
RATIONALE: The nurse should monitor the patient for a metallic taste in the mouth, which is a withdrawal symptom of alprazolam. Diarrhea, dizziness, and dry mouth are adverse effects of the treatment.

CHAPTER 23

SECTION I: ASSESSING YOUR UNDERSTANDING
Activity A MATCHING
1. 1-C, 2-A, 3-D, 4-E, 5-B
2. 1-B, 2-C, 3-A
Activity B FILL IN THE BLANKS
1. Healing
2. Insomnia
3. Valerian
4. Wakefulness
5. Melatonin
6. Barbiturates

SECTION II: APPLYING YOUR KNOWLEDGE
Activity C SHORT ANSWERS
1. Before administering a sedative, the nurse takes and records the patient's blood pressure, pulse, and respiratory rate. The nurse also assesses the patient's needs by asking the following questions:
   - Is the patient uncomfortable with the idea of administering the sedative or hypnotic drug?
   - Is it too early for the patient to receive the drug? Is a later hour preferred?
   - Does the patient receive an opioid analgesic every 4 to 6 hours?
   - Are there environmental disturbances that may keep the patient awake and decrease the effectiveness of the drug?
   - If the sedative is for a surgical procedure, then is its administration correctly timed?
   - Has the patient signed a consent form for the procedure before administration of the drug?
2. Nursing diagnoses particular to a patient taking a sedative or hypnotic are as follows:
   - Risk for Injury: Related to drowsiness or impaired memory
   - Ineffective Breathing Pattern: Related to respiratory depression
   - Ineffective Individual Coping: Related to excessive use of medication

Activity D DOSAGE CALCULATION

1. 4 tablets
2. 3 tablets
3. 2 tablets
4. 2 tablets
5. 2 tablets

SECTION III: PRACTICING FOR NCLEX

Activity E

1. **Answer: a, c, d**
   RATIONALE: Back rubs, night lights, and darkened rooms can help to provide optimal response to sedative therapy. Bedtime coffee would promote wakefulness. Alcohol has an additive effect that, in combination with a sedative, can cause central nervous system depression and even result in death.

2. **Answer: c**
   RATIONALE: The nurse can evaluate the effectiveness of the treatment being given to the patient by observing an improvement in the patient's sleep pattern. An improvement in the patient's consciousness level, normalcy in the patient's respiration rate, and a decrease in the patient's restlessness do not indicate effective treatment.

3. **Answer: b**
   RATIONALE: The nurse should record the patient's blood pressure before administration of the sedative. Platelet count, hematocrit, and blood sugar are not altered by the sedative; hence these factors are not necessarily recorded before administration of the sedative.

4. **Answer: a**
   RATIONALE: The nurse should monitor the patient for nausea, which is an adverse reaction of sedatives. Headache, restlessness, and anxiety are causes of insomnia, for which a sedative may be prescribed.

5. **Answer: d**
   RATIONALE: Sedatives must be administered cautiously to patients with renal impairment. Patients with hearing impairment, hyperglycemia, or glucose intolerance are not high-risk candidates for sedative administration.

6. **Answer: b**
   RATIONALE: The interaction between antihistamines and sedatives causes increased sedation. Restlessness, headache, and chronic pain are symptoms of insomnia that may require treatment with sedatives.

7. **Answer: b**
   RATIONALE: Respiratory depression is a symptom of acute toxicity caused by barbiturates. Increased blood pressure, lowered blood sugar, and frequent micturition are not symptoms of toxicity. Instead, lowered blood pressure and oliguria are symptoms of toxicity. Blood sugar may not be affected by barbiturates.

8. **Answer: c**
   RATIONALE: When barbiturates are administered in the presence of pain, the patient could have delirium. Administration of barbiturates in the presence of pain does not cause an allergic reaction, increased body temperature, or increased blood sugar. Allergic reactions have been reported with the administration of melatonin. Lowered body temperature is an adverse effect of sedatives. Blood sugar may not be affected by barbiturates.

9. **Answer: a, b, d**
   RATIONALE: Restlessness, euphoria, and confusion are withdrawal symptoms of barbiturates. Barbiturates may be used as a sedative for convulsions and seizures.

10. **Answer: a, c, e**
    RATIONALE: Sedatives create relaxation, a calming effect, and drowsiness. Nausea and dizziness are adverse reactions of sedatives and hypnotics.

CHAPTER 24

SECTION I: ASSESSING YOUR UNDERSTANDING

Activity A MATCHING

1. 1-D, 2-C, 3-B, 4-A
2. 1-D, 2-A, 3-B, 4-C

Activity B FILL IN THE BLANKS

1. Psychotherapy
2. Tyramine
3. Priapism
4. Tricyclic
5. Gluteus

SECTION II: APPLYING YOUR KNOWLEDGE

Activity C SHORT ANSWERS

1. Clinical depression is treated with antidepressant drugs. Psychotherapy is used with antidepressants in treating major depressive episodes.
2. There are four types of antidepressants: tricyclic antidepressants, monoamine oxidase (MAO) inhibitors, selective serotonin reuptake inhibitors (SSRIs), and miscellaneous unrelated drugs.
3. Treatment with antidepressants increases the sensitivity of postsynaptic alpha-adrenergic and serotonin receptors and decreases the sensitivity of the presynaptic receptor sites. This enhances recovery from the depressive episode by making neurotransmission activity more effective.
4. Tricyclic antidepressant drugs are used to treat depressive episodes, bipolar disorder, obsessive-compulsive disorders, chronic neuropathic pain, depression accompanied by anxiety disorders, and enuresis. The unapproved uses include treating peptic ulcer disease, sleep apnea, panic disorder,

bulimia nervosa, premenstrual symptoms, and some dermatologic problems. These drugs may be used with psychotherapy in severe cases.

Activity D DOSAGE CALCULATION

1. 3 tablets
2. 6 tablets
3. 2.5 tablets
4. 6 hours
5. 6 tablets
6. 2 tablets

SECTION III: PRACTICING FOR NCLEX

Activity E

1. **Answer: a**
   RATIONALE: Photosensitivity is one of the adverse reactions to tricyclic antidepressant drugs. Hypertensive episodes and severe convulsions are the effects observed when tricyclic antidepressants are administered along with MAO inhibitors. Nervous system depression may result when tricyclic antidepressants interact with sedatives, hypnotics, and analgesics.

2. **Answer: d**
   RATIONALE: The nurse should screen the patient for cerebrovascular diseases when administering MAO inhibitors. Patients with seizure disorder and myocardial infarction are contraindicated in the use of maprotiline. Urinary retention is observed when cimetidine used for gastric upsets interacts with SSRI antidepressant drugs.

3. **Answer: a**
   RATIONALE: The nurse should monitor the patient for an increased risk of bleeding. Increased risk for hypotension is observed when antihypertensive drugs interact with antidepressants. Increased anticholinergic symptoms are observed when cimetidine, used for gastrointestinal upset, interacts with antidepressants. Increased risk for nervous system depression is observed in patients when an analgesic interacts with antidepressants.

4. **Answer: c**
   RATIONALE: The nurse should monitor the patient for somnolence, a possible neuromuscular reaction of SSRIs. Vertigo and blurred vision are adverse reactions observed when MAO inhibitors are administered. Other miscellaneous antidepressants can cause tremor.

5. **Answer: a**
   RATIONALE: Extremely high blood pressure results in hypertensive crisis. The medical intervention involves lowering the blood pressure. Blood sugar and temperature levels and respiration rates do not cause hypertensive crisis.

6. **Answer: a**
   RATIONALE: The nurse should instruct the patient to report priapism or inappropriate penile erection, which is an adverse reaction observed in patients who receiving trazodone. Orthostatic

hypotension or unsteadiness when changing position is observed in patients administered mirtazapine. Sertraline can cause insomnia and diarrhea.

7. **Answer: a, b, e**
   RATIONALE: The nurse should obtain a complete medical history, blood pressure measurements, and pulse and respiratory rates as a part of the preadministration assessment. Antidepressant drugs do not adversely affect complete blood counts and blood sugar levels.

8. **Answer: b**
   RATIONALE: The nurse should closely monitor the patient for hypertensive crisis, a life-threatening adverse effect of tyramine interacting with MAO inhibitor antidepressants. Orthostatic hypotension and blurred vision are adverse effects of MAO inhibitors. Photosensitivity is an adverse reaction of tricyclic antidepressants.

9. **Answer: a**
   RATIONALE: The nurse should instruct the patient to change positions slowly and assist the patient if required. Instructing the patient to drink plenty of fluids, monitoring changes in vital signs, or monitoring for hyperglycemia will not help the patient overcome orthostatic hypotension.

10. **Answer: c**
    RATIONALE: The nurse should administer fluoxetine in the morning, which is the best time for its administration. Most antidepressant drugs, except SSRIs, are best administered at night before bedtime, rather than with lunch or dinner, so that the sedative effects promote sleep, and the adverse reactions appear less troublesome.

CHAPTER 25

SECTION I: ASSESSING YOUR UNDERSTANDING

Activity A MATCHING

1. 1-B, 2-C, 3-A

Activity B FILL IN THE BLANKS

1. Carotid
2. Narcolepsy
3. Sympathomimetic
4. Medulla
5. Arrhythmias

SECTION II: APPLYING YOUR KNOWLEDGE

Activity C SHORT ANSWERS

1. The nursing interventions for a patient with an ineffective breathing pattern who is being administered CNS stimulants are as follows:
   • Record blood pressure, pulse, and respiratory rates.

- Before administering the drug, ensure a patent airway.
- Monitor respirations closely after administration.
- Record the effects of therapy.

2. The nursing interventions for a patient experiencing nausea and vomiting from an analeptic are as follows:
   - The nurse should keep a suction machine nearby in case the patient vomits.
   - In case of urinary retention, the nurse should measure intake and output.
   - The nurse should notify the primary health care provider if the patient cannot void or the bladder appears to be distended on palpation.

Activity D DOSAGE CALCULATION

1. 4 tablets
2. 4 mL
3. 4 tablets
4. 3 tablets
5. 1 tablet

SECTION III: PRACTICING FOR NCLEX

Activity E

1. **Answer: b**
   RATIONALE: Hyperactivity is one of the adverse reactions of CNS stimulants that a nurse should monitor in a patient. Tachycardia, not bradycardia, is a reaction of CNS stimulants. Fever or high blood pressure are not adverse effects generally associated with CNS stimulants.

2. **Answer: a**
   RATIONALE: The nurse should instruct the parents of the patient to give the drug in the morning, 30 to 45 minutes before breakfast, and before lunch. Specify that the drug should not be given in the late afternoon. It should be taken with water, not milk, and it should be consumed directly and not dissolved in water or milk first.

3. **Answer: c**
   RATIONALE: The CNS stimulants are contraindicated in patients with ventilation mechanism disorders (such as chronic obstructive pulmonary disease [COPD]). The drug is not contraindicated in patients with bone marrow suppression, severe liver disease, or ulcerative colitis.

4. **Answer: c**
   RATIONALE: Combining theophylline with CNS stimulants may result in increased risk of hyperactive behaviors. Combining the two does not lead to decreased effectiveness of the CNS stimulant or theophylline. Anesthetics, when taken with CNS stimulants, increase the risk for cardiac arrhythmias.

5. **Answer: c**
   RATIONALE: The nurse should monitor consciousness levels every 5 to 15 minutes. The nurse may send the blood sample for an arterial blood gas analysis but not for a platelet count. Pulse rate and blood pressure should be monitored every 5 to 15 minutes, not every hour. The nurse should carefully monitor the respiratory rate until it returns to normal—not just for 5 minutes after administration.

6. **Answer: a**
   RATIONALE: The nurse should encourage the patient to avoid napping during daytime. In patients with insomnia, the drug should be administered early in the day, not evening, whenever possible. Stimulants such as coffee or tea should be avoided. The nurse should not administer any over-the-counter sleeping pills.

7. **Answer: a, b, e**
   RATIONALE: The nurse should instruct the parents to monitor the eating patterns of the child and check height and weight measurements to monitor growth. The nurse should also stress the importance of preparing nutritious meals and snacks. The child should be encouraged to have a substantial breakfast as he or she may be in school during lunchtime and may not feel hungry. Sleeping pills should be avoided.

8. **Answer: a, c, e**
   RATIONALE: When an amphetamine is used as part of obesity treatment, the nurse obtains and records the blood pressure, pulse, respiratory rate, and weight before therapy is started. There is no need to observe the urinary output or measure blood glucose.

CHAPTER 26

SECTION I: ASSESSING YOUR UNDERSTANDING

Activity A MATCHING

1. 1-B, 2-D, 3-A, 4-C
2. 1-C, 2-A, 3-D, 4-B

Activity B FILL IN THE BLANKS

1. Bipolar
2. Dopamine
3. Serotonin
4. Flattened
5. Extrapyramidal

SECTION II: APPLYING YOUR KNOWLEDGE

Activity C SHORT ANSWERS

1. Before administering antipsychotics for the first time, a nurse should perform the following assessments:
   - The nurse should obtain a complete mental health, social, and medical history.
   - In the case of psychosis, the nurse should obtain the mental health history from a family member or friend.
   - The nurse should observe the patient for any behavior patterns that appear to be deviations from normal.

- Assessment should include obtaining blood pressure, pulse, respiratory rate, and weight.
2. When caring for a patient who is being administered Risperdal and is showing signs of acute psychosis, a nurse should perform the following interventions:
   - Repeat parenteral administration every 1 to 4 hours until the desired effects are obtained.
   - Monitor the patient closely for cardiac arrhythmias or rhythm changes, or hypotension.

Activity D DOSAGE CALCULATION

1. 4 tablets
2. 2.5 mL
3. 4 tablets
4. 5 mL
5. 5 mL

SECTION III: PRACTICING FOR NCLEX

Activity E

1. **Answer: b**
   RATIONALE: The nurse should ask the patient to avoid sunlight as photosensitivity can result in severe sunburn when the patient is taking Haldol. Tanning beds should also be avoided. Minimizing alcohol use or drinking five glasses of water a day will not have a significant impact on photosensitivity.

2. **Answer: b**
   RATIONALE: The nurse should monitor the patient for polyuria or excessive urination. Rashes or dystonia are not symptoms generally associated with lithium carbonate. Also, lithium carbonate causes drowsiness, not insomnia.

3. **Answer: d**
   RATIONALE: The nurse observes the patient for any behavior patterns that appear to be deviating from normal, such as poor eye contact. Inappropriate responses to questions, not brief replies, constitute deviations from normal behavior. The nurse should record instances of laughter only if inappropriate in the given situation. Shyness or timidity may be a personality trait and should not be considered deviant behavior.

4. **Answer: d**
   RATIONALE: The nurse should ensure that assistance is available for securing the patient as the patient is displaying markedly violent behavior patterns. The drug should be given intramuscularly, not intravenously, and preferably in a large muscle mass. The nurse should keep the patient lying down, not upright, for about 30 minutes after administering the drug.

5. **Answer: c**
   RATIONALE: The nurse can mix the oral drugs in liquids such as fruit juice, tomato juice, or milk. The nurse can administer the drug in divided doses, and not just a single daily dose. To confirm whether the patient has swallowed the drug, the

nurse should inspect the patient's mouth because the patient may lie when questioned. The nurse should not compel the patient to swallow the drug and should instead report this to the primary care provider.

6. **Answer: b**
   RATIONALE: The nurse should immediately report rhythmic, involuntary movements of the tongue, face, mouth, jaw, or the extremities as they may indicate that the patient has developed tardive dyskinesia. Dry mouth, orthostatic hypotension, or drowsiness are reactions that are commonly observed in patients who have been administered antipsychotics and need not be reported.

7. **Answer: d**
   RATIONALE: The nurse should monitor the patient for bone marrow suppression and other adverse reactions. The patient should be informed that only a 1-week supply of this drug is dispensed at a time. WBC count tests should be scheduled every week, not every 2 weeks, and the testing should continue for 4 weeks, not 1 week, after therapy is discontinued.

8. **Answer: b**
   RATIONALE: The nurse should continually monitor patients taking lithium for signs of toxicity, such as muscular weakness. The nurse should obtain the sample at least 8–12 hours after the last dose, not 5 hours. The nurse should also ensure that the sample is drawn immediately before the next dose, not 1 hour before. In the acute phase, serum lithium levels should be monitored twice every week, not once every 2 weeks.

9. **Answer: d**
   RATIONALE: The nurse should administer the drug at bedtime to minimize risk of injury to the patient. Providing the drug with food or a calcium supplement or administering the drug every 8 hours won't help in minimizing the risk of injury to the patient.

10. **Answer: a, b, e**
    RATIONALE: The nurse should include the following points in her education plan: Report any unusual changes or physical effects; inform the patient about the risks of extrapyramidal symptoms (EPS) and TD; and avoid exposure to the sun. Altering the dosage if the symptoms increase and taking the drug on an empty stomach are not the instructions provided in the nurse's education plan for patients undergoing antipsychotic drug therapy.

CHAPTER 27

SECTION I: ASSESSING YOUR UNDERSTANDING

Activity A MATCHING

1. 1-B, 2-C, 3-D, 4-A
2. 1-C, 2-A, 3-D, 4-B

Activity B FILL IN THE BLANKS

1. Myocardial
2. Parasympathetic
3. Hypertension
4. C
5. Vasopressors

SECTION II: APPLYING YOUR KNOWLEDGE

Activity C SHORT ANSWERS

1. Before administering metaraminol for the first time, a nurse should perform the following assessments:
   - Obtain the patient's complete medical history, including mental status.
   - Obtain the blood pressure, pulse rate and quality, and respiratory rate and rhythm.
   - Assess the patient's symptoms, problems, or needs.
   - Record any subjective or objective data on the patient's chart.
2. The following nursing interventions are involved during the ongoing administration of metaraminol:
   - Observe the patient for the effect of the drug.
   - Evaluate and document the drug's effect.
   - Obtain and document vital signs.
   - Compare assessments made before and after drug administration.
   - Report adverse drug reactions to the primary health care provider.

Activity D DOSAGE CALCULATION

1. 2 tablets
2. 3 tablets
3. 2 tablets
4. 1 mL
5. 2 tablets

SECTION III: PRACTICING FOR NCLEX

Activity E

1. **Answer: c**
   RATIONALE: When caring for a patient who has been administered metaraminol and is taking digoxin, the nurse should monitor for cardiac arrhythmias. The interaction of digoxin and metaraminol is not known to cause epigastric distress or a decrease in blood pressure; although an increase in blood pressure is an adverse reaction caused by the action of adrenergic drugs. Dopamine, which is an adrenergic drug, is contraindicated in those with pheochromocytoma. However, pheochromocytoma is not an adverse reaction caused by the interaction between digoxin and metaraminol.

2. **Answer: b**
   RATIONALE: Isoproterenol is contraindicated in patients with tachyarrhythmias, tachycardia, or heart block caused by digitalis toxicity, ventricular arrhythmias, and angina pectoris, but not in patients with narrow-angle glaucoma, hypotension, or pheochromocytoma. Dopamine is contraindicated in those with pheochromocytoma (adrenal gland tumor). Epinephrine is contraindicated in patients with narrow-angle glaucoma. Norepinephrine is contraindicated in patients who are hypotensive from blood volume deficits.

3. **Answer: b**
   RATIONALE: The nurse should immediately report any changes in the pulse rate or rhythm as older adults are more likely to have preexisting cardiovascular disease that predisposes them to potentially serious cardiac arrhythmias. Nausea, headache, or urinary urgency are not known to occur in older clients because of the administration of adrenergic drugs and therefore need not be reported to the primary health care provider.

4. **Answer: a**
   RATIONALE: The nurse should monitor for supine hypertension while caring for a patient who is being administered midodrine. Midodrine causes bradycardia, not tachycardia. Orthostatic hypotension is not an adverse effect of midodrine; instead, the drug is taken to reduce orthostatic hypotension. Midodrine is not known to cause respiratory distress.

5. **Answer: a, c, e**
   RATIONALE: The nurse should perform the following interventions: administer only through the intravenous (IV) route, use an electronic infusion pump to administer these drugs, and inspect the needle site and surrounding tissues at frequent intervals. The nurse should not mix dopamine with other drugs unless specifically instructed. The nurse should monitor blood pressure every 2 minutes, not every 30 minutes, from the beginning of therapy until the desired blood pressure is achieved.

6. **Answer: a**
   RATIONALE: The nurse should immediately report a consistent fall in blood pressure, especially if the systolic blood pressure is below 100 mm Hg. Decrease in gastric motility and increase in the heart rate are desirable outcomes of administering metaraminol. Blood glucose levels are not known to increase with the administration of metaraminol.

7. **Answer: a, b, c**
   RATIONALE: The nurse should identify circumstances that disturb sleep and work towards minimizing their effect. Curtains can be drawn over windows to filter light. The nurse can also provide bedtime snacks to the patient. Caffeinated beverages such as tea and coffee should be avoided. Administering drugs only during daytime will not have a significant effect in restoring the patient's sleep pattern.

8. **Answer: a**
   RATIONALE: The nurse should discontinue the old IV line immediately and establish another IV line immediately before calling the primary care provider. Moving the head of the bed to an elevated

position will not help minimize the effect of tissue perfusion. Norepinephrine should not be diluted with alkaline solutions.

CHAPTER 28

SECTION I: ASSESSING YOUR UNDERSTANDING

Activity A MATCHING

1. 1-B, 2-D, 3-A, 4-C
2. 1-C, 2-D, 3-B, 4-A

Activity B FILL IN THE BLANKS

1. Norepinephrine
2. Sympatholytic
3. Phentolamine
4. Blockers
5. Glaucoma
6. Sotalol

SECTION II: APPLYING YOUR KNOWLEDGE

Activity C SHORT ANSWERS

1. The nurse should perform the following preadministration assessments before administering an adrenergic blocking drug:
   - Establish a patient database before administering the adrenergic blocking drug.
   - For a patient with peripheral vascular disease, record the symptoms of the disorder.
   - For a patient with hypertension, take blood pressure and pulse in both arms in sitting, standing, and supine positions before therapy.
   - For patients with cardiac arrhythmia, take the pulse rate, determine the pulse rhythm, and note the patient's general appearance.
   - Obtain subjective data of patient, including his or her complaints/description
2. When caring for a patient receiving adrenergic blocking drug therapy for hypertension, the nurse's role is to:
   - Take blood pressure before each dose.
   - Observe these patients for unusual responses.
   - Take blood pressure on both arms and in sitting, standing, and supine positions during the first week or more of therapy.
   - After blood pressure is stable, take the blood pressure before each drug administration, using the same arm and position for each reading.

Activity D DOSAGE CALCULATION

1. 4 tablets
2. 18 tablets
3. 9 tablets
4. 50 tablets
5. 2 tablets

SECTION III: PRACTICING FOR NCLEX

Activity E

1. **Answer: b**
   RATIONALE: The nurse needs to monitor for orthostatic hypotension in a patient who is treated with phentolamine. This drug is unlikely to cause nausea and diarrhea, bradycardia, and bronchospasm, adverse reactions that are caused by betaxolol or hydrochloride.
2. **Answer: c**
   RATIONALE: Coronary artery disease is a contraindication that the nurse must consider when assessing a patient for alpha-adrenergic blocking drug therapy. The drug is not contraindicated in patients with sinus bradycardia, heart failure, or emphysema, which are contraindications to be considered when assessing a patient for beta-adrenergic blocking drug therapy.
3. **Answer: d**
   RATIONALE: The nurse should discontinue the drug when a patient receiving adrenergic blocking drugs shows a decrease in blood pressure. The nurse need not monitor for excessive perspiration or confusion, considering these conditions do not occur with the administration of adrenergic blocking drugs. Shifting the patient into a more conducive position is not the most appropriate intervention because it will not provide comfort to the patient or reduce the symptoms of a decreased blood pressure.
4. **Answer: a**
   RATIONALE: The nurse should monitor vascular insufficiency in the elderly patient when administering a beta-adrenergic blocking drug. The nurse need not monitor occipital headache, dizziness, and central nervous system (CNS) depression in the elderly patient when administering a beta-adrenergic blocking drug because these conditions are not known to occur in older patients on the administration of beta-adrenergic blocking drugs.
5. **Answer: b**
   RATIONALE: Interaction of lidocaine with beta-adrenergic blockers causes an increase in the serum level of the beta-blocker. Increased risk of hypotension is the result of the interaction between loop diuretics and beta-adrenergic blockers. Interaction between clonidine and beta-adrenergic blockers increases the risk of paradoxical hypertensive effect. Similarly, the effect of the beta-blocker increases when antidepressants interact with beta-adrenergic blockers.
6. **Answer: d**
   RATIONALE: The nurse should monitor for lightheadedness as the adverse reaction in a patient who is administered peripherally acting antiadrenergic drugs. The nurse need not monitor for dry mouth, drowsiness, or malaise; these are generalized reactions associated with centrally acting

anti-adrenergic drugs, not peripherally acting anti-adrenergic drugs.

7. Answer: a

RATIONALE: The nurse should measure the apical pulse rate when the patient is administered a sympatholytic drug. If the pulse is below 60 beats per minute (bpm), if there is any irregularity in the patient's heart rate or rhythm, or if systolic blood pressure is less than 90 mm Hg, the nurse should withhold the drug and contact the primary health care provider. The nurse need not measure the body temperature, heart rate, or respiratory rate of the patient who is to be administered the sympatholytic drug because they are not likely to be affected.

8. Answer: c

RATIONALE: The teaching plan of the patient who is prescribed adrenergic blocking drugs for glaucoma should include contacting the primary health care provider if changes in vision occur. Directions to monitor his or her own pulse and blood pressure and take drugs as directed are included in the teaching plan of a patient with hypertension, angina, or arrhythmia. The nurse need not instruct the patient who is being treated for glaucoma to ambulate often.

9. Answer: a

RATIONALE: The nurse should measure the patient's intraocular pressure to determine the effectiveness of drug therapy. The nurse need not monitor the blood pressure, respiratory rate, or pulse rate of the patient who is receiving beta-adrenergic blocking ophthalmic preparations such as timolol because monitoring these will not determine the effectiveness of the therapy.

10. Answer: b

RATIONALE: The nurse should assess the patient for psychotic behavior caused by the interaction of an anti-adrenergic drug with haloperidol. Interaction of an anti-adrenergic drug with lithium causes increased risk of lithium toxicity. An increased risk of hypertension is the result of interaction between anti-adrenergic drugs and beta-blockers. Interaction between anti-adrenergic drugs and anesthetic agents can increase the effect of the anesthetic.

CHAPTER 29

SECTION I: ASSESSING YOUR UNDERSTANDING

Activity A MATCHING

1. 1-B, 2-C, 3-A
2. 1-B, 2-C, 3-A

Activity B FILL IN THE BLANKS

1. Muscarinic
2. Parasympathetic

3. Acetylcholine
4. Anticholinesterases
5. Nicotinic

SECTION II: APPLYING YOUR KNOWLEDGE

Activity C SHORT ANSWERS

1. Before administering ambenonium for the first time, a nurse should perform the following assessments:
   - A complete neurologic assessment
   - Signs of muscle weakness, such as drooling, inability to chew and swallow, drooping of the eyelids, inability to perform repetitive movements, difficulty breathing, and extreme fatigue

2. The nurse should explain that myasthenia gravis is a disease that involves rapid fatigue of skeletal muscles because of the lack of acetylcholine released at the nerve endings of parasympathetic nerves. Cholinergic drugs that prolong the activity of acetylcholine by inhibiting the release of acetylcholinesterase are called indirect-acting cholinergics or anticholinesterase muscle stimulants. Drugs used to treat this disorder act indirectly to inhibit the activity of acetylcholinesterase and promote muscle contraction.

Activity D DOSAGE CALCULATION

1. 7 tablets
2. 2 tablets
3. 1 vial
4. 2 tablets per dose
5. 0.5 mL

SECTION III: PRACTICING FOR NCLEX

Activity E

1. **Answer: a**

   RATIONALE: The nurse should observe for temporary reduction of visual acuity and headache as adverse reactions of the topical administration of cholinergic drugs. Increased ocular tension, decreased sweat production, and anaphylactic shock are not related adverse reactions. Increased ocular tension, decreased sweat production, and anaphylactic shock are adverse reactions of cholinergic blocking drugs.

2. **Answer: a**

   RATIONALE: The nurse should instruct the patient to remove and replace the system every 7 days. Replacement is best during bedtime and not daytime. The nurse should notify the primary health care provider if eye secretions are excessive or irritation occurs, and he or she should not instruct the patient to change the system every day if eye secretions are excessive. It is important for the patient to carry identification indicating that the patient has myasthenia gravis, not glaucoma.

3. **Answer: d**
RATIONALE: The nurse should check the patient for mechanical obstruction of the gastrointestinal (GI) or genitourinary tracts before administration of bethanechol. Tachyarrhythmias, myocardial infarction, and coronary occlusion are not related disorders that a nurse needs to check before the administration of bethanechol. Cholinergic drugs are used cautiously in patients with recent coronary occlusion, but not bethanechol.

4. **Answer: b**
RATIONALE: The nurse should anticipate the decreased effect of the cholinergic as the effect of the interaction between ambenonium and corticosteroids. Increased neuromuscular blocking effect, increased absorption of the cholinergic, and decreased serum levels of corticosteroids are not related effects of the interactions between ambenonium and corticosteroids. Increased neuromuscular blocking effect results from interaction of aminoglycoside antibiotics with cholinergic drugs.

5. **Answer: c**
RATIONALE: The nurse should remove excessive secretions with a cotton ball or gauze soaked in normal saline or other cleansing solution recommended by the primary health care provider as part of the ongoing assessment for the patient. Assessing for signs of muscle weakness is the preadministration nursing assessment for a patient with myasthenia gravis. Drying of upper respiratory and oral secretions and measuring and recording fluid intake and output are not ongoing assessments for a patient with glaucoma; measuring and recording fluid intake and output is the ongoing assessment for a patient with urinary retention.

6. **Answer: c**
RATIONALE: The nurse caring for a patient who is being administered a cholinergic drug should ensure that aminoglycoside antibiotics are administered cautiously because they increase the risk of neuromuscular blocking effects. Salicylates, analgesics, and antidiabetics need to be administered cautiously to the patient undergoing anticonvulsant drug therapy.

7. **Answer: a, b, c**
RATIONALE: The nurse should instill the drug in the lower conjunctival sac, avoid the tip of the dropper touching the eye, and support the hand by holding the dropper against the patient's forehead while managing a patient who is being prescribed Miostat. The nurse need not advise the patient to wear or carry identification about glaucoma.

8. **Answer: c, d, e**
RATIONALE: The nurse should observe the patient for salivation, clenching of the jaw, and muscle rigidity and spasm as symptoms of drug overdose in order to make frequent dosage adjustments. Drooping of the eyelids and rapid fatigability of the muscles are symptoms of drug underdose.

9. **Answer: c**
RATIONALE: The nurse should place the call light and items that the patient might need within easy reach while managing the care of patient-administered cholinergic therapy for urinary retention. Instructing the patient to void before the drug is administered, encouraging the patient to take the drug with milk, and encouraging the patient to drink five to seven glasses of water after drug administration are not nursing activities specifically related to caring for a patient receiving cholinergic therapy.

10. **Answer: a, c, e**
RATIONALE: The nurse should ensure that bedpan or bathroom is readily available, encourage the patient to ambulate to assist the passing of flatus, and keep a record of the number, consistency, and frequency of stools if the patient develops diarrhea after taking Urecholine orally. Checking for bloodstains in the stool and encouraging the patient to increase the fibrous food intake are not related nursing activities.

CHAPTER 30

SECTION I: ASSESSING YOUR UNDERSTANDING

Activity A MATCHING

1. 1-D, 2-C, 3-A, 4-B
2. 1-C, 2-A, 3-D, 4-B

Activity B FILL IN THE BLANKS

1. Acetylcholine
2. Parasympathetic
3. Cycloplegia
4. Atropine
5. Idiosyncrasy

SECTION II: APPLYING YOUR KNOWLEDGE

Activity C SHORT ANSWERS

1. The nurse should include the following when evaluating the patient's treatment plan:
   - Therapeutic effect is achieved.
   - Adverse reactions are identified, reported, and managed successfully.
   - Oral mucous membranes remain moist.
   - Patient complies with the prescribed drug regimen.
   - Patient and family demonstrate an understanding of the drug regimen.
   - Patient verbalizes the importance of complying with the prescribed therapeutic regimen.
2. The nurse should offer the following instructions to an elderly patient's family when caring for the patient receiving cholinergic blocking drugs for treatment:

- Inform the family of an elderly patient of possible visual and mental impairments (e.g., blurred vision, confusion, or agitation) that may occur during therapy with these drugs. Caution them to remove or avoid objects or situations that may cause falls, such as throw rugs, footstools, and wet or newly waxed floors, whenever possible.
- Instruct the family to place against walls any items of furniture (e.g., footstools, chairs, stands) that obstruct walkways.
- Alert the family to the dangers of heat prostration and explain the steps to avoid this problem.
- Advise the family to closely observe the patient during the first few days of therapy, and notify the primary health care provider if mental changes occur.

Activity D DOSAGE CALCULATION

1. 3 tablets
2. 2 tablets
3. 1.25 mL
4. 3 tablets

SECTION III: PRACTICING FOR NCLEX

Activity E

1. **Answer: d**
   RATIONALE: A nurse should use atropine cautiously in patients with asthma. The nurse should not administer cholinergic blocking drugs for patients with tachyarrhythmias, myasthenia gravis, and glaucoma, considering the presence of these conditions contraindicates the use of these drugs.

2. **Answer: b**
   RATIONALE: When caring for a patient on cholinergic drugs complaining of constipation, the nurse should suggest that the patient increase his or her consumption of food rich in fiber. The nurse should also instruct the patient to increase fluid intake up to 2000 mL daily (if health conditions permit), and obtain adequate exercise. The nurse should instruct the patient to increase fluid intake, which will help minimize the adverse reactions of constipation and dry mouth, while the cholinergic blocking drug would help to eliminate the sensations of urinary frequency and urgency. The nurse should not instruct the patient to take antacids or increase the consumption of citrus fruits because these actions will not help relieve the patient's constipation.

3. **Answer: d**
   RATIONALE: The nurse should monitor for a change in pulse rate or rhythm when caring for a patient receiving atropine for third-degree heart block. The nurse should place the patient on a cardiac monitor during and after administration of the drug—not before the drug administration. The nurse need not provide oxygen support to the patient every hour in this case. Symptoms of mydriasis and cycloplegia are visual impairments

that are not known to occur with the administration of atropine for third-degree heart block.

4. **Answer: a, b, d**
   RATIONALE: The nurse should suggest that the patient wear loose clothes, sponge the skin with cool water, and use a fan to cool the body to lessen the intensity of heat prostration. The nurse need not suggest that the patient apply sunscreen to reduce the discomfort or symptoms of heat prostration. Patients with photophobia should wear sunglasses when moving outdoors, but not patients with heat prostration.

5. **Answer: c**
   RATIONALE: The nurse should assess for increased atropine effects resulting from the interaction between atropine and the tricyclic antidepressant. This interaction is not known to cause decreased effectiveness of the antidepressant, increased respiratory rate, or decreased blood pressure.

6. **Answer: a, b, e**
   RATIONALE: The nurse should monitor for nausea, altered taste perceptions, and dysphagia when caring for a patient who is receiving glycopyrrolate. The administration of glycopyrrolate will not cause tachycardia or mydriasis. Tachycardia does occur with the administration of mepenzolate bromide, and mydriasis occurs with trihexyphenidyl.

7. **Answer: a**
   RATIONALE: The nurse should ensure that a cholinergic drug is not administered preoperatively for this 65-year-old patient because cholinergic blocking drugs are usually not included in preoperative drugs of patients older than 60 years. Cholinergic blocking drugs may affect their eyes and central nervous system. The nurse should monitor the patient's pulse rate or rhythm when caring for a patient receiving atropine for a third-degree heart block. It is not necessary to place the patient in Fowler's position, but it is mandatory to instruct the patient to remain in bed with the side rails raised after the drug is administered. The nurse need not ensure that the patient has received antibiotics preoperatively.

8. **Answer: c**
   RATIONALE: The nurse should administer the drug at the exact time prescribed by the physician to allow the drug to produce the greatest effect before administration of the anesthetic. The nurse need not administer the drug at the exact time to avoid abdominal cramping in the patient after drug administration, to ensure the effectiveness of the drug after the administration of anesthetic, nor to avoid excessive salivation and make the patient feel comfortable.

9. **Answer: b**
   RATIONALE: The nurse should monitor for signs of mouth dryness after the oxybutynin drug is administered to the patient. Mydriasis is an adverse reaction related to trihexyphenidyl.

Blurred vision and hesitancy are adverse reactions associated with administration of atropine, belladonna alkaloids, glycopyrrolate, dicyclomine HCl, mepenzolate bromide, methscopolamine, propantheline bromide, and scopolamine hydrobromide.

10. **Answer: d**

RATIONALE: The nurse should identify drowsiness as part of the desired response for the patient who has been administered atropine preoperatively. Vomiting, elevated temperature, and low pulse rate are not known to be the desired responses to the administration of atropine when it is administered preoperatively.

CHAPTER 31

SECTION I: ASSESSING YOUR UNDERSTANDING

Activity A MATCHING

1. 1-C, 2-A, 3-D, 4-B
2. 1-C, 2-D, 3-B, 4-A

Activity B FILL IN THE BLANKS

1. Convulsion
2. Hydantoins
3. Oxazolidinediones
4. Succinimides
5. Barbiturates

SECTION II: APPLYING YOUR KNOWLEDGE

Activity C SHORT ANSWERS

1. The nurse should perform the following preadministration assessments before administering an anticonvulsant drug:
   - Check for abnormal behavior in the patient.
   - Check the type of seizure disorder in the patient.
   - Document the type of seizure, frequency, length, description of aura, degree of impairment of consciousness, known triggers, family history of seizures, and recent drug therapy.
   - Obtain vital signs to provide baseline data of the patient.
   - Perform various types of laboratory and diagnostic tests to identify the cause of seizures and to confirm diagnosis.
2. When caring for a patient on anticonvulsant drug therapy, the nurse's role is to:
   - Frequently adjust the dosage of anticonvulsants based on patient response to therapy and the occurrence of adverse reactions during initial treatment of the patient
   - Add a second anticonvulsant to the therapeutic regimen depending on the patient's response to therapy

   - Measure regular serum levels of anticonvulsants for toxicity
   - Document time and duration of seizure, and psychic or motor activity occurring before, during, and after seizure of the patient
   - Assist primary health care provider in his or her evaluation of drug therapy

Activity D DOSAGE CALCULATION

1. 24 capsules
2. 4 capsules
3. 2 tablets
4. 4 tablets
5. 2 tablets
6. 2 tablets

SECTION III: PRACTICING FOR NCLEX

Activity E

1. **Answer: a**

   RATIONALE: While administering trimethadione, the nurse should monitor for eye disorders in the patient. The nurse need not monitor for bone marrow depression, hypotension, and myocardial insufficiency in the patient while administering trimethadione. The nurse should monitor for hypotension and myocardial insufficiency while administering phenytoin and bone marrow depression while administering succinimides.

2. **Answer: d**

   RATIONALE: The nurse should monitor for palpitations in the patient who has been prescribed with tranxene anticonvulsant. The nurse need not monitor for dyspepsia, vomiting, and fatigue in the patient with tranxene anticonvulsant; these are adverse reactions that a nurse should monitor in a patient who has received Felbatol.

3. **Answer: b, c, e**

   RATIONALE: The nurse should include brushing and flossing teeth after each meal, considering long-term administration of the hydantoins can cause gingivitis and gingival hyperplasia (overgrowth of gum tissue), in the teaching plan of the patient undergoing hydantoin drug therapy, along with avoiding consumption of discolored capsules and taking the medication with food. Avoiding taking drugs during pregnancy is included in the teaching plan of the patient on anticonvulsant therapy with oxazolidinediones, not in the teaching plan of the patient undergoing hydantoin drug therapy. Notifying the health care provider if blurred vision occurs is included in the teaching plan of the patient undergoing succinimide drug therapy.

4. **Answer: c**

   RATIONALE: The nurse should immediately report to the primary health care provider incidence of thrombocytopenia in the patient. The nurse need not report to the primary healthcare provider for sinus bradycardia, sinoatrial block or Adams-

Stokes syndrome as they are not the hematologic changes but contraindications for phenytoin.

5. **Answer: a, b, c**
   RATIONALE: The nurse should instruct the patient to stay out of the sun, apply sunscreen, and wear protective clothes. Wearing light colored clothes and placing cotton pads soaked in rose water on the eyes will not help in reducing the symptoms or the discomforts associated with disturbed sensory perception.

6. **Answer: c**
   RATIONALE: The nurse should know that phenytoin is contraindicated in a patient with hepatic abnormalities. The drug phenytoin is not contraindicated in patients with cardiac problems, history of asthma, and liver dysfunction.

7. **Answer: d**
   RATIONALE: The nurse should carefully observe for apnea and cardiac arrest in a patient undergoing diazepam therapy. The nurse should examine mouth and gums of patient with impaired oral mucous membranes and the affected areas of the skin in the patient with impaired skin integrity—not in the patient receiving diazepam. This drug is also not known to cause throat irritation, and therefore, the nurse need not observe the patient for symptoms of throat irritation.

8. **Answer: d**
   RATIONALE: The nurse should be aware of increasing the depressant effect of the analgesics as a possible effect of the interaction of analgesics with anticonvulsants. Administering protease inhibitors with anticonvulsants increases the carbamazepine levels. Administering antiseizure medications with anticonvulsants increases seizure activity. Administering antidiabetic medications with anticonvulsants increases blood glucose levels.

9. **Answer: b**
   RATIONALE: The nurse should identify that phenytoin plasma levels are greater than 20 mcg/mL if the patient exhibits signs of drug toxicity. Patients with plasma levels greater than 20 mcg/mL may exhibit nystagmus. Patients with plasma levels greater than 30 mcg/mL may develop ataxia and mental changes. Phenytoin plasma levels between 10 and 20 mcg/mL give the optimal anticonvulsant effect.

10. **Answer: b, d, e**
    RATIONALE: The nurse should document each seizure's time of occurrence and duration, as well as the psychic or motor activity occurring before, during, and after the seizure. The nurse should also measure serum plasma levels of the anticonvulsant for a patient on barbiturate therapy. The nurse need not document the vital signs of the patient every 4 hours and measure blood pressure every hour for patients undergoing barbiturate therapy.

CHAPTER 32

SECTION I: ASSESSING YOUR UNDERSTANDING

Activity A MATCHING

1. 1-B, 2-D, 3-A, 4-C
2. 1-C, 2-A, 3-D, 4-B

Activity B FILL IN THE BLANKS

1. Parkinson's
2. Achalasia
3. On-off
4. Choreiform
5. Pyridoxine

SECTION II: APPLYING YOUR KNOWLEDGE

Activity C SHORT ANSWERS

1. The nurse should monitor the following for the neuromuscular evaluation of the patient:
   - Tremors of the hands or head while the patient is at rest
   - A masklike facial expression
   - Changes (from normal) in walking
   - Type of speech pattern (halting, monotone)
   - Postural deformities
   - Muscular rigidity
   - Drooling, difficulty chewing or swallowing
   - Changes in thought processes
   - Ability of the patient to carry out any or all of the activities of daily living (e.g., bathing, ambulating, dressing)

2. The nurse should keep the following factors in mind when evaluating the patient's treatment plan:
   - The therapeutic effect is achieved and the symptoms of parkinsonism are controlled.
   - Adverse reactions are identified, reported to the primary health care provider, and managed successfully through appropriate nursing interventions.
   - No evidence of injury is seen.
   - The patient verbalizes an understanding of the treatment modalities, adverse reactions, and importance of continued follow-up care.
   - The patient and family demonstrate an understanding of the drug regimen.

3. The nurse should not abruptly discontinue use of the antiparkinsonism drugs. Neuroleptic malignant syndrome may occur when antiparkinsonism drugs are discontinued or the dosage of levodopa is reduced abruptly. The nurse should carefully observe the patient and report the symptoms of muscular rigidity, elevated body temperature, and mental changes when caring for a patient showing an on-off phenomenon on the administration of levodopa.

4. The nurse should perform the following interventions when caring for a patient taking antiparkin-

sonism drugs and experiencing gastrointestinal (GI) disturbances:
- Create a calm environment.
- Serve small, frequent, and nutritious meals.
- Monitor the patient's weight.
- Discontinue the drug or change the antiparkinsonism drug in cases of severe nausea and vomiting.

5. The nurse should include the following information in the patient and family teaching plan:
- Take the drug as prescribed. Increase, decrease, or omit a dose only as directed by the primary health care provider. If gastrointestinal upset occurs, take the drug with food.
- If dizziness, drowsiness, or blurred vision occurs, avoid driving or performing other tasks that require alertness.
- Avoid the use of alcohol unless a primary health care provider has approved it.
- Relieve dry mouth by sucking on hard candy (unless the patient has diabetes) or taking frequent sips of water. Consult a dentist if dryness of the mouth interferes with wearing, inserting, or removing dentures or causes other dental problems.
- Inform patients that orthostatic hypotension may develop with or without symptoms of dizziness, nausea, fainting, and sweating. Caution the patient against rising rapidly after sitting or lying down.
- Notify the primary health care provider if any of these problems occur: severe dry mouth, inability to chew or swallow food, inability to urinate, feelings of depression, severe dizziness or drowsiness, rapid or irregular heartbeat, abdominal pain, mood changes, and unusual movements of the head, eyes, tongue, neck, arms, legs, feet, mouth, or tongue.
- Keep all appointments with the primary health care provider or clinic personnel because close monitoring of therapy is necessary.
- When taking levodopa, avoid vitamin B_6 (pyridoxine) because this vitamin may interfere with the action of levodopa.

Activity D DOSAGE CALCULATION

1. 4 capsules
2. 62.5 mg of Lodosyn
3. 10 increments
4. 5 tablets

SECTION III: PRACTICING FOR NCLEX

Activity E

1. **Answer: b**
   RATIONALE: When caring for a patient exhibiting choreiform and dystonic movement, the nurse should withhold the next dose of the drug and notify the primary health care provider because it may be necessary to reduce the dosage of lev-

odopa or discontinue use of the drug. The nurse should offer frequent sips of water to the patient throughout the day when caring for a patient experiencing dry mouth. The nurse should monitor the patient for persistent nausea, fatigue, lethargy, and anorexia when caring for a patient experiencing constipation. The nurse need not monitor vital signs frequently when caring for a patient exhibiting choreiform and dystonic movement caused by use of carbidopa.

2. **Answer: b, c, d**
   RATIONALE: The nurse should instruct the patient to increase the intake of fiber and fluids and use a stool softener to help prevent constipation. The nurse need not suggest that the patient decrease the intake of carbohydrates or increase the intake of vitamin C, because this will not help reduce the patient's constipation or the discomfort caused by it.

3. **Answer: a, b, c**
   RATIONALE: The nurse should carefully monitor for muscular rigidity, elevated body temperature, and mental changes in the patient with neuroleptic malignant syndrome, which occurs when the antiparkinsonism drugs are discontinued or the dosage of levodopa is reduced abruptly. The nurse need not monitor for tachycardia or orthostatic hypotension because these conditions are not known to occur with an abrupt reduction of levodopa. Tachycardia is an adverse reaction caused by cholinergic blocking drugs. Orthostatic hypotension is an adverse reaction associated with the use of catechol-O-methyltransferase (COMT) inhibitors.

4. **Answer: c**
   RATIONALE: The nurse should anticipate the increased effect of levodopa caused by the interaction between levodopa and antacids. Increased risk of hypertension and dyskinesia is the effect of levodopa interacting with tricyclic antidepressants. Interaction between COMT inhibitors and adrenergic drugs increases the risk of cardiac symptoms.

5. **Answer: a**
   RATIONALE: The nurse should know that COMT inhibitors should be used with caution in patients with decreased renal function. The nurse should use cholinergic blocking drugs with caution in patients with tachycardia, cardiac arrhythmias, and GI tract problems.

6. **Answer: a, b, c**
   RATIONALE: When preparing a discharge care plan for a patient who has had antiparkinsonism drugs, the nurse should instruct the patient to avoid taking vitamin B_6 with levodopa. The nurse should instruct the patient to avoid consuming alcohol and to contact the primary health care provider in case the patient experiences any symptoms of severe dry mouth, inability to chew or urinate, depression, severe dizziness, or unusual muscle

movement. The nurse should instruct the patient to have small and frequent meals if the patient is experiencing constipation due to the drug therapy. The nurse need not instruct the patient to increase their intake of vitamin C.

7. **Answer: a**

   RATIONALE: When caring for a patient on antiparkinsonism drugs experiencing GI disturbances such as nausea and vomiting, the nurse should discontinue the antiparkinsonism drug or change it. Severe nausea or vomiting may necessitate discontinuing the drug and changing to a different antiparkinsonism drug. Administering the drug before meals, administering antacids after meals, or refraining from giving liquids after meals are not appropriate interventions when caring for a patient who is vomiting or experiencing other GI disturbances.

8. **Answer: c**

   RATIONALE: When caring for a patient on antiparkinsonism drugs who is responding to therapy, the nurse should closely monitor the patient's behavior at frequent intervals. Antiparkinsonism drugs can exacerbate mental symptoms and precipitate a psychosis. If sudden behavioral changes are noted, the nurse should withhold the next dose of the drug and report to the primary health care physician immediately. The nurse could observe a drug holiday in case the patient is experiencing an on-off phenomenon and should discontinue the antiparkinsonism drug or change it when the patient experiences GI disturbances.

9. **Answer: a**

   RATIONALE: The nurse observes the patient with parkinsonism for outward changes that may indicate one or more adverse reactions, such as a sudden change in facial expression or changes in posture that may indicate abdominal pain or discomfort, which may be caused by urinary retention, paralytic ileus, or constipation. The nurse need not monitor for changes in the style of walking, diet intake, or sleeping patterns, considering these are not known to indicate abdominal pain.

10. **Answer: d**

    RATIONALE: The use of cholinergic blocking drugs is contraindicated in patients with prostatic hypertrophy. It is not known to be contraindicated in patients with bone marrow depression, cardiac disorders, and visual impairment.

CHAPTER 33

SECTION I: ASSESSING YOUR UNDERSTANDING

Activity A MATCHING

1. 1-D, 2-C, 3-B, 4-A
2. 1-B, 2-C, 3-A

Activity B FILL IN THE BLANKS

1. Alzheimer's
2. Cholinergic
3. Liver
4. Brain
5. Hepatotoxicity

SECTION II: APPLYING YOUR KNOWLEDGE

Activity C SHORT ANSWERS

1. The nurse should assess the following in patients who are prescribed cholinesterase inhibitors:
   - Cognitive ability such as orientation, calculation, recall, and language, and functional ability such as performance of activities of daily living and self care
   - Agitation and impulsive behavior
   - Mental health and medical history, including a history of symptoms of Alzheimer's disease
   - Physical assessments, such as blood pressure measurements (on both arms with the patient in a sitting position), pulse, respiratory rate, and weight
   - Patient's vital signs and body weight

2. **a.** The nurse should perform the following interventions when caring for a patient receiving tacrine:
   - Monitor the patient for liver damage by monitoring levels of alanine aminotransferase (ALT)
   - Obtain ALT levels weekly
   - Monitor transaminase levels every 3 months from at least week 4 to week 16

   b. When caring for patients receiving tacrine, the nurse should monitor for adverse reactions that include nausea, vomiting, diarrhea, dizziness, and headache.

Activity D DOSAGE CALCULATION

1. 9 tablets
2. 2 tablets
3. 2 capsules
4. 3 capsules

SECTION III: PRACTICING FOR NCLEX

Activity E

1. **Answer: a**

   RATIONALE: The nurse should monitor the patient for diarrhea as an adverse reaction of cholinesterase inhibitors. High blood pressure, seizure disorders, and renal dysfunction are not adverse reactions to cholinesterase inhibitors.

2. **Answer: d**

   RATIONALE: Tacrine should be used cautiously in the case of patients with bladder obstruction. Tacrine need not be used cautiously in patients with vaginitis, diabetes mellitus, and cardiovascular problems.

3. **Answer: a, b, c**

   RATIONALE: When performing a physical assessment before administering cholinesterase inhibitors, the nurse should monitor the pulse, respiratory rate, and weight of the patient. The nurse need not monitor brain waves and hepatic function before administering cholinesterase inhibitors.

4. **Answer: b**

   RATIONALE: The nurse should immediately report any elevated ALT levels to the primary health care provider, who may want to continue monitoring the ALT level or discontinue use of the drug because of the danger of hepatotoxicity. However, abrupt discontinuation may cause a decline in cognitive functioning. Abrupt discontinuation of tacrine does not lead to a loss of functional ability, impulsive behavior, or nervous breakdown.

5. **Answer: c**

   RATIONALE: Increased risk of gastrointestinal bleeding is the effect when nonsteroidal anti-inflammatory drugs interact with cholinesterase inhibitors. Asthma, sick sinus syndrome, and increased risk of theophylline toxicity do not result from nonsteroidal anti-inflammatory drugs interacting with cholinesterase inhibitors. Increased risk of theophylline toxicity is the effect of the interaction of theophylline with cholinesterase inhibitors. Asthma and sick sinus syndrome are contraindications in the use of tacrine.

6. **Answer: c**

   RATIONALE: When administering tacrine to a patient, the nurse should monitor the patient for liver damage. Cardiovascular disease, pulmonary disease, and goiter are not associated with the administration of tacrine.

7. **Answer: a, c, e**

   RATIONALE: When caring for a patient receiving cholinesterase inhibitors, the nurse should use side rails, keep the bed in a low position, or use night lights in order to reduce the risk of injury in the patient. The nurse should monitor the patient frequently to reduce the risk of injury, instead of monitoring every 12 hours. The nurse does not need to use soft bedding as it may not help reduce the risk of injury in the patient.

8. **Answer: b**

   RATIONALE: The nurse should administer tacrine to the patient on an empty stomach. The nurse need not administer this drug 30 minutes before meals, 1 hour after meals, or around the clock intravenously to the patient. Instead, the nurse should administer tacrine 1 hour before or 2 hours after meals and around the clock orally.

9. **Answer: a**

   RATIONALE: Ginkgo is contraindicated in patients receiving monoamine oxidase inhibitors because of the risk of a toxic reaction. Ginkgo is not contraindicated in patients receiving sedatives and hypnotics, opioid analgesics, or anticholinergic drugs.

10. **Answer: a**

    RATIONALE: It is important for the nurse to provide proper attention to medication dosing because it helps to decrease adverse gastrointestinal reactions. Proper attention to the dosing of medication is not related to patient's faster recovery, maintenance of the patient's normal body temperature, or decreased variations in the patient's pulse rate.

CHAPTER 34

SECTION I: ASSESSING YOUR UNDERSTANDING

Activity A MATCHING

1. 1-C, 2-D, 3-A, 4-B
2. 1-B, 2-A, 3-D, 4-C

Activity B FILL IN THE BLANKS

1. Bisphosphonates
2. Allopurinol
3. Immunosuppression
4. Gout
5. Colchicine

SECTION II: APPLYING YOUR KNOWLEDGE

Activity C SHORT ANSWERS

1. Preadministration assessments that the nurse should conduct before administration of a musculoskeletal drug are as follows:
   - Obtain the patient's history of disorders, onset, symptoms, and current treatment or therapy.
   - Appraise the patient's physical condition and limitations.
   - Examine affected joints in extremities for appearance of the skin over the joint, evidence of joint deformity, and mobility of the affected joint.
   - Assess for pain in the upper and lower back or hip.
   - Document vital signs and weight.
   - Perform laboratory tests and bone scans to measure bone density, as ordered by the primary health care provider.

2. The ongoing assessments that a nurse should perform when caring for a patient receiving a musculoskeletal drug are as follows:
   - Evaluate the patient periodically for musculoskeletal disorders.
   - Inquire about pain relief and adverse reactions.
   - Evaluate the patient daily or weekly depending on patient's condition and drug.
   - Administer more toxic drugs if first-line treatments are not successful, as ordered by the primary health care provider.

- Closely observe the patient for the development of adverse reactions and report these to the primary health care provider if they occur.

Activity D DOSAGE CALCULATION

1. 3 tablets
2. 4 tablets
3. 3 tablets
4. 2 tablets
5. 6 tablets

SECTION III: PRACTICING FOR NCLEX

Activity E

1. **Answer: a**
   RATIONALE: Dyspepsia is the adverse reaction that the nurse should monitor for in the patient. Sleepiness, lethargy, and constipation are adverse reactions of the skeletal muscle reactant diazepam.

2. **Answer: b**
   RATIONALE: The use of alendronate is contraindicated in hypocalcemic patients. The use of alendronate is not contraindicated in patients with hypertension, insomnia, or diabetes.

3. **Answer: c**
   RATIONALE: The nurse should monitor for methotrexate toxicity in the patient when sulfa antibiotics interact with disease-modifying, antirheumatic drugs. Theophylline toxicity occurs when theophylline interacts with the uric acid inhibitor allopurinol. A rash occurs when ampicillin interacts with allopurinol. However, hepatotoxicity does not occur when disease-modifying antirheumatic drugs are administered along with sulfa antibiotics.

4. **Answer: a, b, c**
   RATIONALE: The nurse should monitor hematology, liver function, and renal function in patients administered methotrexate every 1 to 3 months. The nurse should notify the primary care provider of any abnormal hematology, liver function, or kidney function findings. However, the nurse need not monitor pancreatic and cardiovascular functions in patients administered methotrexate, considering these conditions are not known to occur as adverse reactions to this drug.

5. **Answer: d**
   RATIONALE: After administering DMARDs, the patient should notify the primary health care provider in the case of diarrhea. Administering drugs with food, drinking 10 glasses of water a day, and avoiding driving or hazardous tasks in case of drowsiness are instructions that a patient should follow when on drugs used to treat gout.

6. **Answer: b**
   RATIONALE: The nurse should closely monitor the patient for adverse reactions as an ongoing assessment for patients receiving bisphosphonates for musculoskeletal disorders. Obtaining the patient's history of disorders, appraising the patient's physical condition and limitations, and assessing for pain in the upper and lower back or hip are preadministration assessments for patients receiving drugs for musculoskeletal disorders.

7. **Answer: a, b, e**
   RATIONALE: Reporting adverse reactions, especially vision changes; being alert to reactions such as skin rash, fever, cough, or easy bruising; and being attentive to the patient's complaints such as tinnitus, or hearing loss, are the appropriate nursing interventions when a patient is receiving hydroxychloroquine for a musculoskeletal disorder. A nurse encourages liberal fluid intake and measures intake and output when using uric acid inhibitors. The nurse need not ask the patient to compensate for missed dosages.

8. **Answer: a**
   RATIONALE: Use of sulfinpyrazone is contraindicated in patients with peptic ulcer disease. The use of colchicine and not sulfinpyrazone is contraindicated in patients with renal, hepatic, and cardiac diseases.

9. **Answer: a**
   RATIONALE: When a patient with rheumatic arthritis is administered the uric acid inhibitor sulfinpyrazone along with oral anticoagulants, the interaction between the two can lead to an increased risk of bleeding in the patient. Interaction of tolbutamide with the uric acid inhibitor sulfinpyrazone can lead to an increased risk of hypoglycemia. Increased effect of verapamil is caused when verapamil interacts with sulfinpyrazone. Probenecid's effectiveness decreases when it is administered along with salicylates.

10. **Answer: a**
    RATIONALE: The nurse should examine the appearance of the skin over joints in patients with gout. Patients with arthritis will have affected joint mobility, patients with osteoporosis may suffer from pain in the upper and lower back or hip, and patient's with rheumatoid arthritis may display evidence of hearing loss.

CHAPTER 35

SECTION I: ASSESSING YOUR UNDERSTANDING

Activity A MATCHING

1. 1-C, 2-B, 3-D, 4-A
2. 1-B, 2-D, 3-C, 4-A

Activity B FILL IN THE BLANKS

1. Expectorant
2. Opioid
3. Dextromethorphan
4. Atelectasis
5. Lozenges
6. Respiratory

SECTION II: APPLYING YOUR KNOWLEDGE

Activity C SHORT ANSWERS

1. The nurse should perform the following preadministration assessments:
   - Document the type of cough (productive, nonproductive).
   - Describe the color and amount of sputum present.
   - Assess and record vital signs.
2. The nurse's role after he or she administers antitussives to the patient includes:
   - Monitoring for a therapeutic effect
   - Auscultating the lung
   - Taking vital signs periodically
   - Recording the type of cough in the chart
   - Recording the frequency of coughing in the patient's chart
   - Noting and recording whether the cough interrupts sleep or causes pain in the chest or other parts of the body

Activity D DOSAGE CALCULATION

1. 4 capsules
2. 6 tablets
3. 4 gelcaps
4. 6 tablets

SECTION III: PRACTICING FOR NCLEX

Activity E

1. **Answer: b, c, e**
   RATIONALE: When caring for a patient who has been prescribed an expectorant for the treatment of a cough, the nurse should assess the respiratory status of the patient, document lung sounds, and record consistency of sputum. The nurse need not ask the patient about throat infection or examine the patient's pulse rate every 30 minutes.

2. **Answer: b, c, e**
   RATIONALE: The nurse should include instructions in the teaching plan, such as avoiding irritants including cigarette smoke, avoiding drinking fluids for 30 minutes after taking the drug, and avoiding chewing or breaking open the oral capsules for a patient undergoing antitussive drug therapy. This patient need not take the medicine 1 hour before meals or take the medicine with milk to enhance absorption.

3. **Answer: b**
   RATIONALE: The nurse should monitor the patient for sedation as a reaction associated with antitussive administration. The nurse need not monitor the patient for diarrhea, somnolence, and dehydration because these are not reactions associated with antitussive administration.

4. **Answer: d**
   RATIONALE: The nurse should know that antitussives are contraindicated in the patient with hypersensitivity to the drug. Antitussives are not contraindicated in patients with cardiac problems, asthma, or liver dysfunction.

5. **Answer: a**
   RATIONALE: The nurse should be aware that hypokalemia is a possible effect of potassium-containing medication interacting with iodine products. Hypoglycemia, hypertension, and hemorrhage are not effects of the interaction of potassium-containing medication with iodine products.

6. **Answer: b**
   RATIONALE: The nurse should encourage fluid intake of up to 2000 mL per day, if this amount is not contraindicated by the patient's condition or disease process, to promote effective airway clearance. The nurse need not monitor fluid intake of the patient every 8 hours, encourage taking mucolytics after each coughing episode, or suggest avoiding the consumption of milk products.

7. **Answer: b**
   RATIONALE: The nurse should instruct the patient to dilute the medicine before use. The nurse need not instruct the patient to take the medicine on an empty stomach, take the drug with warm milk, or warm the medicine before use.

8. **Answer: a**
   RATIONALE: The nurse should instruct the patient to consult the primary health care provider if the cough lasts more than 10 days. The nurse need not instruct the patient to consult the primary health care provider if the patient's cough is accompanied by dizziness, the frequency of coughing is 20 minutes, or the cough is accompanied by vomiting.

9. **Answer: b**
   RATIONALE: The nurse should ensure that suction equipment is at the patient's bedside, immediately available for the aspiration of secretions. The nurse need not ensure that the patient is taking only this drug therapy, gets continuous oxygen supply, or keeps drinking warm water.

10. **Answer: a**
    Rationale: The nurse should monitor for hypotension in the patient. The nurse need not monitor the patient for dyspepsia, bronchitis, or opisthotonos as risks associated with the interaction of dextromethorphan with monoamine oxidase inhibitors.

CHAPTER 36

SECTION I: ASSESSING YOUR UNDERSTANDING

Activity A MATCHING

1. 1-C, 2-E, 3-B, 4-A, 5-D
2. 1-D, 2-E, 3-A, 4-B, 5-C

Activity B FILL IN THE BLANKS

1. Mast

2. Decongestant
3. Vasoconstriction
4. Histamine
5. Sedating

SECTION II: APPLYING YOUR KNOWLEDGE

Activity C SHORT ANSWERS

1. The nurse should include the following points in the teaching plan for a patient who is prescribed antihistamines to combat the symptoms of angioneurotic edema:
   - If there is drowsiness, do not drive or perform hazardous tasks. The drowsiness may diminish with continued use.
   - While taking the drug, avoid the use of alcohol and other drugs that can cause drowsiness.
   - Take frequent sips of water, suck on hard candy, or chew gum (preferably sugarless) to relieve the dryness of mouth and throat that may be caused by antihistamine use.
   - If gastric upset occurs, take the drug with food. If the gastric upset is not relieved, talk to the primary health care provider.
   - Avoid taking fexofenadine within 2 hours of taking an antacid.
   - Do not crush or chew the sustained-release preparations.
2. The decongestant used for sinusitis may be a topical or oral medication. The nurse should assure the patient that topical decongestants have minimal systemic effects in most individuals. Occasional side effects seen with topical decongestants include:
   - Nasal burning
   - Nasal stinging
   - Dryness of the nasal mucosa
   On frequent use or swallowing of the topical decongestant liquid, similar side effects are seen as those with oral decongestants. Use of oral decongestants may result in the following side effects:
   - Tachycardia and other cardiac arrhythmias
   - Nervousness, restlessness, and insomnia
   - Blurred vision
   - Nausea and vomiting

Activity D DOSAGE CALCULATION

1. 2 teaspoonfuls
2. 3 tablets
3. 4 tablets
4. 2.5 teaspoonfuls
5. 4 tablets
6. 2 tablets

SECTION III: PRACTICING FOR NCLEX

Activity E

1. **Answer: a, b, d**
   RATIONALE: The nurse should inform the patient taking prescribed antihistamines about the possible side effects, such as thickening of the bronchial mucosa, disturbed coordination and anaphylactic shock or urticaria (hives). Though antihistamines are used to treat allergies, they themselves can cause allergic reactions, including anaphylactic shock and urticaria. Increased frequency of micturition and excessive sweating and salivation are not seen with antihistamines. They can cause dryness of the oral mucosa.

2. **Answer: c**
   RATIONALE: The nurse should administer the antihistamine with caution if there is angle-closure glaucoma. Acute conjunctivitis and allergic rhinitis are indications for the use of antihistamines. Precaution is also needed when the drug is given in a hypertensive patient, but not in a hypotensive patient.

3. **Answer: a, c, d**
   RATIONALE: When caring for an elderly patient on decongestant therapy, the nurse should monitor for symptoms of overdosage, such as hallucination, convulsion, and central nervous system (CNS) depression. Dyspnea and fatigue are not seen commonly with the use of decongestants.

4. **Answer: d**
   RATIONALE: The nurse should tell the patient to administer the drug via inhaler by warming it in his or her hand before use. The nasal spray should be administered by sitting upright and sniffing hard. The tip of the container should not touch the nasal mucosa. Nasal drops should be administered by reclining on the bed with the head hanging.

5. **Answer: c**
   RATIONALE: The nurse should assess blood pressure before administering promethazine in a patient who is also taking an opioid analgesic. Bone density, urine output, and skin turgidity need not be assessed.

6. **Answer: b**
   RATIONALE: The nurse should choose the deep intramuscular route for administering antihistamines because certain antihistamines may irritate the skin and the subcutaneous tissue. Intravenous, intradermal, and subcutaneous routes are, therefore, not preferred.

7. **Answer: c–a–e–b–d–f**
   RATIONALE: In response to injury, histamine is first released. It produces dilatation of the arterioles, which results in localized redness and increased capillary permeability. This leads to escape of fluids from the blood vessels, producing localized swelling.

8. **Answer: c**
   RATIONALE: The nurse should inform the patient that magnesium-based antacids could reduce the

effects of antihistamines by reducing their absorption. Beta-blocking agents and opioid analgesics enhance the effects of antihistamines. Monoamine oxidase inhibitors do not reduce the effects of antihistamines.

9. **Answer: a, b, e**
RATIONALE: The nurse should administer decongestants cautiously in patients with hypertension, hyperthyroidism, or glaucoma. No extra caution is required when the drug is used with conjunctivitis or nephropathy.

10. **Answer: b, d, e**
RATIONALE: The nurse should instruct the patient taking antihistamines to avoid the use of alcohol and other sedatives as they can increase the CNS depressant action of antihistamines. The drug should be taken with food to avoid gastric upset. Frequent sips of water or sucking on hard candy can help relieve the dryness of mouth, nose, and throat seen with the use of these drugs. Antihistamines should not be taken within 2 hours of taking an antacid. Aluminum- and magnesium-based antacids decrease the absorption of the medication. Sustained-release tablets should never be crushed or chewed before use; they should be taken whole.

CHAPTER 37

SECTION I: ASSESSING YOUR UNDERSTANDING

Activity A MATCHING

1. 1-D, 2-C, 3-E, 4-A, 5-B
2. 1-B, 2-E, 3-A, 4-C, 5-D

Activity B FILL IN THE BLANKS

1. Dilatation
2. Mucus
3. Wheezing
4. Calcium
5. Agonist

SECTION II: APPLYING YOUR KNOWLEDGE

Activity C SHORT ANSWERS

1. a. The nurse should inform the patient about the following possible adverse effects of theophylline:
   - Restlessness
   - Nervousness
   - Tachycardia
   - Tremors
   - Headache
   - Palpitations
   - Increased respirations
   - Nausea
   - Vomiting
   - Fever
   - Hyperglycemia
   - Electrocardiographic changes
   b. The nurse should include the following points in the patient teaching plan:
   - Take the drug exactly as ordered.
   - Do not increase the dose or frequency on your own. Consult the health care provider if symptoms become worse.
   - Follow your primary health care provider's instructions concerning the monitoring of theophylline serum levels.
   - If gastric upset occurs, take the drug with food or milk.
   - Do not chew or crush sustained-release tablets.
   - Drink plenty of water each day to decrease the thickness of secretions.
   - Do not use any over-the-counter drugs unless approved by the health care provider.
   - Avoid smoking while on the drug.
   - Avoid cola, coffee, chocolate, and charcoal-prepared foods.
   - Do not change to any other brand of drug without consulting the physician.

2. The nurse needs to carefully observe a patient with chronic bronchitis before administrating bronchodilator therapy. All preadministration assessments must be carefully documented. These assessments should include the following:
   - Assess vital signs, including blood pressure, pulse, and respiratory rate. A respiratory rate less than 12 breaths/minute or greater than 24 breaths/minute is considered abnormal.
   - Assess the lung fields and properly document the sounds heard.
   - Note any difficulty in breathing, coughing, wheezing, "noisy" respirations, or use of accessory muscles when breathing.
   - If there is expectoration, record a description of the sputum.
   - Note and record the patient's general physical condition.
   - Record any signs of hypoxia-like mental confusion, restlessness, anxiety, and cyanosis.
   - Note that the health care provider may order arterial blood gas analysis or pulmonary function tests.
   - Ask the patient questions concerning allergies, frequency of attacks, severity of attacks, factors that cause or relieve attacks, and any antiasthmatic drugs used currently or taken previously.

Activity D DOSAGE CALCULATION

1. 2 teaspoonfuls
2. 0.25 mL
3. 0.5 mL of the diluted solution
4. 0.25 mL
5. 300 mg
6. 0.1 mL

SECTION III: PRACTICING FOR NCLEX

Activity E

1. **Answer: c**
   RATIONALE: Terbutaline is a safer drug to administer to a pregnant patient with acute respiratory distress. Terbutaline comes under U.S. Food and Drug Administration (FDA) Pregnancy Category B and can be used with caution. All other sympathomimetic bronchodilators, including albuterol, epinephrine, and salmeterol, are under Pregnancy Category C. These drugs can be used only if the expected benefits clearly outweigh the potential risks to the fetus.

2. **Answer: d**
   RATIONALE: The nurse should inform the patient that beta-blockers could increase the effects of aminophylline. Ketoconazole, rifampin, and loop diuretics decrease the effects of theophyllines, including aminophylline.

3. **Answer: a**
   RATIONALE: The nurse should assess the electrocardiographic changes to check for the occurrence of adverse effects with aminophylline. Aminophylline belongs to the theophylline group, which causes electrocardiographic changes as side effects. Changes in blood hemoglobin, fluid intake and output, or the consistency of stool are not adverse effects associated with aminophylline.

4. **Answer: b**
   RATIONALE: The nurse may observe increased sweating, or diaphoresis, in a patient with asthma. Increased micturition, decreased pulse rate, or decreased blood pressure is not seen in patients with asthma. During an asthmatic attack, there may be an increased pulse rate.

5. **Answer: b**
   RATIONALE: When zafirlukast is given to a patient on aspirin, there may be an increase in the plasma levels of zafirlukast. The absorption of zafirlulast does not decrease in a patient taking aspirin along with zafirlulast. Similarly, there is no decrease in the plasma levels or increase in the thrombolytic effects of aspirin because of such an interaction.

6. **Answer: c–d–b–e–a**
   RATIONALE: In asthma, the mast cells release histamine. This causes increased mucus formation and edema of the airway, leading to bronchospasm and inflammation. This leads to narrowing of the airway along with clogging caused by extra mucus. When the airways are narrowed, the airflow to the lungs decreases.

7. **Answers: a, b, d**
   RATIONALE: Corticosteroids, leukotriene formation inhibitors, and mast cell stabilizers may be used as adjunct therapy, along with bronchodilators in asthmatic patients. They relieve the inflammation associated with asthma. Uricosuric agents and leukotriene receptor antagonists are not used as adjunct therapy to treat asthma. Uricosuric agents are used in the treatment of gout. Leukotriene receptor agonists may be used as adjunct therapy to treat asthma.

8. **Answers: b, c, e**
   RATIONALE: Flunisolide, beclomethasone, and triamcinolone are inhalational corticosteroid agents used in the treatment of asthma. Cromolyn and ipratropium are not used in the treatment of asthma. Cromolyn is a mast cell stabilizer. Ipratropium is an anticholinergic drug.

9. **Answers: b, d, e**
   RATIONALE: When a patient on antiasthmatic drugs experiences nausea, the nurse should instruct the patient to eat small frequent meals, limit fluids with meals, and rinse the mouth properly after eating. These interventions will help alleviate the symptoms of nausea. Keeping the head end of the bed elevated helps in preventing the symptoms of heartburn and not nausea. Sucking on sugarless candy may help alleviate the unpleasant taste sensation experienced with certain antiasthmatic drugs and may not alleviate the symptoms of nausea.

10. **Answer: a**
    RATIONALE: The nurse should instruct the patient to take montelukast orally only once in the evening. This drug should be taken even when there are no symptoms. The health care provider should be contacted if asthma is not well controlled, even with therapy. The patient should not take the drug more than once daily.

CHAPTER 38

SECTION I: ASSESSING YOUR UNDERSTANDING

Activity A MATCHING

1. 1-C, 2-A, 3-D, 4-B
2. 1-D, 2-F, 3-A, 4-C, 5-B, 6-E

Activity B FILL IN THE BLANKS

1. Intravenous
2. Left
3. Neonatal
4. Bradycardia
5. Digitalized

SECTION II: APPLYING YOUR KNOWLEDGE

Activity C SHORT ANSWERS

1. Before starting digoxin administration, the nurse should make the following physical assessments:
   - Record the patient's blood pressure, apical-radial pulse rate, and respiratory rate.
   - Measure the patient's weight.

- Check for distension of the jugular veins.
- Examine for edema in the extremities.
- Look for cyanosis, dyspnea, and mental changes.
- Auscultate the lungs for any unusual sounds during inspiration or expiration.
- Inspect any sputum expelled and note its appearance.

2. The nurse should include the following points in the teaching plan for patients taking digitalis:
   - Take the drug at the same time every day.
   - Record the pulse before taking the drug. Withhold the drug and notify the primary health care provider if the pulse is less than 60 or more than 100 beats per minute.
   - Do not discontinue the drug or take an extra dose without consulting the primary health care provider.
   - Report to the health care center any signs of digitalis toxicity, such as nausea, vomiting, diarrhea, unusual fatigue, weakness, and vision changes.
   - Carry or wear a medical alert band.
   - Do not take over-the-counter drugs unless the health care provider approves them.
   - Keep the drug in its original container.

Activity D DOSAGE CALCULATION

1. 2 tablets
2. 5 ampoules
3. 10 vials
4. 5 mL
5. 8 vials
6. 3 ampoules

Section III: PRACTICING FOR NCLEX

Activity E

1. **Answer: a**
   RATIONALE: These signs and symptoms indicate that the patient is experiencing heart failure. The symptoms of heart failure are cough, dyspnea, weakness, anorexia, and unusual fatigue. Signs of heart failure include pitting edema and distended jugular veins. There is also reduced ejection fraction. These signs and symptoms are not seen in glomerulonephritis, pulmonary disease, or hypothyroidism.

2. **Answer: b**
   RATIONALE: The nurse should monitor for signs of digoxin toxicity. The effect of benzodiazepine–digoxin interaction results in increased plasma digoxin levels. Increasing the dosage of digoxin or the benzodiazepine will result in digoxin toxicity. Signs of reduced effectiveness of digoxin are seen with thyroid hormone administration and not with benzodiazepines.

3. **Answer: c**
   RATIONALE: Digitalis can be used in atrial fibrillation. Digitalis is contraindicated in ventricular tachycardia, atrioventricular block, and ventricular failure.

4. **Answer: d**
   RATIONALE: The nurse should withhold the drug and notify the practitioner. A pulse rate less than 60 beats per minute indicates digoxin toxicity. Increasing the infusion rate will augment the toxicity. Gastrointestinal suctioning causes hypokalemia, which sensitizes the heart to digoxin toxicity. Milrinone lactate is given in unresponsive cases of heart failure, not in toxic states.

5. **Answer: b**
   RATIONALE: The nurse should administer approximately half the total dose as the first dose. During rapid digitalization, several doses are administered over a period of time. The first dose is approximately half the total dose. Additional doses are administered at intervals of 6–8 hours.

6. **Answer: a, d, e**
   RATIONALE: The signs of digoxin toxicity that the nurse should assess for are anorexia, blurred vision, and vomiting. Headache and weakness are adverse effects of digoxin, even at normal dosage, and do not signify digoxin toxicity.

7. **Answer: b, c, d**
   RATIONALE: The nurse should report electrolyte changes such as hypokalemia, hypomagnesemia, and hypocalcemia to the practitioner. These changes increase the sensitivity of the heart muscle to the effects of digitalis. This, in turn, increases the risk for developing digitalis toxicity. Hyponatremia and hypophosphatemia do not increase the risk of digitalis toxicity.

8. **Answer: b, d, e**
   RATIONALE: Appropriate interventions include ensuring that the patient consumes small frequent meals, restricts fluid intake at meals, and rinses mouth after meals. These are techniques that help control nausea and vomiting. Fluid intake at meals will increase the feeling of nausea and should be avoided 1 hour before meals. Doubling the drug dosage will worsen the condition.

9. **Answer: c, d, e**
   RATIONALE: The adverse effects of digitalis administration that the nurse should assess for are drowsiness, vomiting, and arrhythmias. Hepatotoxicity is the adverse effect of inamrinone administration, not digitalis administration. Similarly, angina is the adverse effect of milrinone administration, not digitalis administration.

10. **Answer: b–c–d–a–e**
    RATIONALE: The nurse should teach the steps involved in the calculation of the pulse. Place the nondominant arm on the table or arm of the chair. Place the index and third fingers of the other hand on the wrist bone. Feel for a beating or pulsing sensation, which is the pulse. Record the number of times the pulse beats in a minute. If the pulse beats more than 100 beats per minute, notify the practitioner.

CHAPTER 39

SECTION I: ASSESSING YOUR UNDERSTANDING

Activity A MATCHING

1. 1-D, 2-A, 3-E, 4-B, 5-C
2. 1-C, 2-A, 3-D, 4-E, 5-B

Activity B FILL IN THE BLANKS

1. Threshold
2. Sympathetic
3. Proarrhythmic
4. Sodium
5. Hypertension

SECTION II: APPLYING YOUR KNOWLEDGE

Activity C SHORT ANSWERS

1. a. When a patient is prescribed an antiarrhythmic agent, the nurse should inform him about the following possible adverse effects that are common to most antiarrhythmic agents:
   - Central nervous system effects
     - Light-headedness
     - Weakness
     - Somnolence
   - Cardiovascular effects
     - Hypotension
     - Arrhythmia
     - Bradycardia
   - Other effects
     - Urinary retention
     - Local inflammation
   All of the antiarrhythmic drugs need to be used cautiously in cases of:
   - Renal disease
   - Hepatic disease
   - Electrolyte imbalance
   - Congestive heart failure (CHF)
   - Pregnancy
   - Lactation
   - Children
   b. The drug disopyramide is used cautiously in those with:
   - Myasthenia gravis
   - Urinary retention
   - Glaucoma
   - Prostate enlargement
2. Before administering an antiarrhythmic agent, the nurse should perform the following assessments:
   - Assess and record the blood pressure, apical and radical pulses, and respiratory rate for comparison during therapy.
   - Assess and record the patient's general condition, including skin color, orientation, level of consciousness, and general status.
   - Record any symptoms described by the patient.
   - Review and report any abnormalities in any laboratory and diagnostic tests, renal and hepatic function tests, complete blood count, and serum enzymes and electrolyte analyses, as directed by the health care provider.
   - Possibly put the patient on a cardiac monitor before initiating therapy.
   - Ensure an electrocardiogram (ECG) is performed, if ordered by the primary health care provider, to provide baseline data for comparison during therapy.

Activity D DOSAGE CALCULATION

1. 1.5 tablets per dose
2. 2 tablets per dose
3. 5.5 mL
4. 80 mg in each dose
5. 3500 mg
6. 195 mg

SECTION III: PRACTICING FOR NCLEX

Activity E

1. **Answer: b**
   RATIONALE: Disopyramide is an example of a class IA antiarrhythmic drug. Disopyramide decreases the depolarization of myocardial fibers during the diastolic phase of the cardiac cycle, prolongs the refractory period, and increases the action potential duration of normal cardiac cells. Lidocaine belongs to class IB drugs, propafenone to class IC drugs, and amiodarone to class III antiarrhythmic drugs.

2. **Answer: d**
   RATIONALE: Flecainide depresses the sodium channels in the heart. It is an antihypertensive belonging to the class IC drugs. It depresses fast sodium channels, decreases the height and rate of rise of action potentials, and slows conduction of all areas of the heart. It does not depress the calcium, chloride, or oxygen channels of the heart.

3. **Answer: c**
   RATIONALE: Light-headedness is a possible adverse effect seen with antiarrhythmic drug therapy. Other adverse effects include hypotension, somnolence, and urinary retention. Hypertension, insomnia, and frequent urination are not adverse effects of antiarrhythmic drugs.

4. **Answer: c**
   RATIONALE: Amiodarone belongs to U.S. Food and Drug Administration (FDA) pregnancy category D. Drugs in this category have demonstrated a risk to the fetus in adequate, well-controlled, or observational studies in pregnant women. However, the drug may be given in a life-threatening situation if safer drugs cannot be used or are ineffective. The category B drugs show a risk to the fetus in animal studies. Either there are no controlled human studies or well-controlled human studies fail to show any risk to the fetus. These drugs may be used cautiously in pregnancy. The category C

drugs may be used in pregnancy only if the possible benefits clearly outweigh the potential hazards to the fetus. In category X drugs, the risks clearly outweigh the benefits. Therefore these drugs are clearly contraindicated in pregnancy.

5. **Answer: d**

RATIONALE: The nurse should immediately notify the primary health care provider when the pulse rate is below 60 beats per minute or above 120 beats per minute. Pulse rates of 82 beats per minute, 92 beats per minute, and 102 beats per minute fall within the controllable range of patients with tachycardia.

6. **Answer: c**

RATIONALE: The nurse should instruct the patient to eat small, frequent meals instead of a few large ones. This will help alleviate nausea, which is a common adverse effect seen with the use of antiarrhythmic drugs. The nurse should instruct the patient to avoid lying flat for at least 2 hours after meals in order to prevent nausea. The drug should be administered with meals to avoid gastric upset. Drinking lots of fluid after the drug may lead to vomiting if there is nausea.

7. **Answer: d**

RATIONALE: When taken concurrently with disopyramide, rifampin can decrease the serum levels of disopyramide. When taken concurrently with disopyramide, erythromycin and quinidine increase the levels of disopyramide in the serum. Thioridazine increases the risk of life-threatening arrhythmias and does not decrease the serum levels of disopyramide if the drugs are taken concurrently.

8. **Answer: d**

RATIONALE: The nurse should report a lidocaine blood level of 6.0 mcg/mL to the health care provider. A blood level higher than that is associated with an increased risk of central nervous system and cardiovascular depression. Blood lidocaine levels of 1.5 mcg/mL, 3.0 mcg/mL, and 4.5 mcg/mL are not a cause of alert and need not be reported immediately to the health care provider.

9. **Answer: a, d, e**

RATIONALE: Weakness, arrhythmias, and light-headedness are possible adverse effects of antiarrhythmic drugs. Another possible adverse effect is hypotension, not hypertension. Somnolence, and not insomnia, may also occur as an adverse effect associated with antiarrhythmic drugs.

10. **Answer: b**

RATIONALE: Shortness of breath may be seen as a sign of heart failure in elderly patients on antiarrhythmic drug therapy. Other signs include an increase in weight and decrease in urine output. Heart failure does not cause a decrease in weight or an increase in urine volume. Chills and fever may be seen with antiarrhythmic drug therapy, but they are not caused by heart failure. Rather,

they may result from agranulocytosis, an adverse reaction to antiarrhythmic drugs.

CHAPTER 40

SECTION I: ASSESSING YOUR UNDERSTANDING

Activity A MATCHING

1. 1-B, 2-D, 3-A, 4-C, 5-F, 6-G, 7-E
2. 1-B, 2-C, 3-A

Activity B FILL IN THE BLANKS

1. Coronary
2. Calcium
3. Smooth
4. Dermatitis
5. Claudication

SECTION II: APPLYING YOUR KNOWLEDGE

Activity C SHORT ANSWERS

1. The nurse should educate patients having anginal attacks about certain aspects of the disease and also about the use of antianginal drugs. The teaching plan should include the following:
   - Take the drug regularly, as recommended by the health care provider.
   - Notify the health care provider if the pain worsens or is not relieved by the medication.
   - Take the oral medications on an empty stomach, unless told otherwise by the health care provider.
   - Avoid the consumption of alcohol, unless directed otherwise by the health care provider.
   - Keep an additional supply of the drug for events such as vacations and bad weather conditions.
   - Maintain a record of acute anginal attacks. This should include the date, time of the attack, and dose used to relieve pain.

2. The nurse should make certain the following assessments of a patient receiving vasodilator therapy.
   - Assess the involved extremity daily for color and temperature changes.
   - Record the patient's comments regarding pain improvement or relief following therapy.
   - Monitor the pulse and blood pressure once or twice a day. This is to detect any fall in the blood pressure, which occurs with the use of these drugs.
   - When cilostazol is used for treating intermittent claudication, assess for improvement in the walking distance.

Activity D DOSAGE CALCULATION

1. 2 tablets
2. 2 tablets
3. 2 tablets
4. 2.5 mL
5. 2 tablets
6. 7 tablets

SECTION III: PRACTICING FOR NCLEX

Activity E

1. **Answer: a**
   RATIONALE: After three doses of sublingual nitroglycerin given every 5 minutes, the nurse should report to the practitioner of no improvement. The nurse should administer three doses of sublingual nitroglycerin in a 15-minute period. If the pain worsens or if there is no improvement in the pain, he or she should notify the primary health care provider. In such cases, a change of dosage or alternate drug therapy may be required.

2. **Answer: d**
   RATIONALE: The nurse should administer cilostazol 30 minutes before food or 2 hours after food to ensure optimal absorption of the drug. Cilostazol should not be administered with grape juice as it increases the blood concentration of the drug. Antianginal drugs and not cilostazol need to be given in the supine position to prevent postural hypotension.

3. **Answer: b**
   RATIONALE: The nurse should identify that L-arginine brings about its action by increasing the nitric oxide concentration. L-arginine is a herb used in the treatment of heart failure, hypertension, and peripheral vascular diseases (PVDs). Abnormalities of the vascular endothelium cause the degradation of nitric oxide. L-arginine is used in vascular conditions because it increases nitric oxide levels. Calcium channel blockers, and not L-arginine, are involved in blocking calcium channels. L-arginine is not involved in promoting sodium retention or in blocking alpha-adrenergic receptors.

4. **Answer: c**
   RATIONALE: Isoxsuprine is the drug that is not given in the immediate postpartum period. Isoxsuprine, a vasodilator used in to treat PVDs, should not be given in the immediate postpartum period as it causes the uterus to relax. Nitroglycerin and isosorbide dinitrate are nitrates used to treat angina. These drugs are used cautiously in pregnancy and lactation. Nifedipine is a calcium channel-blocking drug, which is used cautiously in pregnancy and lactation. Nitroglycerin, isosorbide dinitrate, and nifedipine are not used in the treatment of PVD.

5. **Answer: b**
   RATIONALE: Papaverine can be given in the management of PVDs. Papaverine is a vasodilating drug, which acts on the smooth muscle layers of the blood vessel. Nitroglycerin, isosorbide mononitrate, and amyl nitrite are vasodilating drugs used in the management of angina, not for PVDs.

6. **Answer: b, c, e**
   RATIONALE: The effects of calcium channel blockers on the heart include retarding the conduction velocity, dilating the coronary arteries, and depressing myocardial contractility. Calcium channel blockers act by blocking the calcium channel present in the cardiac and vascular smooth muscle layers. By depressing the myocardial contractility, these drugs do not increase, but rather decrease, the heart rate. Some of the calcium channel blockers are used in atrial fibrillation, which is rapid contractions occurring in the atrial muscle. Calcium channel blockers do not cause rapid atrial contractions.

7. **Answer: c, d, e**
   RATIONALE: The nurse should monitor for asthenia, arrhythmia and flushing in patients receiving diltiazem. Diltiazem is a calcium channel blocker used in the treatment of angina. The adverse effects occurring with diltiazem therapy include dizziness, peripheral edema, headache, nausea and constipation. It also causes hypotension and bradycardia. Hypertension and tachycardia do not occur with diltiazem use.

8. **Answer: b, c, e**
   RATIONALE: An increase in painless walking distance, decrease in leg pain and cramping, and reduced scaling of the affected area indicate improvement with cilostazol therapy. During such therapy, the nurse should assess for decreased pain and cramping, improvement of skin color and temperature, and an increase in painless walking distance. Warmth and not coldness will increase in the extremities on improvement following therapy. The amplitude of the peripheral pulse will also increase, not decrease.

9. **Answer: b, c, e**
   RATIONALE: The nurse should assess for adverse effects such as sedation, flushing, and headache in patients taking isoxsuprine, which is a vasodilating drug used in the treatment of PVD. Hypotension and tachycardia are the other adverse effects caused by use of peripheral vasodilators. Hypertension and bradycardia are not adverse effects associated with isoxsuprine.

10. **Answer: b–d–c–a**
    Rationale: The nurse should instruct the patient taking translingual nitrates to read the instructions supplied with the product properly before using nitrates. The drug should be used prophylactically 5–10 minutes before engaging in strenuous activities. The patient should be instructed to spray one or two metered doses of nitrate under or onto the tongue when chest pain occurs. If the pain does not subside after taking three metered doses in a 15-minute period, the patient should report to the health care provider.

CHAPTER 41

SECTION I: ASSESSING YOUR UNDERSTANDING

Activity A MATCHING

1. 1-C, 2-A, 3-E, 4-B, 5-D
2. 1-B, 2-D, 3-E, 4-A, 5-C

Activity B FILL IN THE BLANKS

1. Vasoconstrictor
2. Diuretic
3. Hypertensive
4. Sodium
5. Hyponatremia

SECTION II: APPLYING YOUR KNOWLEDGE

Activity C SHORT ANSWERS

1. When caring for a patient on captopril therapy, the nurse should perform the following assessments:
   - Monitor the blood pressure in the same arm in the same position every time. The blood pressure should be recorded every 15–30 minutes for at least 2 hr after the first dose of captopril is administered. The nurse is monitoring for hypotension, which occurs with angiotensin converting enzyme (ACE) inhibitors. Notify the health care provider if the blood pressure increases or decreases.
   - Weigh the patient regularly during the initial period of the therapy. A weight gain of 2 lb or more per day should be reported.
   - Assess for edema of the extremities and also in the sacral area. If edema is present, the nurse should notify the health care provider.
2. When caring for a patient taking antihypertensive drugs, the nurse should include the following points in the patient teaching plan:
   - Take the drug regularly and do not discontinue or stop the drug. Notify the health care provider before doing so.
   - Have regular blood pressure checkups and record the readings.
   - Avoid over-the-counter drugs, unless approved by the health care provider.
   - Avoid the consumption of alcohol, unless approved by the practitioner.
   - Educate the patient about precautions to be taken to prevent dizziness or lightheadedness.
   - Avoid performing hazardous tasks or tasks involving the need for alertness if drowsiness occurs.
   - Educate the patient about the adverse effects occurring with the therapy.
   - Inform the patient to contact the health care provider if adverse effects occur.
   - Implement diet recommendations given.

Activity D DOSAGE CALCULATION

1. 8 tablets
2. 2 ampoules
3. 2 tablets
4. 3 tablets
5. 4 tablets
6. Half a tablet

SECTION III: PRACTICING FOR NCLEX

Activity E

1. **Answer: a**
   RATIONALE: Systolic pressure between 120 and 139 mm Hg is indicative of prehypertension, which poses a risk for the development of hypertension. Individuals with such blood pressure changes should practice certain lifestyle changes.
2. **Answer: b**
   RATIONALE: Captopril is an ACE inhibitor, which is contraindicated in patients with renal impairment. Hydralazine and minoxidil are vasodilating drugs used for hypertension management and are administered to patients with renal impairment after dose adjustments. Doxazosin is an alpha-adrenergic blocker used for the treatment of hypertension, and it may be administered with caution to patients with renal impairment.
3. **Answer: d**
   RATIONALE: Nitroprusside is the drug that should be administered in hypertensive emergencies. Nitroprusside, which is a potent vasodilator, should be given IV to bring down the blood pressure rapidly. If the blood pressure is not lowered, it damages the kidneys, eyes, and heart. Amlodipine, acebutolol, and diltiazem are not the preferred drugs in hypertensive emergencies.
4. **Answer: c**
   RATIONALE: The risk of hypoglycemia increases with the simultaneous use of insulin and ACE inhibitors like enalapril. Use of potassium-sparing diuretics along with ACE inhibitors increases the risk of electrolyte imbalance. Concomitant allopurinol usage increases the risk of hypersensitivity reactions. There is increased risk of hypotensive effects occurring with the concomitant use of diuretics. However, increased risk of hypersensitivity, hypotensive effect, and electrolyte imbalance do not occur when both the drugs are used.
5. **Answer: c, d, e**
   RATIONALE: Headache is a common adverse effect of antiadrenergic drugs. The nurse should instruct the patient to apply a cool cloth over the forehead, to engage in progressive body relaxation, and to take an analgesic drug. Elevating the legs above the head in a supine position increases the blood gushing to the head and worsens the headache. Stopping prazosin will not relieve the headache.
6. **Answer: a, d, e**
   RATIONALE: The nurse should report changes such as swelling of the face, difficulty in breathing, and angina or severe indigestion, to the practitioner in patients receiving minoxidil. Minoxidil is a vasodilating drug used in the treatment of hypertension. Minoxidil causes a rapid rise in the heart rate. A rise in the heart rate of 20 beats per minute or more should be reported. Weight gain of 5 lb or more, not 1 lb, should also be reported.

7. Answer: a

RATIONALE: The nurse should ensure that captopril is taken 1 hour before or 2 hours after food to enhance the absorption of the drug. Captopril should not be given along with food. This will retard absorption. Rubbing the patient's back prior to administration and engaging the patient in exercise will not affect absorption. Hence, the nurse need not be involved in such activities.

8. Answer: a, d, e

RATIONALE: Orthostatic hypotension is common during the initial therapy with antihypertensives such as terazosin. The nurse should instruct the patient experiencing orthostatic hypotension to rise slowly from a sitting or lying position, rest on the bed for 1 or 2 minutes before rising, and stand still for a few minutes after rising. Increasing the fluid intake or applying a cool cloth over the forehead will not relieve dizziness.

9. Answer: b, c, d

RATIONALE: Heart disease, blindness, and stroke will occur as a consequence of hypertension. Hypertension causes the heart to work harder and leads to the production of atherosclerosis. Obesity and adrenal tumors are risk factors for the development of hypertension, not the consequences.

10. Answer: a, b, e

RATIONALE: The nurse should inform the patient that hypotension, sedation, and arrhythmia are adverse effects seen with hawthorn use. Hawthorn is a natural agent used to treat cardiovascular problems. Neutropenia and pruritus are the adverse effects of ACE inhibitors and not of hawthorn use.

CHAPTER 42

SECTION I: ASSESSING YOUR UNDERSTANDING

Activity A   MATCHING

1. 1-D, 2-A, 3-B, 4-C
2. 1-C, 2-A, 3-D, 4-B

Activity B   FILL IN THE BLANKS

1. Hyperlipidemia
2. Lipid
3. Liver
4. Catalyst
5. Rhabdomyolysis

SECTION II: APPLYING YOUR KNOWLEDGE

Activity C   SHORT ANSWERS

1. The nurse should perform the following preadministration assessments before administering an antihyperlipidemic drug:
   - Document serum cholesterol levels and liver function tests.

- Note dietary history, focusing on the types of foods normally included in the diet.
- Record vital signs and weight.
- Inspect skin and eyelids for evidence of xanthomas.

2. The nurse's role after he or she administers an antihyperlipidemic drug includes:
   - Frequently monitoring blood cholesterol and triglyceride levels
   - Checking vital signs and assessing bowel functions
   - Notifying the primary health care provider of changes in serum transaminase levels

Activity D   DOSAGE CALCULATION

1. 4 packets
2. 5 tablets
3. 2 tablets
4. 3 capsules
5. 4 tablets

SECTION III: PRACTICING FOR NCLEX

Activity E

1. Answer: a

RATIONALE: The nurse should instruct the patient to take the drug 2 hours before cholestyramine, a bile acid sequestrant. The nurse need not instruct the patient to ensure a time gap of 1 hour when taking these drugs, take both the drugs 30 minutes before the meals, or take a bile acid sequestrant with warm water as these are not the appropriate instructions.

2. Answer: c

RATIONALE: The atorvastatin drug is contraindicated in patients with serious liver disorders. The atorvastatin drug should be used cautiously in patients with visual disturbances. Bile acid sequestrants are contraindicated in patients with complete biliary obstruction. The fibric acid derivatives are contraindicated in patients with renal dysfunction.

3. Answer: d

RATIONALE: The nurse should monitor for arthralgia in the patient. Vertigo, headache, and cholelithiasis are the adverse reactions to gemfibrozil drug administration.

4. Answer: c

RATIONALE: The nurse should observe enhanced effects of the anticoagulant in the patient as the effect of clofibrate interacting with anticoagulants. Increased hypoglycemic effect is a result of the interaction between sulfonylureas and fibric acid derivatives (particularly with gemfibrozil). Increased risk of severe myopathy is an effect of the interaction of hydroxymethylglutaryl-coenzyme A (HMG-CoA) inhibitors with macrolides, erythromycin, clarithromycin, amiodarone, niacin, and verapamil. Increased risk of hypertension is not an effect of the interaction of clofibrate with anticoagulants.

5. Answer: b, c, e

RATIONALE: The nurse should use HMG-CoA reductase inhibitors with caution in patients with a history of acute infection, visual disturbances, endocrine disorders, alcoholism, hypotension, trauma, and myopathy. Fibric acid derivatives should be used cautiously in patients with peptic ulcer disease. Niacin is used cautiously in patients with unstable angina.

6. **Answer: a**

   RATIONALE: The nurse should monitor for bleeding in the patient who is receiving garlic therapy along with warfarin. The nurse need not monitor the patient for irritation as it is an adverse reaction to garlic and is not caused by the interaction of warfarin with garlic. The nurse need not monitor the patient receiving garlic therapy for peptic ulcers and skin rashes.

7. **Answer: a, b, c**

   RATIONALE: The nurse should monitor for difficulty in passing stools, hard dry stools, and complaints of constipation when caring for an elderly patient on bile acid sequestrants. The nurse need not monitor the patient for mouth dryness or urinary hesitancy as these are adverse reactions to antispasmodic drugs.

8. **Answer: a**

   RATIONALE: In case of a paradoxical elevation of blood lipid levels in the patient receiving an anti-hyperlipidemic drug, the nurse should notify the primary health care physician for a different anti-hyperlipidemic drug. The nurse need not collect the blood samples for further examination, administer the next dose of the drug with milk, or record the fluid intake and output every hour as these interventions will not help to improve the patient's condition.

9. **Answer: b**

   RATIONALE: The nurse should inform the patient that dyspnea is a toxic reaction to flax consumption. Abdominal pain, cramps, and dyspepsia are adverse reactions to atorvastatin and are not toxic reactions associated with the consumption of flax powder.

10. **Answer: a, b, d**

    RATIONALE: The nurse should instruct the patient to increase fluid intake, eat foods high in dietary fiber, and exercise daily to help prevent constipation. The nurse should instruct the patient to take oral vitamin K supplements to prevent the deficiency of vitamin K. The nurse need not instruct the patient to take the drug 1 hour after meals as this will not help the patient prevent constipation.

CHAPTER 43

SECTION I: ASSESSING YOUR UNDERSTANDING

Activity A MATCHING

1. 1-D, 2-C, 3-A, 4-B
2. 1-B, 2-D, 3-A, 4-C

Activity B FILL IN THE BLANKS

1. Prothrombin
2. Thrombus
3. Arterial
4. Thrombolytics
5. Enzyme
6. Heparin

SECTION II: APPLYING YOUR KNOWLEDGE

Activity C SHORT ANSWERS

1. The nurse should consider the following factors to determine the success of the treatment plan:
   - The therapeutic drug effect is achieved.
   - Adverse reactions are identified, reported to the primary health care provider, and managed successfully using appropriate nursing interventions.
   - The patient demonstrates an understanding of the drug regimen.
   - The patient verbalizes the importance of complying with the prescribed therapeutic regimen.
   - The patient lists or describes early signs of bleeding.

2. The nurse should offer the following instructions to the patient:
   - Follow the dosage schedule prescribed by the primary health care provider, and report any signs of active bleeding immediately.
   - Use a soft toothbrush, and consult a dentist regarding routine oral hygiene, including the use of dental floss.
   - Use an electric razor when possible to avoid small skin cuts.
   - Take the drug at the same time each day.
   - Avoid changing brands of anticoagulants without consulting a physician or pharmacist.
   - Contact the primary health care provider in case of bleeding and bruising on any part of the body.
   - Limit foods high in vitamin K.
   - Avoid alcohol unless use has been approved by the primary health care provider.

Activity D DOSAGE CALCULATION

1. 5 tablets
2. 3 tablets
3. 4 tablets
4. 4 tablets
5. 6 tablets

SECTION III: PRACTICING FOR NCLEX

Activity E

1. **Answer: a, c, d**

   RATIONALE: The nurse should monitor the patient receiving alteplase for gingival bleeding, epistaxis, and ecchymosis. Thrombolytic drugs such as alteplase will dissolve all clots encountered, both occlusive clots and those repairing vessel leaks; hence, bleeding is a great concern when using these agents. Erythema is an adverse reaction to phytonadione, sodium, and heparin administration. Anemia is the adverse effect of reteplase and tenecteplase administration.

2. **Answer: c**
   RATIONALE: The nurse should observe for an increased risk of bleeding as the effect of the interaction of abciximab with aspirin. Decreased effectiveness of aspirin, increased effectiveness of abciximab, and decreased absorption of abciximab are not the effects of interaction between abciximab and aspirin.

3. **Answer: b, d, e**
   RATIONALE: Anticoagulants are contraindicated in patients with tuberculosis, leukemia, and hemorrhagic disease. Thrombolytics should be used with caution in patients with diabetic retinopathy and gastrointestinal (GI) bleeding.

4. **Answer: d**
   RATIONALE: The nurse should continually assess the patient for any signs of bleeding after the anisindione drug is administered. Blood for a complete blood count is usually drawn before the administration of the thrombolytic agents. The international normalized ratio (INR) is determined before an anticoagulant or thrombolytic therapy begins. Blood for a baseline PT/INR test is drawn before the first dose of warfarin is given.

5. **Answer: a**
   RATIONALE: The nurse should instruct the patient to use a soft toothbrush, and consult a dentist regarding routine oral hygiene, including the use of dental floss. The nurse should not include instructions such as eating foods high in vitamin K, taking medication with food, and taking the drug at different time each day in the teaching plan for the patient. Instead, the nurse should instruct the patient to limit foods high in vitamin K and take the drug at the same time each day.

6. **Answer: c**
   RATIONALE: The nurse should inspect for bright red to black stools, which is an indication of GI bleeding. The nurse need not inspect the urine for a red-orange color. Oral anticoagulants may impart a red-orange color to alkaline urine, making it difficult to detect hematuria; in such conditions, a urinalysis would be necessary to detect hematuria. The nurse need not monitor the patient's fluid intake and output. If bleeding occurs, the nurse should stop the drug and monitor the vital signs every hour or more frequently for at least 48 hours after the drug is discontinued, instead of monitoring them every 4 hours.

7. **Answer: a**
   RATIONALE: The nurse should monitor the patient for internal and external bleeding after the administration of heparin. The nurse need not monitor for difficulty in breathing, excessive perspiration, or skin rash. Difficulty in breathing and skin rash are the signs of an allergic (hypersensitivity) reaction when thrombolytic drugs are administered.

8. **Answer: d**
   RATIONALE: The nurse should avoid the intramuscular (IM) administration of heparin to avoid the possibility of local irritation, pain, or hematoma. The application of firm pressure after injection helps to prevent hematoma formation. The nurse need not avoid administration sites such as the buttocks and lateral thighs as these are also areas of heparin administration by the subcutaneous (SC) route. When heparin is given by the SC route, the nurse should avoid areas within 2 inches of the umbilicus because of the increased vascularity of that area.

9. **Answer: c**
   RATIONALE: The nurse should observe the patient for new evidence of bleeding if administration of the drug is necessary. The nurse need not measure the patient's body temperature every hour, monitor the patient's pulse rate every 2 hours, or administer the drug to the patient via the IV route. The nurse should monitor the patient's blood pressure and pulse rate every 15 to 30 minutes for 2 hours or more after administration of the heparin antagonist. Protamine sulfate, which is used to treat overdosage of low molecular weight heparins (LMWHs), is given slowly via the IV route over 10 minutes.

10. **Answer: a, b, e**
    RATIONALE: The nurse should observe the patient for symptoms such as abdominal pain, coffee-ground emesis, black tarry stools, hematuria, joint pain, and spitting or coughing up blood. Developing petechiae is a symptom of warfarin overdosage. Chest pain is an adverse effect of clopidogrel.

CHAPTER 44

SECTION I: ASSESSING YOUR UNDERSTANDING

Activity A MATCHING

1. 1-D, 2-C, 3-B, 4-A
2. 1-D, 2-C, 3-B, 4-A

Activity B FILL IN THE BLANKS

1. Erythropoiesis
2. Anemia
3. Leucovorin
4. Megaloblastic
5. Macrocytic

SECTION II: APPLYING YOUR KNOWLEDGE

Activity C SHORT ANSWERS

1. Before administering the first dose of ferrous gluconate, the nurse should perform the following assessments in the patient:
   - Obtain a general health history and ask about the symptoms of anemia.
   - Take vital signs to provide a baseline during therapy.
   - Perform other physical assessments, which may include evaluating the patient's general appearance and, in the severely anemic, the patient's ability to carry out the activities of daily living.
   - If iron dextran is to be given, obtain an allergy history because this drug is given with caution to those with significant allergies or asthma.
   - Take the patient's weight and hemoglobin level to calculate the dosage.

2. The nurse should monitor for the following adverse reactions in a patient who is receiving sodium ferric gluconate complex for the treatment of iron deficiency anemia:
   - Flushing
   - Hypotension
   - Syncope
   - Tachycardia
   - Dizziness
   - Pruritus
   - Dyspnea
   - Conjunctivitis
   - Hyperkalemia

Activity D DOSAGE CALCULATION

1. 1.5 mL
2. 1 mL
3. 14 tablets
4. 2 mL

SECTION III: PRACTICING FOR NCLEX

Activity E

1. **Answer: b**
   RATIONALE: The nurse should monitor for allergic hypersensitivity in the patient administered a Folvite injection. The nurse need not monitor the patient for anorexia, arthralgia, or adrenal hyperplasia. Arthralgia is an adverse reaction associated with the use of epoetin alfa. Adrenal hyperplasia is caused by an unusual increase in the production of androgens by the adrenal glands. Anorexia nervosa is an eating disorder characterized by voluntary starvation and exercise stress.

2. **Answer: a**
   RATIONALE: Epoetin alfa is contraindicated in patients with hypersensitivity to human albumin. Epoetin alfa is not contraindicated in patients with an allergy to cyanocobalamin, patients undergoing treatment for pernicious anemia, or patients with

hemolytic anemia. Vitamin B_{12} is contraindicated in patients who are allergic to cyanocobalamin. Folic acid and leucovorin are contraindicated in patients undergoing treatment for pernicious anemia, and iron supplements are contraindicated in patients with hemolytic anemia.

3. **Answer: a, c, e**
   RATIONALE: Patients who consume alcohol, neomycin, or colchicine show a reduced absorption of vitamin B_{12} when they are administered vitamin B_{12} to counter its deficiency. Caffeine and nicotine are not known to reduce the absorption of vitamin B_{12} in patients taking vitamin B_{12} supplements for its deficiency.

4. **Answer: a**
   RATIONALE: The nurse should obtain the patient's weight and hemoglobin level to calculate the dosage of iron dextran to be administered. The patient's heart rate, blood pressure, and body temperature are not required for calculating the dosage of iron dextran. Heart rate, blood pressure, and body temperature are the patient's vital signs, which the nurse has to take when conducting preadministration and ongoing assessments.

5. **Answer: c**
   RATIONALE: When a patient is administered iron supplements along with methyldopa, the nurse should monitor him or her for a decreased effect of Parkinson's medication. The interaction of iron supplements with methyldopa is not known to decrease blood pressure or increase heart rate. Increased absorption of iron is observed in patients taking iron supplements with ascorbic acid or vitamin C.

6. **Answer: a, b, c**
   RATIONALE: To fulfill the nutritional deficiency of vitamin B_{12} through a balanced diet, the nurse should ask the patient to consume a diet consisting of seafood, meat, eggs, and dairy products, which are rich sources of vitamin B_{12}. The nurse need not instruct the patient to consume leafy vegetables, breads, and cereals to increase the intake of vitamin B_{12} in the body. Leafy vegetables are rich in iron and fiber, and breads and cereals are rich in carbohydrates and proteins—but not in vitamin B_{12}.

7. **Answer: b**
   RATIONALE: In the teaching plan, the nurse should instruct the patient receiving ferrous fumarate to take the drug with water on an empty stomach or to take the drug with food or meals if the patient experiences gastrointestinal upset. The nurse should ask the patient not to take antacids because they may interfere with the absorption of iron. The nurse should not ask the patient to drink the liquid iron preparation directly from a glass because doing so can stain the patient's teeth. Instead, the patient should use a straw while drinking. The patient should avoid multivitamin preparations, unless the primary health care provider approves them, in case the patient is taking folic acid. Otherwise, the patient need not avoid taking

multivitamin preparations when taking ferrous fumarate.

8. **Answer: a, b, e**
   RATIONALE: The nurse should monitor for adverse reactions such as urticaria, dyspnea, and rashes in patients receiving parenteral administration of iron for the treatment of anemia. Insomnia and diabetes are not known to occur from the parenteral administration of iron.

9. **Answer: a**
   RATIONALE: When conducting the ongoing assessment for a patient receiving oral iron supplements, the nurse should inform the patient that the color of his or her stools will be black. Administering oral supplements does not result in high palpitations, weight gain, or the development of rashes.

10. **Answer: a**
    RATIONALE: The nurse should instruct patients receiving iron supplements to avoid milk because it interferes with the absorption of iron. The nurse need not ask the patients to avoid poultry, meat, and fish as these products do not interfere with the absorption of iron.

CHAPTER 45

SECTION I: ASSESSING YOUR UNDERSTANDING

Activity A MATCHING

1. 1-E, 2-A, 3-B, 4-C, 5-D
2. 1-C, 2-A, 3-D, 4-B

Activity B FILL IN THE BLANKS

1. Edema
2. Carbonic
3. Potassium
4. Paresthesias
5. Dermatologic

SECTION II: APPLYING YOUR KNOWLEDGE

Activity C SHORT ANSWERS

1. The nurse should perform the following preadministration assessments before administering a diuretic drug to a patient:
   - Take vital signs and weigh the patient.
   - Carefully review current laboratory test results, especially the levels of serum electrolytes.
   - Monitor blood urea nitrogen (BUN) and creatinine clearance levels in patients with renal dysfunction.
   - If the patient has peripheral edema, inspect the involved areas and record in the patient's chart the degree and extent of edema.
   - Obtain the patient's description of pain and vital signs if the patient is receiving a carbonic anhydrase inhibitor for increased intraocular pressure.

- Take vital signs and weight during the preadministration physical assessment of the patient receiving a diuretic for epilepsy. Review the patient's chart for a description of the seizures and their frequency.
- If the patient is to receive an osmotic diuretic, focus the assessment on the patient's disease or disorder and the symptoms being treated. For example, if the patient has a low urinary output and the osmotic diuretic is given to increase urinary output, then review the intake-and-output ratio and the patient's symptoms. In addition, weigh the patient and take vital signs as part of the preadministration physical assessment.

2. The nurse should perform the following assessments after the administration of a diuretic drug:
   - During initial therapy, observe the patient for the effects of drug therapy. The type of assessment will depend on such factors as the reason for the administration of the diuretic, the type of diuretic administered, the route of administration, and the condition of the patient.
   - Measure and record fluid intake and output, and report to the primary health care provider any marked decrease in output.
   - During ongoing therapy, weigh the patient at the same time daily, making certain that the patient is wearing the same amount or type of clothing.
   - Depending on the specific diuretic, perform frequent serum electrolyte, uric acid, and liver and kidney function tests during the first few months of therapy, and perform periodic tests thereafter.

Activity D DOSAGE CALCULATION

1. 3 tablets
2. 4 tablets
3. 3 tablets
4. 20 mL
5. 2.5 tablets

SECTION III: PRACTICING FOR NCLEX

Activity E

1. **Answer: a, c, d**
   RATIONALE: The nurse should measure and record the patient's weight daily to monitor fluid loss. The nurse should measure the fluid intake and output every 8 hr and assess the respiratory rate every 4 hr to ensure that the patient is receiving optimal response to therapy. The nurse need not check the patient's pupils every 2 hours for dilation or his or her response to light; these interventions are done for patients with acute closed-angle glaucoma.

2. **Answer: b**
   RATIONALE: When caring for a patient receiving diuretics and experiencing gastrointestinal (GI) upset, the nurse should instruct the patient to take the drug with food or milk. The nurse need not instruct the patient to take the drug on an empty stomach or avoid intake of fibrous food because these interventions will not reduce the

symptoms or discomforts of GI upset. The nurse should not instruct the patient to reduce fluid intake to prevent discomfort associated with GI upset. Patients exhibit anxiety with the frequent need to urinate as a result of the diuretic therapy, but the nurse should not reduce their fluid intake to reduce the need to urinate. The nurse should explain that the need to urinate frequently will decrease after a few weeks of therapy.

3. **Answer: c**
   RATIONALE: The nurse should closely observe the patient receiving spironolactone for signs of hyperkalemia, which is a serious and potentially fatal electrolyte imbalance. This drug is a potassium sparing medication. The nurse should closely observe the patient for paresthesias and anorexia after administering acetazolamide to the patient. Vertigo may result from administration of bendroflumethiazide.

4. **Answer: b**
   RATIONALE: The nurse should monitor the patient for an increased risk of hyperglycemia as a result of interaction between chlorothiazide and the antidiabetic drug. The patient will not develop hypersensitivity to the antidiabetic as a result of this interaction. The nurse should monitor for an increased risk of ototoxicity when loop diuretics are administered with cisplatin or aminoglycosides; however, it is not known to occur when chlorothiazide and an antidiabetic drug interact. An increase in the effect of chlorothiazide is also not known to occur because of the interaction of chlorothiazide and the antidiabetic drug.

5. **Answer: a, b, d**
   RATIONALE: The nurse should inform the patient that herbal diuretics should not be taken unless approved by the primary health care provider. The nurse should also inform the patient that while most plant and herbal extracts available as over-the-counter diuretics are nontoxic, most of them are either ineffective or no more effective than caffeine. The nurse should not encourage the patient to consume diuretic teas like those made from juniper berries because they are contraindicated; juniper berries have been associated with renal damage. Horsetail contains severely toxic compounds, and teas with ephedrine should be avoided, especially by individuals with hypertension.

6. **Answer: a**
   RATIONALE: The nurse should know that endocrine disturbances, heart failure, and kidney and liver diseases cause excess fluid retention in the body. Hematologic changes, gastric distress, and hyperkalemia are adverse reactions to bendroflumethiazide and are not known to cause excess fluid retention in the body. Hyperkalemia is most likely to occur in patients with diabetes.

7. **Answer: b, d, e**
   RATIONALE: The nurse should monitor serum electrolyte, blood urea nitrogen (BUN), and creatinine clearance levels before administering metolazone to a patient with renal dysfunction. Patients with edema caused by heart failure should be weighed daily to monitor fluid loss. Serum potassium levels are monitored for patients at risk for hypokalemia.

8. **Answer: b**
   RATIONALE: The nurse should know that the patient is experiencing an electrolyte imbalance. Warning signs of a fluid and electrolyte imbalance include dry mouth, thirst, weakness, lethargy, drowsiness, restlessness, muscle pains or cramps, confusion, GI disturbances, hypotension, oliguria, tachycardia, and seizures. Hyperkalemia, hypercalcemia, and hyponatremia are characterized by high levels of potassium and calcium and low levels of sodium ions circulating in the blood, respectively. Symptoms of hyperkalemia include paresthesia (numbness, tingling, or prickling sensation), muscular weakness, fatigue, flaccid paralysis of the extremities, bradycardia, shock, and electrocardiographic abnormalities. Hypercalcemia and hyponatremia are not characterized by muscle pain, cramps, oliguria, hypotension, and GI disturbances.

9. **Answer: c**
   RATIONALE: If the serum potassium levels in the patient exceed 5.3 mEq/mL, the nurse should discontinue the drug and notify the physician immediately, considering this could be a sign of hypokalemia. The drug should not be discontinued if the patient experiences gout attacks, if the patient's urine tests positive for glucose, or if excess fluid has been removed from the patient's body. Thiazide diuretics may cause gout attacks, during which patients could experience joint pain. Patients who have diabetes mellitus and take loop or thiazide diuretics may test positive for the presence of glucose in their urine, in which case the primary health care provider has to be contacted immediately. The patient who has had excess fluid removed from the body because of drug therapy needs to continue diuretic drug therapy to prevent further accumulation of fluid.

CHAPTER 46

SECTION I: ASSESSING YOUR UNDERSTANDING

Activity A MATCHING

1. 1-B, 2-A, 3-D, 4-C
2. 1-C, 2-A, 3-D, 4-B

Activity B FILL IN THE BLANKS

1. Cystitis
2. Antispasmodic
3. Neurogenic

4. Nocturia
5. Urge

SECTION II: APPLYING YOUR KNOWLEDGE

Activity C SHORT ANSWERS

1. The nurse should consider the following factors to determine the success of the treatment plan:
   • Achievement of the therapeutic effect
   • Identification, reporting, and successful management of adverse reactions through appropriate nursing interventions
   • Demonstration of the understanding of the drug regimen by the patient and family
   • Patient verbalization of the importance of complying with the prescribed therapeutic regimen
2. The nurse should include the following points in the teaching plan:
   • Take the drug with food or meals (nitrofurantoin must be taken with food or milk). If gastrointestinal (GI) upset occurs despite taking the drug with food, contact the primary health care provider.
   • Take the drug at the prescribed intervals and complete the full course of therapy. Do not discontinue taking the drug even though the symptoms have disappeared unless directed to do so by the primary health care provider.
   • If drowsiness or dizziness occurs, avoid driving and performing tasks that require alertness.
   • During therapy with this drug, avoid alcoholic beverages and do not take any nonprescription drug unless the primary health care provider has approved it.
   • Notify the primary health care provider immediately if symptoms do not improve after 3 or 4 days.
   • Take nitrofurantoin with food or milk to improve absorption. Continue therapy for at least 1 week or for 3 days after the urine shows no signs of infection. Notify the primary health care provider immediately if any of the following occur: fever, chills, cough, shortness of breath, chest pain, or difficulty breathing. Do not take the next dose of the drug until the primary health care provider has been contacted. The urine may appear brown during therapy with this drug; this is not abnormal.

Activity D DOSAGE CALCULATION

1. 3 tablets
2. 10 tablets
3. 8 tablets
4. 8 capsules

SECTION III: PRACTICING FOR NCLEX

Activity E

1. **Answer: a**
   RATIONALE: When caring for a patient experiencing dry mouth, the nurse should instruct the patient to suck on sugarless lozenges. Sucking on

hard candy can also bring relief to patients with dry mouth, and so the nurse need not instruct the patient to refrain from consuming hard candy. The nurse need not instruct the patient to increase the intake of fibrous foods because doing so will not bring relief to the discomfort of dry mouth. The nurse instructs the patient to take nitrofurantoin with food or milk to improve absorption of the drug. Taking Enablex with milk will not lessen the discomforts or the symptoms of dry mouth.

2. **Answer: b**
   RATIONALE: The nurse should monitor for dry eyes in the patient on solifenacin drug therapy. Dry eyes, blurred vision, and dry mouth are common adverse reactions to antispasmodic drugs. Headache, pruritus, and rash are the adverse reactions to phenazopyridine and are not known to occur with the administration of solifenacin.

3. **Answer: a**
   RATIONALE: The nurse should monitor the patient for an increased risk of bleeding when sulfamethoxazole is administered with oral anticoagulants. Delay in gastric emptying is observed in the patient when anticholinergics are administered with nitrofurantoin. Decreased effect of the sulfamethoxazole is not known to occur as a result of interaction with oral anticoagulants. Urinary tract excretion of the anti-infective, particularly fosfomycin, and lowered plasma concentrations occur when metoclopramide is administered with fosfomycin.

4. **Answer: c**
   RATIONALE: The nurse should know that antispasmodics are contraindicated in patients with myasthenia gravis. Antispasmodics are not contraindicated in patients with hepatic impairment, cerebral arteriosclerosis, or convulsive disorders. Anti-infectives should be used cautiously in those with renal or hepatic impairment. Nalidixic acid (NegGram), an anti-infective, is contraindicated in patients who have convulsive disorders. Nitrofurantoin, an anti-infective, and nalidixic acid are used cautiously in patients with cerebral arteriosclerosis.

5. **Answer: c**
   RATIONALE: The nurse should administer the urinary tract anti-infective with prune juice to decrease the pain experienced by the patient on voiding. The nurse can also administer cranberry juice to the patient. Even other fluids, preferably water, are encouraged during drug administration, though the nurse need not administer the drug strictly with warm water. The nurse should not administer the drug after meals or strictly with milk to prevent pain experienced by the patient on voiding. Nitrofurantoin is generally administered with milk to prevent the irritation it causes in the stomach.

6. **Answer: c**

   RATIONALE: The nurse should avoid administering phenazopyridine for more than 2 days when the patient is also receiving an antibacterial drug for the urinary tract infection. When used for more than 2 days, the drug may mask symptoms of a more serious disorder. The nurse should encourage the patient to drink at least 2000 mL of fluid daily and administer the urinary tract anti-infectives with cranberry or prune juice to dilute urine and decrease pain on voiding. The nurse need not administer phenazopyridine 2 hours before giving the antibacterial drug as this is not an appropriate intervention.

7. **Answer: a**

   RATIONALE: The nurse should instruct the patient to increase the intake of fluids to alleviate the effect of constipation caused by flavoxate. The nurse need not increase the patient's intake of citrus fruits, decrease the patient's consumption of milk products, or administer the drug with warm water as these interventions will not help alleviate the effect of constipation.

8. **Answer: b**

   RATIONALE: The nurse should administer the drug with milk to prevent irritation in the stomach of the patient receiving a nitrofurantoin urinary tract anti-infective. The nurse need not administer the drug with apple juice, at bedtime, or 1 hour before meals as these interventions will not prevent irritation in the stomach of the patient receiving nitrofurantoin.

9. **Answer: b, c, d**

   RATIONALE: During preadministration assessment, the nurse should question the patient regarding symptoms of infection before instituting therapy, take and record the vital signs, and record the color and appearance of the urine. The nurse also assesses for and documents pain, urinary frequency, bladder distension, or other symptoms associated with the urinary system. The nurse constantly monitors the patient's body temperature as part of the ongoing assessment. Any significant rise in body temperature should be reported to the primary health care provider because methods of reducing the fever may need to be altered, or culture and sensitivity tests may need to be repeated. Though urine culture and sensitivity tests are performed to determine bacterial sensitivity to the drugs before drug administration, periodic urinalysis and culture and sensitivity tests are performed only during ongoing assessments to monitor the effects of drug therapy.

10. **Answer: c**

    RATIONALE: The nurse should use anti-infective drugs cautiously in patients with renal impairment. Antispasmodic drugs are used cautiously in patients with gastrointestinal infections, urinary retention, and hypertension.

CHAPTER 47

SECTION I: ASSESSING YOUR UNDERSTANDING

Activity A MATCHING

1. 1-C, 2-E, 3-A, 4-B, 5-D
2. 1-B, 2-C, 3-A, 4-E, 5-D

Activity B FILL IN THE BLANKS

1. Gastrointestinal
2. Esophagus
3. Vomiting
4. Dronabinol
5. Duodenal

SECTION II: APPLYING YOUR KNOWLEDGE

Activity C SHORT ANSWERS

1. The nurse should perform the following preadmission assessments:
   - Question the patient regarding the type and intensity of symptoms.
   - Document the number of vomiting experiences and approximate amount of fluid lost.
   - Record vital signs and assess signs of fluid and electrolyte imbalances.
   - Explain the rationale for preventing an episode of vomiting.

2. The nurse's role after the administration of the drug includes:
   - Monitoring the patient frequently for continued complaints of pain, sour taste, or spitting of blood or coffee–ground-colored emesis
   - Keeping suction equipment available in case insertion of a nasogastric tube or suctioning is warranted to prevent aspiration of the emesis
   - Observing the patient for signs and symptoms of electrolyte imbalance if vomiting is severe
   - Monitoring the blood pressure, pulse, and respiratory rate every 2 to 4 hours
   - Carefully measuring intake and output until vomiting ceases
   - Documenting on the chart each case of vomiting
   - Notifying the primary health care physician if there is blood in the emesis or if vomiting suddenly becomes more severe
   - Measuring the patient's weight daily to weekly in those with prolonged and repeated episodes of vomiting
   - Assessing the patient at frequent intervals for effectiveness of the drug to relieve symptoms
   - Notifying the primary health care provider if the drug fails to relieve or diminish symptoms

Activity D DOSAGE CALCULATION

1. 6 capsules
2. 2 capsules
3. 4 tablets

4. 4 tablets
5. 6 capsules

SECTION III: PRACTICING FOR NCLEX

Activity E

1. **Answer: c**
   RATIONALE: The nurse should monitor the patient for euphoria, which is an adverse reaction to dronabinol. Sedation and hypoxia are adverse reactions to ondansetron HCl. Asthenia is an adverse reaction to granisetron HCl.

2. **Answer: a**
   RATIONALE: The nurse should observe an increased risk of respiratory depression in the patient as the interaction between antacids and opioid analgesics. The white blood cell count will decrease when the antacid is administered with carmustine. Bleeding may increase when antacids are administered with oral anticoagulants. Also, there is an increased risk of dehydration if the patient suffers from vomiting and diarrhea.

3. **Answer: a, b, d**
   RATIONALE: The nurse should administer promethazine with caution to patients with hypertension, sleep apnea, or epilepsy. Trimethobenzamide is used cautiously in children with a viral illness. Cholinergic blocking antiemetics are used cautiously in patients with glaucoma.

4. **Answer: b**
   RATIONALE: The nurse should monitor the patient for coffee–ground-colored emesis after the administration of aluminum hydroxide gel. The nurse need not monitor for headache, signs of electrolyte imbalances, or the amount of fluid lost. The nurse should assess for signs of electrolyte imbalances before starting antiemetic therapy. He or she should document the approximate amount of fluid lost as part of the preadministration assessment for a patient receiving a drug for nausea and vomiting.

5. **Answer: d**
   RATIONALE: The nurse should instruct the patient to avoid driving or performing other hazardous tasks when taking the drug because drowsiness may occur with use. The nurse need not instruct the patient to increase the frequency of the dose if symptoms worsen, avoid direct exposure to sunlight, or take other drugs 1 hr before taking the antacid. The nurse should instruct the patient not to increase the frequency of use or the dose if symptoms become worse; instead, the patient should see the primary health care provider as soon as possible. Considering the antacids impair the absorption of some drugs, the other drugs should not be taken within 2 hours before or after taking the antacid.

6. **Answer: a, c, e**
   RATIONALE: Before an emetic is given to the patient, the nurse should obtain information such as substances that have been ingested, the time the substances were ingested, and symptoms noted before seeking medical treatment. Cause for ingesting the poison and the patient's mental status before taking the poison are not related to the administration of the emetic.

7. **Answer: b, c, e**
   RATIONALE: The nurse should monitor the patient for symptoms of dehydration, such as decreased urinary output, concentrated urine, dry mucous membranes, poor skin turgor, restlessness, irritability, and confusion. Increased respiratory rate is also a symptom of dehydration. White streaks in stools are a normal observation when the patient is taking antacids.

8. **Answer: a**
   RATIONALE: The nurse should monitor the patient for rate of infusion at frequent intervals during administration through IV because too rapid an infusion may induce cardiac arrhythmias. Recording body temperature every hour, observing for irritation caused by drug administration, or taking blood pressure every 2 hours are not relevant interventions in this case.

9. **Answer: d**
   RATIONALE: The nurse should record the fluid intake and output of the patient who experiences diarrhea after taking the antacid drug to monitor dehydration in the patient. The nurse removes items with a strong odor from the room if the patient has nausea and a vomiting sensation. Changing to a different antacid usually alleviates the problem. Recording the patient's temperature every hour will not help when caring for the patient with diarrhea.

10. **Answer: c**
    RATIONALE: The nurse should remove items with a strong smell and odor to prevent sensations of vomiting and to enhance the patient's appetite. Suggesting that the patient consume milk products or perform physical exercises will not help the patient improve his or her appetite. The nurse should give frequent oral rinses to the patient to remove the disagreeable taste that accompanies vomiting.

CHAPTER 48

SECTION I: ASSESSING YOUR UNDERSTANDING

Activity A MATCHING

1. 1-C, 2-A, 3-D, 4-B
2. 1-D, 2-B, 3-A, 4-C

Activity B FILL IN THE BLANKS

1. Diarrhea
2. Chamomile
3. Laxative
4. Pruritus
5. Aminosalicylates

SECTION II: APPLYING YOUR KNOWLEDGE

Activity C SHORT ANSWERS

1. The nurse should perform the following preadministration assessment:
   - Question the patient regarding the type and intensity of symptoms, such as pain, discomfort, diarrhea, or constipation.
   - Listen to bowel sounds and palpate the abdomen
   - Monitor the patient for signs of guarding or discomfort.

2. The nurse's role after the administration of the drug to the patient includes:
   - Assessing the patient for relief of symptoms such as diarrhea, pain, or constipation
   - Notifying the primary health care provider if the drug fails to relieve symptoms
   - Monitoring vital signs on a daily basis or more frequently
   - Observing the patient for adverse drug reactions
   - Evaluating the effectiveness of drug therapy
   - Evaluating the patient's response to therapy

Activity D DOSAGE CALCULATION

1. 168 capsules
2. 2 tablets
3. 2 capsules
4. 24 tablets
5. 2 tablets

SECTION III: PRACTICING FOR NCLEX

Activity E

1. **Answer: c**
   RATIONALE: The nurse should monitor for increased blood glucose levels as a result of mesalamine interacting with hypoglycemic drugs. When the patient receives warfarin with mesalamine, the risk of bleeding increases. Neither decreased absorption of hypoglycemic drugs nor a reduced effect of mesalamine will result from the interaction of the two drugs.

2. **Answer: b**
   RATIONALE: The nurse should monitor for constipation, dry skin and mucous membranes, nausea, and light-headedness on administering loperamide to a patient with acute diarrhea. Cramping is an adverse reaction to olsalazine. Infliximab could cause sore throat, and anorexia is an adverse reaction to sulfasalazine.

3. **Answer: a**
   RATIONALE: The nurse should administer bismuth subsalicylate with caution to patients with severe hepatic impairment. Aminosalicylates are contraindicated in patients with intestinal obstruction. Laxatives are contraindicated in patients with signs of acute appendicitis and rectal bleeding.

4. **Answer: b**
   RATIONALE: The nurse should instruct the patient to chew the drug thoroughly because complete particle dispersion enhances antiflatulent action. The nurse need not instruct the patient to take the drug early in the morning. Instead, the nurse should instruct the patient to take the drug after each meal and at bedtime. The nurse should give a bulk-producing or stool-softening laxative with a full glass of juice, followed by an additional full glass of water.

5. **Answer: a**
   RATIONALE: The nurse should encourage the patient with chronic diarrhea to drink extra fluids. The nurse need not instruct the patient to avoid the use of commercial electrolytes or encourage the patient to eat foods high in fiber. When diarrhea is severe, the nurse should use commercial electrolytes. The nurse should encourage patients with constipation to eat high-fiber foods and to exercise often.

6. **Answer: b, c, e**
   RATIONALE: The nurse should instruct an outpatient undergoing antidiarrheal therapy to observe caution when driving as the drug may cause drowsiness. The patient should also avoid the use of alcohol and other nonprescription drugs unless the primary health care provider has approved them. The nurse instructs the patient who has been prescribed laxatives to eat foods high in roughage and get sufficient exercise.

7. **Answer: d**
   RATIONALE: The nurse should instruct the patient to take mineral oil in the evening on an empty stomach for optimal response to therapy. The nurse should not instruct the patient to take it half an hour after a meal, take it before breakfast, or take it at bedtime or after dinner as these methods will not promote an optimal response to therapy.

8. **Answer: c**
   RATIONALE: The nurse should instruct the patient to eat foods high in bulk or roughage, drink plenty of fluids, and perform exercise to avoid constipation. The nurse need not instruct the patient to take commercial electrolytes, take the drug with food, or avoid milk products as these interventions are not appropriate and will not help in preventing constipation.

9. **Answer: b**
   RATIONALE: The nurse should monitor the patient for serious electrolyte imbalances, an effect of the prolonged use of laxatives. Obstruction of the small intestine occurs when bulk-forming laxatives are administered without adequate fluid intake or in patients with intestinal stenosis. Renal impairment and fecal impaction do not result from the prolonged use of laxatives.

10. **Answer: c**
    RATIONALE: Antidiarrheals are contraindicated in patients with obstructive jaundice, pseudomem-

branous colitis, and abdominal pain of unknown origin. Constipation, nausea, and abdominal distention are adverse reactions associated with the administration of antidiarrheals.

CHAPTER 49

SECTION I: ASSESSING YOUR UNDERSTANDING

Activity A MATCHING

1. 1-B, 2-C, 3-A
2. 1-C, 2-D, 3-A, 4-B

Activity B FILL IN THE BLANKS

1. Insulin
2. Polyuria
3. Glycogen
4. Hypokalemia
5. Hyperglycemia
6. Hemoglobin
7. Ketoacidosis

SECTION II: APPLYING YOUR KNOWLEDGE

Activity C SHORT ANSWERS

1. The nurse should consider the following factors when evaluating the success of the treatment plan:
   - The therapeutic drug effect is achieved and normal or near-normal blood glucose levels are maintained.
   - Hypoglycemic reactions are identified, reported to the primary health care provider, and managed successfully.
   - Anxiety is reduced.
   - The patient begins to demonstrate the ability to cope with the disorder and its required treatment.
   - The patient demonstrates a positive outlook and adjustment to the diagnosis.
   - The patient verbalizes a willingness to comply with the prescribed treatment regimen.
   - The patient demonstrates an understanding of the drug regimen.
   - The patient demonstrates an understanding of the information presented in teaching sessions.
   - The patient is able to monitor blood glucose levels or test urine for glucose and ketones.
2. The nurse should provide the following instructions to the patient and family:
   - Take the drug exactly as directed on the container.
   - Exactly follow the diet and drug regimen prescribed by the primary health care provider.
   - Never stop taking the drug or increase or decrease the dose unless told to do so by the primary health care physician.
   - Take the drug at the same time or times each day.
   - Avoid alcohol, dieting, commercial weight-loss products, and strenuous exercise programs.

- Maintain good foot and skin care and routine eye and dental examinations for early detection of problems.
- Notify the primary health care provider if any of the following occur: episodes of hypoglycemia, apparent symptoms of hyperglycemia, elevated blood glucose levels, positive results of urine tests for glucose or ketone bodies, or pregnancy.
- Note that an antidiabetic drug is not oral insulin and cannot be substituted for insulin.
- Test blood for glucose and urine for ketones, as directed by the primary health care provider.
- Wear identification, such as a MedicAlert bracelet, to inform medical personnel and others of diabetes and the drug or drugs currently being used to treat the disease.

Activity D DOSAGE CALCULATION

1. 4 tablets
2. 5 tablets
3. 6 tablets
4. 3 tablets
5. 6 tablets

SECTION III: PRACTICING FOR NCLEX

Activity E

1. **Answer: b**
   RATIONALE: The nurse should monitor for myalgia, headache, pain, aggravated diabetes, infections, and fatigue in the patient receiving pioglitazone HCl drug therapy. The nurse need not monitor for congestive heart failure, sodium retention, and glycosuria; these are the adverse reactions observed in patients receiving diazoxide drug therapy.

2. **Answer: a**
   RATIONALE: Chlorpropamide, a sulfonylurea, is contraindicated in patients with coronary artery disease and liver or renal dysfunction. Alpha glucosidase inhibitors are contraindicated in patients with colonic ulceration, chronic intestinal diseases, and inflammatory bowel disease.

3. **Answer: c**
   RATIONALE: The nurse informs the patient that the need for insulin is greatest during the third trimester of pregnancy. Insulin requirements usually decrease in the first trimester, increase during the second and third trimester, and decrease rapidly after delivery. Insulin is not required before conception as gestational diabetes occurs during pregnancy.

4. **Answer: b**
   RATIONALE: The nurse should administer regular insulin to the patient 30 to 60 minutes before a meal to achieve optimal results. Insulin aspart is administered within 5 to 10 minutes of a meal. Insulin lispro is administered 15 minutes before a meal, and insulin glargine is administered once at bedtime via the subcutaneous (SC) route.

5. Answer: c
RATIONALE: The nurse should administer dextrose to the patient rather than sugar if the administration of miglitol results in hypoglycemia. The nurse should discuss the disease and methods of controlling it with the patient after he or she is diagnosed as diabetic. The nurse should not administer acetohexamide with insulin to the patient as it may enhance the hypoglycemic effect. The nurse obtains the capillary blood specimens of the patient when he or she has deficient fluid volume.

6. Answer: b
RATIONALE: When preparing an insulin mixture, the nurse should draw up insulin lispro first in the syringe and then draw up the long-acting insulin. The nurse should confirm if the ratio of insulin NPH to regular insulin should be 70:30 or 50:50. When the patient is to receive regular insulin and NPH insulin, or regular and lente insulin, the nurse must clarify with the primary health care provider whether two separate injections are to be given or if the insulins may be mixed in the same syringe. Premixed solutions may not be effective in patients who have difficulty controlling their diabetes, and hence, the nurse need not keep the mixture for 1 hour.

7. Answer: c
RATIONALE: The nurse should instruct the patient receiving α-glucosidase inhibitors to keep a source of glucose ready for signs of low blood glucose. Patients prescribed meglitinides therapy should avoid drug administration in case of a skipped meal. The nurse should instruct the patient prescribed metformin to report respiratory distress or muscular aches to the primary health care provider. Also, the nurse should instruct the patient to take the drug at the same time or times each day.

8. Answer: d
RATIONALE: The insulin pump method is used both for the patient who has undergone renal transplantation and the pregnant women with diabetes and early long-term complications because the drug attempts to mimic the body's normal pancreatic function. The needle and syringe method, using microfine needles; jet injection system method; and syringes with prefilled cartridges are used, in general, for most diabetic patients.

9. Answer: a
RATIONALE: Before insulin administration, the nurse should make sure that air bubbles are eliminated from the syringe barrel and the hub of the needle. The nurse should not shake the vial vigorously just before withdrawal; instead, the vial should be tilted end to end very gently. The nurse need not ensure that the vial has been standing for an hour. If the vial has been standing for an hour, the insulin will be in suspension, and the nurse should tilt the vial gently and rotate it in the palm of the hands. The nurse should not use a syringe labeled with a higher concentration; instead the nurse should always use a syringe marked with the required concentration.

10. Answer: b
RATIONALE: The nurse should instruct the patient to change the needle every 1 to 3 days when administering insulin with an insulin pump. The blood glucose levels should be monitored four to eight times per day. The amount of insulin to be injected is not the same every time; instead it should be adjusted according to blood glucose levels. A mixture of isophane and regular insulin should not be used for the patient; only regular insulin should be administered through the insulin pump.

CHAPTER 50

SECTION I: ASSESSING YOUR UNDERSTANDING

Activity A MATCHING
1. 1-B, 2-A, 3-D, 4-C
2. 1-C, 2-D, 3-B, 4-A

Activity B FILL IN THE BLANKS
1. Corticosteroids
2. Prolactin
3. Gonadotropins
4. Rhinyle
5. Menotropins

SECTION II: APPLYING YOUR KNOWLEDGE

Activity C SHORT ANSWERS
1. The nurse plays the following role in promoting an optimal response to the growth hormone therapy:
   - The nurse should administer the growth hormone subcutaneously.
   - The nurse should not shake the vial containing the hormone.
   - The nurse should swirl the vial containing the hormone.
   - The nurse should not administer the solution if it is cloudy.
   - The nurse should divide the weekly dosage and give it in three to seven doses throughout the week.
   - The nurse should give the drug at bedtime to closely adhere to the body's natural release of the hormone.
   - The nurse should conduct periodic testing of growth hormone levels, glucose tolerance, and thyroid functioning during the treatment.
2. The nurse's role in educating the patient and the family includes the following:
   - The nurse discusses in detail the therapeutic regimen for increasing the growth of the child.
   - The nurse instructs the parents on the proper injection technique if the drug is to be given at bedtime and not in the outpatient clinic.

- The nurse encourages parents to keep all clinic or office visits with the child.
- The nurse explains that the child may experience sudden growth and increase in appetite.
- The nurse instructs the parents to report lack of growth; symptoms of diabetes such as increased hunger, increased thirst, or frequent voiding; or symptoms of hypothyroidism such as fatigue, dry skin, and intolerance to cold.

Activity D DOSAGE CALCULATION

1. 8 tablets
2. 12 tablets
3. 10 tablets
4. 6 tablets
5. 4 tablets

SECTION III: PRACTICING FOR NCLEX

Activity E

1. **Answer: a, c, e**
   RATIONALE: The nurse should cautiously administer corticotropin to patients with diabetes, diverticulosis, renal insufficiencies, myasthenia gravis, tuberculosis, hypothyroidism, cirrhosis, nonspecific ulcerative colitis, heart failure, seizures, or febrile infections. Sinus bradycardia and arthralgia are not adverse reactions of corticotropin. Sinus bradycardia is an adverse reaction to octreotide acetate. Arthralgia is an adverse reaction to somatropin.

2. **Answer: d**
   RATIONALE: The nurse should mention the decreased antidiuretic effect to the patient as the effect of the interaction between vasopressin and oral anticoagulants. Increased risk of hypokalemia, increased need for antidiabetic medication, and decreased muscle function are not effects of the interaction between vasopressin and oral anticoagulants. When the patient is administered a diuretic or amphotericin with adrenocorticotropic hormone (ACTH), the risk of hypokalemia increases. The need for antidiabetic medication increases when the patient is administered insulin or an oral antidiabetic with ACTH. When the patient is administered cholinergic blockers with ACTH, muscle function decreases.

3. **Answer: b, c, d.**
   RATIONALE: The nurse should monitor for adverse reactions such as acneiform eruptions, increased sweating, and perineal itching in patients receiving dexamethasone for mycosis fungoides. Nasal congestion and abdominal cramps are not adverse reactions associated with the use of dexamethasone for mycosis fungoides. They are adverse reactions to desmopressin acetate.

4. **Answer: b**
   RATIONALE: The nurse should monitor for a rise in blood glucose level in a patient receiving adrenocorticotropic hormones for nonsuppurative thyroiditis. The nurse need not record the

patient's abdominal girth, measure specific gravity of the urine, or monitor the bone age in a patient receiving adrenocorticotropic hormones. The nurse records the patient's abdominal girth before administering vasopressin to relieve abdominal distension. Specific gravity of the urine is measured when the patient needs to self-administer vasopressin by the parenteral route. Bone age is monitored periodically as an ongoing assessment of a patient receiving growth hormones.

5. **Answer: a**
   RATIONALE: The nurse should give the drug with food or a full glass of water to minimize gastric irritation. The nurse need not give an enema, supply large amounts of drinking water, or auscultate the abdomen to minimize gastric irritation. An enema may be given when vasopressin is administered before abdominal roentgenography. Patients with diabetes insipidus are continually thirsty and need to be supplied with large amounts of drinking water. The nurse auscultates the abdomen before administering vasopressin to relieve abdominal distension.

6. **Answer: c**
   RATIONALE: The nurse should monitor for hypertension in the patient receiving fludrocortisone acetate for primary adrenocortical deficiency. The nurse need not monitor for joint pain, hyperthyroidism, or insulin resistance in the patient receiving fludrocortisone acetate. Joint pain, hyperthyroidism, and insulin resistance are adverse reactions to growth hormone.

7. **Answer: a**
   RATIONALE: The nurse should discontinue the drug therapy if the infertile patient receiving ganirelix acetate complains of visual disturbances. The nurse need not administer the drug with food, assess the skin integrity, or perform a complete blood count (CBC) in the patient receiving ganirelix. Oral corticosteroids are given with food to minimize gastric irritation. Assessing skin integrity and performing a CBC are preadministration assessments for a patient receiving corticotropin.

8. **Answer: c**
   RATIONALE: The nursing diagnosis checklist for a patient receiving glucocorticoids for systemic lupus erythematosus should include Disturbed Body Image related to adverse reactions, as well as Risk for Infection related to immune suppression or impaired wound healing; Risk for Injury related to muscle atrophy, osteoporosis, or spontaneous fractures; Acute Pain related to epigastric distress of gastric ulcer formation; Excess Fluid Volume related to adverse reactions such as sodium and water retention; and Disturbed Thought Processes related to adverse reactions such as depression, psychosis, and other changes in mental status. The nursing diagnosis checklist for a patient

receiving glucocorticoids need not include Pain related to abdominal distension, Deficient Fluid Volume related to inability to replenish fluid intake, or Risk for Infection related to masking of signs of infection. The diagnosis checklist for a patient receiving vasopressin includes Pain related to abdominal distension and Deficient Fluid Volume related to inability to replenish fluid intake when the patient is administered vasopressin. The nurse should include Risk for Infection related to masking of signs of infection in the diagnosis checklist when the patient is administered ACTH.

9. **Answer: a**
RATIONALE: When the drug is administered before abdominal roentgenography, the nurse should administer two injections of 10 units each. The nurse should give first dose 2 hours before an x-ray examination, and he or she should give an enema before administering the first dose of vasopressin to the patient undergoing abdominal roentgenography. The nurse need not check stools; monitor for rash, urticaria, and hypotension; or ensure that the daily oral doses are given before 9 am for a patient receiving vasopressin and undergoing abdominal roentgenography. The nurse should check stools for evidence of bleeding or monitor the patient for rash, urticaria, and hypotension when the patient is administered ACTH. Daily oral doses of glucocorticoids or mineralocorticoids are generally given before 9 am to minimize adrenal suppression.

10. **Answer: b, d, e**
RATIONALE: The nurse is likely to observe buffalo hump, moon face, oily skin and acne, osteoporosis, purple striae on the abdomen and hips, altered skin pigmentation, and weight gain in the patient experiencing an overdose of prednisone. The nurse need not observe for swelling and muscle pain as these are not adverse reactions to an overdose of prednisone; they are adverse reactions to somatropin.

CHAPTER 51

SECTION I: ASSESSING YOUR UNDERSTANDING

Activity A MATCHING

1. 1-B, 2-C, 3-A
2. 1-C, 2-A, 3-D, 4-B

Activity B FILL IN THE BLANKS

1. Hyperthyroidism
2. Hypothyroid
3. Iodine
4. Euthyroid
5. Antithyroid

SECTION II: APPLYING YOUR KNOWLEDGE

Activity C SHORT ANSWERS

1. The nurse should provide the following information to the patient and family, emphasizing the importance of taking the thyroid hormone replacement therapy:
   - Replacement therapy is for life, with the exception of transient hypothyroidism seen in those with thyroiditis.
   - Do not increase, decrease, or skip a dose unless advised to do so by the primary health care provider.
   - Notify the primary health care provider if any of the following occur: headache, nervousness, palpitations, diarrhea, excessive sweating, heat intolerance, chest pain, increased pulse rate, or any unusual physical changes or events.
   - Weigh yourself weekly and report any significant weight gain or loss to the primary health care provider.
2. The nurse should consider the following factors to determine the success of the therapy:
   - The therapeutic effect is achieved.
   - Adverse reactions are identified and reported to the primary health care provider.
   - The patient verbalizes the importance of complying with the prescribed treatment regimen.
   - The patient verbalizes an understanding of the treatment modalities and importance of continued follow-up care.
   - The patient and family demonstrate an understanding of the drug regimen.

Activity D DOSAGE CALCULATION

1. 3 tablets
2. 6 tablets
3. 3 tablets
4. 2 tablets

SECTION III: PRACTICING FOR NCLEX

Activity E

1. **Answer: b**
RATIONALE: The nurse should notify the primary health care provider if agranulocytosis, an adverse reaction to methimazole, occurs. The nurse need not notify the primary health care provider about tachycardia, weight loss, and fatigue; these are common adverse reactions to levothyroxine sodium (T_4), liothyronine sodium (T_3), sodium iodine (^{131}I), liotrix (T_3, T_4), and desiccated thyroid USP.

2. **Answer: a**
RATIONALE: The nurse should observe decreased effectiveness of the cardiac drug when thyroid hormones are administered with digoxin. The

nurse need not monitor for increased risk of prolonged bleeding, decreased effectiveness of the thyroid drug, or increased potential for bleeding in the patient as the effect of interaction between the thyroid hormones and digoxin. When thyroid hormones are administered with oral anticoagulants, the risk of prolonged bleeding increases. When the patient is administered thyroid hormones with antidepressants, there is an increased—not decreased—effectiveness of the thyroid drug. When the patient is administered antithyroid drugs with propylthiouracil, the potential for bleeding increases.

3. **Answer: c**
   RATIONALE: The nurse should monitor for mild diuresis as a sign of therapeutic response after the thyroid hormone is administered to the patient. The nurse need not monitor for agranulocytosis, headache, and loss of hair as signs of therapeutic response after the thyroid hormone has been administered to the patient. Agranulocytosis, headache, and loss of hair are adverse reactions to antithyroid preparations.

4. **Answer: b, c, e**
   RATIONALE: The nurse should document cold intolerance, confusion, and unsteady gait as the symptoms of hypothyroidism during the preadministration assessment. The nurse need not document weight loss and sweating as the symptoms of hypothyroidism. Weight loss and sweating are the adverse reactions to levothyroxine sodium (T_4).

5. **Answer: a, c, e**
   RATIONALE: The nurse should instruct the patient to take the drug at regular intervals, record his or her weight twice a week, and avoid taking the drug in larger doses. The nurse need not instruct the patient undergoing propylthiouracil therapy to take the drug before breakfast or to notify the primary health care provider if palpitations occur. The nurse should instruct the patient taking thyroid hormones to take the drug before breakfast and notify the primary health care provider if headache, nervousness, palpitations, diarrhea, excessive sweating, heat intolerance, chest pain, increased pulse rate, or any unusual physical change or event occurs.

6. **Answer: b**
   RATIONALE: The nurse should notify the primary health care provider if the patient develops chest pain so that the provider can reduce the dosage of the thyroid hormone. The nurse need not notify the primary health care provider to reduce the dosage of the thyroid hormone if high fever, sweating, or headache develops. High fever is a sign of thyroid storm, which occurs in patients whose hyperthyroidism is inadequately treated. Sweating is the adverse reaction to levothyroxine sodium (T_4), and headache is the adverse reaction to levothyroxine sodium (T_4) and methimazole.

7. **Answer: d**
   RATIONALE: The nurse should monitor the patient for altered mental status, high fever, and extreme tachycardia as signs of thyroid storm. The nurse need not monitor the patient for anxiety, increased pulse rate, or nervousness as signs of thyroid storm during the ongoing assessment. Anxiety and nervousness are signs of hyperthyroidism. Increased pulse rate is the sign of a therapeutic response.

8. **Answer: a**
   RATIONALE: When the patient has been prescribed an iodine procedure, it is essential that the nurse take a careful allergy history, particularly to iodine or seafood, before administering the procedure. The nurse need not monitor for signs of agranulocytosis, assess the patient for mouth infection, or monitor the patient's stool color.

9. **Answer: b**
   RATIONALE: Thyroid hormones are contraindicated in patients with known hypersensitivity to the drug, an uncorrected adrenal cortical insufficiency, or thyrotoxicosis. The drug is not contraindicated in patients with agranulocytosis, granulocytopenia, and hypoprothrombinemia. Agranulocytosis, granulocytopenia, and hypoprothrombinemia are some of the severe systemic reactions to antithyroid drugs.

10. **Answer: a, c, d**
    RATIONALE: The nurse should report signs of hyperthyroidism such as moist skin, moderate hypertension, and increased appetite to the primary healthcare provider before the next dose is due because it may be necessary to decrease the daily dosage. Easy bruising, sore throat, fatigue, fever, or bleeding are the signs and symptoms indicating an adverse reaction related to a decrease in blood cells.

CHAPTER 52

SECTION I: ASSESSING YOUR UNDERSTANDING

Activity A MATCHING

1. 1-C, 2-A, 3-E, 4-B, 5-D
2. 1-E, 2-C, 3-D, 4-A, 5-B

Activity B FILL IN THE BLANKS

1. Menarche
2. Endogenous
3. Catabolism
4. Prostate
5. Androgens

SECTION II: APPLYING YOUR KNOWLEDGE

Activity C SHORT ANSWERS

1. Treatment with androgens may lead to an increase in fluid volume. When a nurse is monitoring

patients on androgen therapy, the following assessments should be made:

- Edema: The nurse should observe the patient for any signs of edema as a result of sodium and water retention. He or she should also note any puffiness of the eyelids. If the patient is ambulatory, there may be dependent swelling of the hands or feet. If the patient is nonambulatory, the nurse may need to look for swelling of the sacral area.
- Weight of the patient: The weight should be noted prior to androgen therapy, and this should serve as a guide. As part of his or her ongoing assessment of the patient, the nurse needs to compare the patient's weight with the preadministration weight on a daily basis.
- Fluid intake and output: The nurse needs to monitor the patient's daily fluid intake and output to calculate the fluid balance. Older adults with heart and kidney diseases pose a greater risk as they are at an increased risk of developing sodium and water retention. The nurse should be alert when caring for such patients.

2. The nurse should include the following points in the teaching plan when educating a patient about oral contraceptives:

- Read the package insert carefully. In case of any questions, discuss them with the primary health care provider.
- Take the first dose as directed by the package insert or as directed by the primary health care provider.
- Take the drug at intervals not exceeding once every 24 hours. It is best taken with the evening meal or at bedtime. The dose schedule has to be followed for proper efficacy of the drug. Failure to comply may lead to pregnancy.
- Until the first week of the next cycle, use an additional method of birth control.
- If one day's dose is missed, take the missed dose as soon as remembered, or take two tablets the next day.
- If 2 days are missed, then take two tablets for the next 2 days and then continue the normal dosing schedule. Use another form of birth control until the cycle is completed and a new cycle has begun.
- If 3 consecutive days or more are missed, discontinue the drug. Use another form of birth control until a new cycle begins. Before restarting the regimen, confirm the absence of pregnancy as a result of the break in regimen.
- If unsure what to do about a missed dose, contact the primary health care provider.
- Avoid both active and passive smoking while taking oral contraceptives.
- Report any adverse reactions, such as fluid retention or edema in the extremities; weight gain; pain, swelling, or tenderness in the legs; blurred vision; chest pain; yellowed skin or eyes; dark urine; or abnormal vaginal bleeding.

- Schedule periodic examinations by the primary health care provider and related laboratory tests during the therapy.

Activity D DOSAGE CALCULATION

1. 4 tablets
2. 3 tablets
3. 2 tablets
4. 1.5 tablets
5. 2 capsules
6. 7.5 tablets in a day

SECTION III: PRACTICING FOR NCLEX

Activity E

1. **Answer: b**
   RATIONALE: The nurse should consider that the androgen therapy might have been prescribed for testosterone deficiency. The male hormone testosterone and its derivatives are collectively called "androgens." Thus, androgen therapy may be prescribed for testosterone deficiency. Adrenal cortical cancer is treated with adrenal steroid inhibitors, such as mitotane, and not by androgen therapy. Symptoms of benign prostatic hypertrophy are treated by androgen hormone inhibitors, not by androgen therapy. Male pattern baldness occurs because of androgens, and androgen hormone inhibitors are used for its prevention.

2. **Answer: d**
   RATIONALE: Anabolic steroids may be used to promote weight gain following profound weight loss caused by surgery, trauma, or infections. Anabolic steroids are not intended to increase muscle mass and strength in young, healthy individuals. Such abuse can cause serious adverse effects and is considered illegal. Androgens, progestins, and conjugated estrogens are not prescribed for promotion of weight gain following profound weight loss; although some of these drugs may cause some weight gain as a side effect.

3. **Answer: a**
   RATIONALE: Increased antidiuretic effects may be seen when androgens or androgen hormone inhibitors are used concomitantly in a patient on oral anticoagulant therapy. Decreased anticoagulant effects are seen when female hormones, and not male hormones, are used with oral anticoagulant therapy. Increased risk of hypoglycemia may be seen when male hormone therapy is used in patients taking sulfonylureas, and not oral anticoagulants. The risk of paranoia increases when imipramine, not oral anticoagulants, is given with male hormones or male-hormone inhibitors.

4. **Answer: b**
   RATIONALE: Gynecomastia, or enlargement of the breast, is a complication of androgen therapy seen among male patients. Testicular atrophy, not enlargement of testes, may be another side effect

of androgen therapy. Virilization is the appearance of male secondary sexual characteristics in females and is seen as a side effect of androgen therapy in females, and not males. Water retention, and not frequent urination, is seen in patients on androgen therapy.

5. Answer: c
RATIONALE: In menopausal women with an intact uterus, progestins are given along with estrogen to reduce the risk of an endometrial carcinoma. Gastrointestinal (GI) irritation may be caused by estrogen. However, taking the medication with food can reduce this. Progestins do not reduce GI irritation caused by estrogen. The associated atrophic vaginitis is treated with estrogen therapy, not progestin therapy. Risk of osteoporosis is also reduced by taking estrogens and not by taking progestins.

6. Answer: c
RATIONALE: Impaired vision may occur as an adverse effect of the herb black cohosh. It may also cause high, not low, blood pressure. It does not cause ringing in the ears, but rather, it is used to treat this symptom seen during menopause. The herb causes weight gain and not weight loss.

7. Answer: b
RATIONALE: The nurse should keep in mind that Depo-Provera is to be shaken vigorously before administration. This ensures a uniform suspension. The drug is not implanted in the subdermal tissue but is given as a deep intramuscular injection. The initial dosage is given within the first 5 days of menstruation or within 5 days postpartum. It is not given on the tenth day of the menstrual cycle. Depo-Provera is given intramuscularly every 3 months, and it does not provide contraceptive protection for as long as 5 years.

8. Answer: a, b, d
RATIONALE: The risk of iron deficiency anemia, ovarian cancer, and osteoporosis decreases with the use of oral contraceptives. The risks of cervical erosion and vaginal candidiasis increase, and not decrease, with the use of oral contraceptive drugs.

9. Answer: d
RATIONALE: If a woman has missed 1 day's dose of an oral contraceptive, she should be advised to take the missed dose as soon as remembered or to take two tablets the next day. When the patient has missed the dose for 3 consecutive days or more, she should discontinue the drug and use another form of birth control until her next cycle begins. Remembering to take one tablet the next day and forgetting about the missed dose does not help as it may reduce the contraceptive's effectiveness and lead to pregnancy.

10. Answer: d
RATIONALE: The nurse should explain that the female hormone estropipate is a synthetic estrogen. Estropipate is not produced endogenously and must be obtained from outside as a drug. Estradiol, estrone, and estriol are estrogens that are produced endogenously in the body. These are not synthetic hormones. Estradiol is available as a drug, but it is also produced endogenously and need not be obtained only as a drug.

CHAPTER 53

SECTION I: ASSESSING YOUR UNDERSTANDING

Activity A   MATCHING

1. 1-C, 2-B, 3-A, 4-E, 5-D
2. 1-B, 2-C, 3-A, 4-E, 5-D

Activity B   FILL IN THE BLANKS

1. Contractions
2. Posterior
3. Eclampsia
4. Ergotism
5. Antidiuretic

SECTION II: APPLYING YOUR KNOWLEDGE

Activity C   SHORT ANSWERS

1. The nurse should immediately discontinue the oxytocin infusion if any of these changes are noted:
   - A significant change in the fetal heart rate (FHR) or rhythm
   - A marked change in the frequency, rate, or rhythm of uterine contractions
   - A marked increase or decrease in the patient's blood pressure or pulse or any significant change in the patient's general condition

2. During the ongoing assessment of a patient receiving a tocolytic drug, the role of a nurse includes:
   - Recording blood pressure, pulse, and respiratory rate
   - Monitoring fetal heart rate (FHR)
   - Checking the intravenous (IV) infusion rate
   - Examining the area around the IV needle insertion site for signs of infiltration
   - Monitoring uterine contractions (frequency, intensity, length)
   - Measuring maternal intake and output

Activity D   DOSAGE CALCULATION

1. 4 ampoules
2. 4 mL
3. 2 tablets
4. 10 mL
5. 0.25 mL
6. 0.5 mL

SECTION III: PRACTICING FOR NCLEX

Activity E

1. **Answer: a**
   RATIONALE: When administering oxytocin intranasally to facilitate the letdown of milk, the nurse should place the patient in an upright position and, with the squeeze bottle held upright, should administer the prescribed number of sprays to one or both nostrils. The supine and lateral positions are not favorable for breastfeeding the infant or collecting milk. The standing position would be inconvenient to the patient and is not an appropriate position when administering oxytocin intranasally.

2. **Answer: a, d, e**
   RATIONALE: The patient receiving oxytocin to induce labor may be concerned about the use of the drug. To reduce the anxiety, the nurse should explain the purpose of the IV infusion and the expected results to the patient. Not explaining the expected results or outcome to the patient will increase her anxiety. The nurse should spend time with the patient and offer encouragement and reassurance. Without prior instructions from the primary health care provider, the nurse should not administer any drug as it might lead to drug interactions and complications.

3. **Answer: c**
   RATIONALE: In some patients who are calcium deficient, the uterus may not respond well to ergonovine. The nurse should immediately report a lack of response to ergonovine. Administering calcium by IV injection usually restores response to the drug. Magnesium sulfate is a tocolytic drug and cannot be used in this condition. Increasing the dosage of the drug might lead to complications such as ergotism. Terbutaline is a tocolytic used to prevent preterm labor and is not used in this situation.

4. **Answer: d**
   RATIONALE: Magnesium sulfate is contraindicated in a patient with eclampsia. Other contraindications include hypersensitivity to the drug, heart block, myocardial damage, and severe preeclampsia within 2 hours of delivery. Oxytocin is contraindicated in conditions such as cephalopelvic disproportion and total placenta previa. Ergonovine is contraindicated in patients with hypertension, not magnesium sulfate.

5. **Answer: c**
   RATIONALE: The nurse should place a cardiac monitor on the patient during administration of magnesium sulfate, as a dosage change might be required. The nurse should check the blood pressure and the pulse range to determine when the IV infusion has to be stopped. Urinary output should be monitored only if the patient develops vomiting. Vaginal bleeding is an adverse effect of indomethacin and not magnesium sulfate; hence, monitoring for vaginal bleeding is not required. Monitoring of urine output, pedal edema, and vaginal bleeding is not required during the administration of magnesium sulfate.

6. **Answer: d**
   RATIONALE: Ergonovine is contraindicated in patients with hypertension, before delivery of the placenta, and in patients with hypersensitivity to the drug. In patients with renal disease or heart disease or those who are lactating, the drug should be used cautiously and is not strictly contraindicated.

7. **Answer: a, c, d**
   RATIONALE: When administering methylergonovine for controlling postpartum bleeding, the nurse should monitor the vital signs every 4 hr and should note the character and amount of vaginal bleeding. The nurse should immediately notify the primary health care provider when abdominal cramping is moderate to severe. The primary health care provider—and not the nurse—decides when to terminate the drug, depending on the patient's condition. The nurse need not put the patient in the lateral position after administration of the drug.

8. **Answer: a**
   RATIONALE: When oxytocin is administered IV, there is a danger of excessive fluid volume (water intoxication) because oxytocin has an antidiuretic effect. Therefore, it is necessary for hourly measurements of fluid intake and output. Ergonovine, methylergonovine, and magnesium sulfate are not associated with water intoxication.

9. **Answer: a, c, e**
   RATIONALE: Symptoms of ergotism include coolness, numbness and tingling of extremities, dyspnea, nausea, confusion, tachycardia or bradycardia, chest pain, hallucinations, and convulsions. Water intoxication and diplopia are not the symptoms of ergotism. Water intoxication may be seen in patients receiving oxytocin, and diplopia is an adverse reaction associated with magnesium sulfate.

10. **Answer: a**
    RATIONALE: Magnesium sulfate is used to manage preterm labor in pregnancies of more than 27 weeks' gestation. It is a calcium antagonist and works to decrease the force of uterine contractions. Indomethacin is a nonsteroidal anti-inflammatory drug (NSAID) that blocks the production of prostaglandins, which contribute to uterine contractions. Magnesium sulfate does not block the production of prostaglandins. Magnesium sulfate, not being an oxytocic drug, does not stimulate the uterus. Oxytocin, and not magnesium sulfate, has an antidiuretic action.

CHAPTER 54

SECTION I: ASSESSING YOUR UNDERSTANDING

Activity A MATCHING

1. 1-C, 2-A, 3-D, 4-B, 5-E
2. 1-E, 2-A, 3-D, 4-B, 5-C

Activity B FILL IN THE BLANKS

1. Reye's
2. Artificially
3. Booster
4. Immunity
5. Cell

SECTION II: APPLYING YOUR KNOWLEDGE

Activity C SHORT ANSWERS

1. The nurse should document the following information in the patient's chart or form provided by the institution:
   - Date of vaccination
   - Route and site of vaccine administration, type, and manufacturer
   - Vaccine expiration date and drug lot number
   - Name, address, and title of individual administering the vaccine
2. When educating the parents of a child receiving a vaccination, the nurse should include the following information:
   - The risks of contracting vaccine-preventable diseases and the benefits of immunization
   - The importance of bringing immunization records during all visits
   - The date for the next vaccination
   - The common adverse reactions (e.g., fever or soreness at the injection site) and methods to combat these reactions (e.g., acetaminophen, warm compresses)
   - Reporting of any adverse reactions after administration of a vaccine

Activity D DOSAGE CALCULATION

1. 7.5 mL
2. 6 patients
3. 3 mL
4. 0.35 mL
5. 8 patients
6. 0.5 mL

SECTION III: PRACTICING FOR NCLEX

Activity E

1. **Answer: a, b, c**
   RATIONALE: The benefits of lentinan, a derivative of the shiitake mushroom, include boosting the body's immune system, lowering blood cholesterol levels, and prolonging the survival time of patients with cancer by increasing immunity. The benefit of this herb in lowering cholesterol levels is achieved by increasing the rate at which cholesterol is excreted from the body. Mild side effects such as skin rashes and gastrointestinal upset have been reported. Lentinan does not help in lowering blood pressure or reducing the risks of heart diseases.

2. **Answer: a**
   RATIONALE: The recommended dosage of shiitake mushrooms is 1–5 capsules per day. This dose is used to maintain general health and also to lower cholesterol levels. The other recommended dosages include 3–4 fresh shiitake mushrooms and 1 dropper two to three times a day. An increase in dosage such as 10 mushrooms and 1 dropper 8 times daily might lead to severe adverse effects, such as skin rashes and gastrointestinal upset. Twelve cups of shiitake juice are not recommended.

3. **Answer: c**
   RATIONALE: Lymphocytes play a major role in providing cellular and humoral immunity. Immunity refers to the ability of the body to identify and resist microorganisms that are potentially harmful. This ability enables the body to inhibit tissue and organ damage. T lymphocytes play a major role in maintaining cellular immunity, as B lymphocytes do in maintaining humoral immunity. Neutrophils, basophils, and eosinophils do not play a major role in humoral immunity.

4. **Answer: a, b, d**
   RATIONALE: Uses of vaccines and toxoids include routine immunization of infants and children and immunization of adults against tetanus. Vaccines and toxoids can also benefit adults at high risk for contracting certain diseases (e.g., pneumococcal and influenza vaccines) and children or adults at risk for exposure to a particular disease (e.g., hepatitis A for those going to endemic areas). The rubella vaccine is never given in pregnant women as it might lead to infection. It is given for immunization of nonpregnant women of childbearing age. Vaccines and toxoids are contraindicated in leukemia.

5. **Answer: d**
   RATIONALE: Antivenins should be administered within 4 hours of exposure to yield the most effective response. Antivenins are used for passive, transient protection from the toxic effects of bites by spiders (black widows and similar spiders) and snakes (rattlesnakes, copperheads, cottonmouths, and corals). The nurse should know that the most effective response is obtained when the drug is administered within 4 hours after exposure. If the drug is administered after 4 hours, it might lessen the therapeutic value and its action against the venom.

6. **Answer: c**
   RATIONALE: The nurse should alert the patient about herpes zoster, which is a complication of

chickenpox. Chickenpox can cause herpes zoster (shingles), which is a painful condition, later in life. When salicylates are administered to patients with chickenpox, they may develop Reye's syndrome. Hepatitis, Reye's syndrome, and acute renal failure are not late complications of chickenpox.

7. **Answer: a, b, d**

   RATIONALE: Diseases that can be prevented by vaccination before traveling to endemic areas include cholera, diphtheria, typhoid, and yellow fever. Other diseases that can be prevented by vaccination before traveling to endemic areas include Japanese encephalitis, Lyme disease, and smallpox. Tetanus and rubella vaccines are not required prior to traveling to endemic areas.

8. **Answer: a, d**

   RATIONALE: To reduce the pain, general interventions such as increasing the fluid intake, allowing for adequate rest, and keeping the atmosphere quiet and unstimulating may be beneficial. The primary health care provider may prescribe acetaminophen every 4 hours to relieve the pain. Local irritation at the injection site may be treated with warm or cool compresses, but they do not help in relieving pain at the injection site. Decreasing fluids in the diet and massaging the injected site also do not help in relieving the pain at the injection site.

9. **Answer: a**

   RATIONALE: With patients who are lactating, vaccines must be used with caution. Other patient conditions that require caution include minor illnesses, allergies, and pregnancy. Contraindications for the use of vaccines include acute febrile illnesses, leukemia, lymphoma, immunosuppressive illness, drug therapy, and nonlocalized cancer.

10. **Answer: a, b, c**

    RATIONALE: After receiving an immunologic agent, patients are usually advised to stay in the clinic for observation for about 30 minutes to assess for signs of hypersensitivity, if any. Signs of hypersensitivity that a nurse should assess for include pruritus, dyspnea, and laryngeal edema. Other signs of hypersensitivity include angioneurotic edema, hives, and severe dyspnea. Renal failure and convulsions are not signs associated with hypersensitivity.

CHAPTER 55

SECTION I: ASSESSING YOUR UNDERSTANDING

Activity A MATCHING

1. 1-B, 2-E, 3-A, 4-C, 5-D
2. 1-C, 2-A, 3-E, 4-B, 5-D

Activity B FILL IN THE BLANKS

1. Malignant
2. Myelosuppression
3. Neutropenia
4. Erythemia
5. Chemotherapy

SECTION II: APPLYING YOUR KNOWLEDGE

Activity C SHORT ANSWERS

1. Nursing care for a patient receiving antineoplastic drugs depends on:
   - Drug or combination of drugs given
   - Dosage of drugs
   - Route of administration
   - Patient's physical response to therapy
   - Response of tumor to chemotherapy
   - Type and severity of adverse reactions
2. The nurse should observe the following guidelines when caring for patients receiving chemotherapeutic drugs:
   - Follow policies established by the health care provider.
   - Increase frequency of assessments if the patient's condition changes.
   - Incorporate health care setting guidelines into the individualized nursing care plan.
   - Review the drugs being given before their administration.
   - Ensure the drugs are prescribed by a provider trained specifically in the care of oncology patients.
   - Consult appropriate references to obtain information on the drug—preparation, administration, average dose ranges, and adverse reactions.

Activity D DOSAGE CALCULATION

1. 2 vials
2. 5 vials
3. 3 vials
4. 2 capsules
5. 2 vials
6. 4 tablets

SECTION III: PRACTICING FOR NCLEX

Activity E

1. **Answer: a, d, e**

   RATIONALE: Chemotherapy is administered in a series of cycles to allow for the recovery of the normal cells, to destroy more of the malignant cells, and to affect cells that rapidly divide and reproduce. Chemotherapy is administered at the time the cell population is dividing as part of a strategy to optimize cell death. Green tea releases antioxidants, polyphenols, and flavonoids into the system.

2. Answer: a, b, d
RATIONALE: The nurse informs the patient with hypertension to drink green tea with caution as it causes nervousness, insomnia, and gastrointestinal (GI) upset. Green tea does not cause mouth ulcers or stomatitis, which may be caused by injury, deficiency in vitamin B_{12}, folic acid or iron, or viral infections.

3. Answer: d
RATIONALE: The nurse should explain that a cell–cycle-specific drug targets the cells in one of the phases of cell division. Cell–cycle-nonspecific drugs target the cells at any phase of the cycle or cells in various stages of cell division. Cell–cycle-specific drugs do not affect only malignant cells; they affect all cells that rapidly divide and reproduce, and in the process, normal cells that line the oral cavity and GI tract and cells of the gonads, bone marrow, hair follicles, and lymph tissue are also affected.

4. Answer: b
RATIONALE: The nurse should explain that an antimetabolite incorporates itself into the cellular components during the S phase of cell division, thus interfering with the synthesis of RNA and DNA. Alkylating agents change the cell to a more alkaline environment, which in turn damages the cell. Plant alkaloids interfere with amino acid production in the S phase and formation of the microtubules in the M phase of cell division.

5. Answer: a, c, d
RATIONALE: When preparing a nursing care plan for ongoing assessment of the patient, the nurse should consider the guidelines established by the health care facility, the patient's general condition, and the patient's individual response to the drug. The patient's appetite is of concern to the nurse after administration of the drug because a decreased appetite could result in imbalanced nutrition. Adequacy of health insurance coverage is of importance to the nurse as part of the preadministration assessment procedure for the patient.

6. Answer: a
RATIONALE: When administering a subcutaneous injection, the nurse should use no more than 1 mL of the drug. An Angiocath is used for intravenous administration. The z-track method of administration is recommended for all intramuscular (IM) injections. The injection for subcutaneous administration should contain no more than 1 mL of the drug; 3 mL is the maximum to administer for IM injections.

7. Answer: c
RATIONALE: The nurse should provide the patient with frequent, small meals, which are better tolerated than three large meals. The nurse should not provide the patient with fatty or greasy foods, which may not be tolerated. The nurse should not provide the patient food without salt; instead these patients tolerate cold, dry, and salty foods better.

8. Answer: b
RATIONALE: The nurse must apply pressure to the injection site for at least 3 to 5 minutes to avoid the formation of a hematoma. The nurse must not use the same site for withdrawals and injections and instead should rotate the site of injections. The nurse must suggest that the patient avoid the use of electric razors and nail trimmers to prevent the occurrence of any injury leading to bleeding.

9. Answer: d
RATIONALE: The nurse should offer consistent and empathetic care to the patient and his or her family; the treatment is spread over time and provides the nurse with several opportunities to help the anxious patient. The health care team, not the nurse alone, assists in making critical decisions regarding treatment, emphasizes safety requirements for chemotherapy, and plans and institutes therapy to control the disease.

10. Answer: b
RATIONALE: The nurse should inform the patient to take the drug as directed on the prescription container. The nurse should instruct the patient to take the exact amount of the drug at the same time every day and to inform the dentist or any other physician of the antineoplastic drug therapy that is being followed. In addition, the nurse should instruct the patient not to decrease the dose as symptoms of the illness decrease and, instead, continue the dose as prescribed by the physician.

CHAPTER 56

SECTION I: ASSESSING YOUR UNDERSTANDING

Activity A MATCHING

1. 1-B, 2-D, 3-A, 4-C
2. 1-D, 2-A, 3-B, 4-C

Activity B FILL IN THE BLANKS

1. Superinfection
2. Immunocompromised
3. Hypersensitivity
4. Antiseptic
5. Germicide
6. Antipsoriatics

SECTION II: APPLYING YOUR KNOWLEDGE

Activity C SHORT ANSWERS

1. The preadministration assessment involves a visual inspection and palpation of the involved area(s). The nurse should carefully record the areas of involvement, including the size, color, and appearance. A specific description is important so that changes can be readily identified, indicating worsening or improvement of the lesions. The nurse should note the presence of scales, crusting, drainage, or any complaint of itching. Some agencies may provide a figure on which the lesions can be drawn, indicating the shape and distribution of the involved areas.

2. At the time of each topical drug application, the nurse inspects the affected area for changes (e.g., signs of improvement or worsening of the infection) and for adverse reactions such as redness or rash. The nurse contacts the primary health care provider and does not apply the drug if these or other changes are noted or if the patient reports new problems such as itching, pain, or soreness at the site.

Activity D **DOSAGE CALCULATION**

1. 56
2. 42

SECTION III: PRACTICING FOR NCLEX

Activity E

1. **Answer: a**
   RATIONALE: Masoprocol is a keratolytic, which are contraindicated in patients with known hypersensitivity to the drugs and for use on moles, birthmarks, or warts with hair growing from them; genital or facial warts; warts on mucous membranes, or infected skin. Masoprocol is not contraindicated as monotherapy for bacterial skin infections; for use on the face, groin, or axilla; or as sole therapy in plaque psoriasis. The topical corticosteroids are contraindicated in patients with known hypersensitivity to the drug or any component of the drug; as monotherapy for bacterial skin infections; for use on the face, groin, or axilla (only the high-potency corticosteroids); and as sole therapy in plaque psoriasis and ophthalmic use.

2. **Answer: b**
   RATIONALE: Alclometasone dipropionate is a topical corticosteroid, which is contraindicated in patients with known hypersensitivity to the drug or any component of the drug; as sole therapy in plaque psoriasis; as monotherapy for bacterial skin infections; for use on the face, groin, or axilla (only the high-potency corticosteroids); and ophthalmic use. Alclometasone dipropionate is not contraindicated for use on moles, birthmarks, or warts with hair growing from them; genital or facial warts; warts on mucous membranes; or on infected skin. However, keratolytics are contraindicated in patients with known hypersensitivity to the drugs and for use on moles, birthmarks, or warts with hair growing from them; genital or facial warts; on warts on mucous membranes; or on infected skin.

3. **Answer: c**
   RATIONALE: Benzocaine is a topical anesthetic, and topical anesthetics are used cautiously in patients receiving Class I antiarrhythmic drugs such as tocainide and mexiletine because the toxic effects are additive and potentially synergistic. Benzocaine need not be used cautiously during pregnancy and lactation. The drug is not associated with immunocompromised patients who have herpes simplex virus infections, cutaneous candidiasis, or tinea pedis. Topical antibiotics are pregnancy category C drugs and are used cautiously during pregnancy and lactation. Immunocompromised patients with herpes simplex virus infections are treated with antiviral drugs. Patients having cutaneous candidiasis or tinea pedis are treated with antifungal drugs.

4. **Answer: d**
   RATIONALE: Anthralin may cause skin irritation, as well as temporary discoloration of the hair and fingernails. Hypothalamic-pituitary-adrenal axis suppression, Cushing's syndrome, hyperglycemia, and glycosuria are not adverse reactions associated with anthralin; these are the systemic adverse reactions to topical corticosteroids.

5. **Answer: a**
   RATIONALE: Alclometasone dipropionate is a topical corticosteroid, and in the use of topical corticosteroids, systemic reactions may occur with hypothalamic-pituitary-adrenal axis suppression, Cushing's syndrome, hyperglycemia, and glycosuria. Numbness and dermatitis, mild and transient pains, and flu-like syndrome are not the adverse reactions associated with alclometasone dipropionate. Numbness, dermatitis, and mild and transient pains are adverse reactions to the application of collagenase. Flu-like syndrome is an adverse reaction to keratolytic drugs.

6. **Answer: b**
   RATIONALE: Numbness, dermatitis, and mild and transient pains are adverse reactions to the application of collagenase. Flu-like syndrome, Cushing's syndrome, hyperglycemia, and glycosuria are not adverse reactions to the application of collagenase. Flu-like syndrome is an adverse reaction to keratolytic drugs. Cushing's syndrome, hyperglycemia, and glycosuria are the systemic adverse reactions to topical corticosteroids.

7. **Answer: c**
   RATIONALE: Salicylic acid is a keratolytic, and flu-like syndrome is an adverse reaction to keratolytic drugs. Numbness and dermatitis, mild and transient pains, temporary discoloration of the hair, hyperglycemia, and glycosuria are not adverse reactions to salicylic acid. Numbness and dermatitis and mild and transient pains are adverse reactions to the application of collagenase. Anthralin may cause skin irritation, as well as temporary discoloration of the hair and fingernails. Hyperglycemia and glycosuria, hypothalamic-pituitary-adrenal axis suppression, and Cushing's syndrome are the systemic adverse reactions to topical corticosteroids.

8. Answer: d

RATIONALE: Accuzyme is a topical enzyme that is used to help remove necrotic tissue from chronic dermal ulcers. Accuzyme is not used for the treatment of psoriasis, eczema, or insect bites. Psoriasis, eczema, or insect bites are treated with topical corticosteroids.

9. Answer: a

RATIONALE: Topical corticosteroids exert localized anti-inflammatory activity. When applied to inflamed skin, they reduce itching, redness, and swelling. Topical corticosteroids do not act to reduce the number of bacteria on the skin surface, to prevent infection in cuts and wounds, or to cleanse the skin thoroughly. Topical antibiotics and germicides are used to reduce the number of bacteria on the skin surface, to prevent infection in cuts and wounds, and to cleanse the skin thoroughly.

10. Answer: b

RATIONALE: Topical antiseptics and germicides are used for washing the hands before and after caring for patients, as a surgical scrub, and as a preoperative skin cleanser. Topical antipsoriatics, topical enzymes and topical antifungals are not used for washing the hands before and after caring for patients. Topical antipsoriatics are drugs used to treat psoriasis. A topical enzyme is used to help remove necrotic tissue from chronic dermal ulcers and severely burned areas. Topical antifungals are used to inhibit the growth of fungi.

CHAPTER 57

SECTION I: ASSESSING YOUR UNDERSTANDING

Activity A MATCHING

1. 1-B, 2-D, 3-A, 4-C
2. 1-C, 2-A, 3-B

Activity B FILL IN THE BLANKS

1. Superinfection
2. Glaucoma
3. Miosis
4. Antibacterial
5. Natamycin
6. Cycloplegia

SECTION II: APPLYING YOUR KNOWLEDGE

Activity C SHORT ANSWERS

1. The nurse may be responsible for examining the outer structures of the ear, namely the earlobe and the skin around the ear. The nurse should document a description of any drainage or impacted cerumen and check with the primary health care provider before administering an otic preparation to a patient with a perforated eardrum.

2. The nurse assesses the patient's response to therapy by confirming whether pain or inflammation has decreased. The nurse should examine the outer ear and ear canal for any local redness or irritation that may indicate sensitivity to the drug.

Activity D DOSAGE CALCULATION

1. 16 drops
2. 24 drops

SECTION III: PRACTICING FOR NCLEX

Activity E

1. Answer: a

RATIONALE: Prolonged use of otic preparations containing an antibiotic such as ofloxacin may result in a superinfection caused by an overgrowth of bacterial or fungal microorganisms not affected by the antibiotic being administered. Systemic effects of cholinesterase inhibitors, exacerbation of existing hypertension, and additive central nervous system (CNS) depressant effects are not related to the use of otic antibiotics. Individuals working with organophosphate insecticides or pesticides are at risk for systemic effects of the cholinesterase inhibitors from absorption through the respiratory tract or the skin. Older adults are at risk for exacerbation of existing disorders such as hypertension if systemic absorption of sympathomimetic ophthalmic drugs occurs. When brimonidine is used with CNS depressants such as alcohol, barbiturates, opiates, sedatives, or anesthetics, there is a risk for an additive CNS depressant effect.

2. Answer: b

RATIONALE: Ofloxacin is a pregnancy category C drug and should be administered in pregnancy only if the potential benefit justifies the risk to the fetus. Brimonidine tartrate, being an alpha 2-adrenergic blocker, is contraindicated in patients taking monoamine oxidase inhibitors. Brimonidine may cause fatigue or drowsiness and therefore must be used cautiously for patients who perform activities requiring mental alertness. Dapiprazole may cause difficulty in dark adaptation and may reduce field of vision; therefore, it must be used cautiously when driving at night or performing activities in dimly lit areas.

3. Answer: c

RATIONALE: Before instilling floxacin otic, the nurse informs the patient that while the solution remains in the ear canal, a feeling of fullness may be felt in the ear and that hearing in the treated ear may be temporarily impaired. Fatigue and drowsiness and local effects, such as headache and visual blurring, may be experienced as systemic effects during treatment with brimonidine tartrate.

4. Answer: d

RATIONALE: The nurse should hold the container in the hand for a few minutes to warm it to body temperature. Cold and warm (above body temperature) preparations may cause dizziness or other sensations after being instilled in the ear. The number of drops needs to be confirmed as per the prescription when being instilled and while the applicator is inside the bottle. The nurse need not hold the container in the hand for a few minutes to confirm if it has been refrigerated. If the drops are in a suspension form, the nurse should shake the container well for 10 seconds before using.

5. **Answer: a**
   RATIONALE: When instilling eardrops, the nurse has the patient lie on his or her side with the ear toward the ceiling. If the patient wishes to remain in an upright position, the head should be tilted toward the untreated side with the ear toward the ceiling. To straighten the ear canal in adults and children ages 3 and older, the nurse should gently pull the cartilaginous portion of the outer ear up and back. The dropper or applicator tip should never be inserted into the ear canal.

6. **Answer: c**
   RATIONALE: The nurse should stop using Cerumenex if ear drainage, discharge, pain, or irritation occurs. Also Cerumenex should not be used for more than 4 days. If excessive cerumen remains, the primary health care provider should be consulted. Cold and warm (above body temperature) preparations may cause dizziness or other sensations after being instilled into the ear; this can be avoided by the nurse holding the container in his or her hand for a few minutes to warm it to body temperature.

7. **Answer: b**
   RATIONALE: Being a sympathomimetic drug, dipivefrin hydrochloride may cause transient local reactions such as brow ache, headache, burning and stinging, eye pain, allergic lip reactions, and ocular irritation. Deposits may occur in the conjunctiva and cornea with prolonged use of adrenochrome (a red pigment contained in epinephrine). Ocular allergic reactions and foreign body sensation are the local effects of the administration of brimonidine tartrate.

8. **Answer: d**
   RATIONALE: Dapiprazole hydrochloride, being an alpha-adrenergic blocker, may cause local effects such as ptosis (drooping of the upper eyelid), burning in the eye, eyelid edema, itching, corneal edema, brow ache, dryness of the eye, tearing, and blurred vision. Abnormal corneal staining and decreased night vision are the local adverse reactions associated with beta-adrenergic blocking drugs. Frequent urge to urinate is a systemic adverse reaction to direct-acting miotic drugs.

9. **Answer: a**
   RATIONALE: Echothiophate iodide is a cholinesterase inhibitor ophthalmic preparation, and therefore, the ophthalmic adverse reactions could include eyelid muscle twitching, iris cysts, burning, lacrimation, conjunctivitis, ciliary redness, brow ache, and headache. Abdominal cramps, cardiac irregularities, and urinary incontinence are systemic adverse reactions to cholinesterase inhibitors.

10. **Answer: b**
    RATIONALE: Travoprost, being a prostaglandin agonist, is likely to cause local adverse reactions that include eyelid discomfort, blurred vision, burning and stinging, foreign body sensation, itching, increased pigmentation of the iris, dry eye, and excessive tearing. Unpleasant taste, asthma, and cold or flu symptoms are the systemic adverse reactions associated with mast cell inhibitors.

CHAPTER 58

SECTION I: ASSESSING YOUR UNDERSTANDING

Activity A MATCHING

1. 1-C, 2-A, 3-D, 4-B

Activity B FILL IN THE BLANKS

1. Electrolyte
2. Alkaline
3. Overload
4. Hyponatremia
5. Substrates

SECTION II: APPLYING YOUR KNOWLEDGE

Activity C SHORT ANSWERS

1. The nurse should consider the following factors when evaluating the intravenous (IV) replacement solution therapy to determine its effectiveness:
   - The therapeutic effect of the drug is achieved.
   - The fluid volume deficit is corrected.
   - The nutrition deficit is corrected.
   - The patient and family demonstrate an understanding of the procedure.
2. The nurse should include the following points in a patient teaching plan for the intake of potassium:
   - Take the drug exactly as directed on the prescription container. Do not increase, decrease, or omit doses of the drug unless advised to do so by the primary health care provider.
   - Take the drug immediately after meals or with food and a full glass of water.
   - Avoid the use of nonprescription drugs and salt substitutes (many contain potassium) unless the primary health care provider has approved use of a specific drug or product.
   - Contact the primary health care provider if tingling of the hands or feet, a feeling of heaviness in the legs, vomiting, nausea, abdominal pain, or black stools should occur.

- If the tablet has a coating (enteric-coated tablets), swallow it whole. Do not chew or crush the tablet.
- If effervescent tablets are prescribed, place the tablet in 4 to 8 oz of cold water or juice. Wait until the fizzing stops before drinking. Sip the liquid during a period of 5 to 10 minutes.
- If an oral liquid or a powder is prescribed, add the dose to 4 to 8 oz of cold water or juice and sip slowly during a period of 5 to 10 minutes. Measure the dose accurately.

Activity D DOSAGE CALCULATION

1. 4 tablets in a day
2. 160 mL
3. 2 tablets
4. 4.8 mL

SECTION III: PRACTICING FOR NCLEX

Activity E

1. **Answer: b**
   RATIONALE: When caring for a patient who needs to receive magnesium, the nurse should confirm that the patient does not have heart block or myocardial damage because presence of these conditions contraindicates the use of magnesium. Potassium is contraindicated in patients who have untreated Addison's disease. Sodium is contraindicated in patients who experience fluid retention. Calcium is contraindicated in patients taking digitalis because risk of digitalis toxicity increases when digitalis preparations are administered with calcium.

2. **Answer: a, b, d**
   RATIONALE: When caring for a patient who is receiving electrolytes and experiencing gastrointestinal (GI) disturbances, the nurse should ensure that the patient takes the drugs with meals to reduce nausea. The meals should be served in smaller quantities more frequently. The nurse should also continue to monitor the patient for signs and symptoms of nausea. The nurse should not administer antacids to the patient. The nurse also need not encourage an increase in the patient's intake of fruit juices because it will not help reduce nausea, nor will it reduce the symptoms and other discomforts associated with GI disturbances.

3. **Answer: c**
   RATIONALE: The nurse should know that if a patient's intake of protein nutrients is significantly less than the amount required by the body to meet energy expenditures, a state of negative nitrogen balance occurs. The body begins to convert protein from muscle into carbohydrate for energy to be used by the body. This results in weight loss and muscle wasting. Metabolic acidosis is an adverse reaction to ammonium chloride and protein substrates. GI disturbances are likely

to occur with administration of electrolytes. Hypotensive episodes occur as adverse reactions to plasma protein fractions.

4. **Answer: c**
   RATIONALE: When caring for a patient who is being administered fat emulsions, the nurse should monitor the patient's ability to eliminate the infused fat from the circulation because the lipidemia must clear between daily infusions. The nurse should not administer an IV solution, which is a little colder than room temperature. The IV solution should be administered at room temperature. Diarrhea is not known to occur with the use of fat emulsions; however, the nurse must monitor the patient for difficulty in breathing, headache, flushing, nausea, vomiting, or signs of a hypersensitivity reaction. The nurse should monitor the patient for signs of hypernatremia if the patient is administered NaCl solution through the IV route. However, hypernatremia is not known to occur with administration of fat emulsions.

5. **Answers: a**
   RATIONALE: When caring for a patient who is being administered plasma proteins, the nurse should monitor for adverse reactions such as urticaria, nausea, chills, fever, and hypotensive episodes. Flushing of skin is an adverse reaction to protein substrates and not plasma protein fractions. Dyspnea and wheezing are the adverse reactions to energy substrates.

6. **Answer: b, c, e**
   RATIONALE: When caring for a patient on sodium electrolyte infusion therapy, the nurse should observe the rate of IV infusion, as ordered by the primary health care provider, every 15 to 30 minutes. The nurse should also observe the patient's condition for signs of pulmonary edema, especially if sodium is given via IV. Patients receiving NaCl by the IV route have their intake and output measured every 8 hours. The nurse should inform the primary health care provider if the patient voids less than 100 mL of urine every 4 hours when caring for a patient who is receiving magnesium. The kidneys eliminate magnesium, so it is used with caution in patients with renal impairment. A microscopic filter is attached to the IV line when amino acid solutions are administered. The filter prevents microscopic aggregates from entering the bloodstream where they could cause massive emboli.

7. **Answer: b**
   RATIONALE: The nurse should know if the patient has congestive heart failure (CHF) before administering bicarbonate. Bicarbonate is used cautiously in patients with CHF, renal impairment, and with glucocorticoid therapy. Bicarbonate is also a pregnancy category C drug and is used cautiously during pregnancy. It is contraindicated in patients with metabolic or respiratory alkalosis,

hypocalcemia, renal failure, or severe abdominal pain of unknown cause, as well as patients on sodium-restricted diets.

8. **Answer: a**

RATIONALE: The nurse should check the patient's pulse rate at regular intervals, usually every 4 hours or more often if an irregularity in the heart rate is observed. Depending on the patient's condition, cardiac monitoring may be indicated so that it can continuously monitor the heart rate and rhythm during therapy. The nurse should discontinue the IV infusion immediately and contact the primary health care provider in case an extravasation occurs during administration. Potassium is irritating to the tissues and may also cause tissue necrosis. The nurse need not monitor the patient for nausea and vomiting, considering they do not occur with a decreased or increased cardiac output. The nurse should not plan to administer a direct IV injection of potassium as it can result in sudden death. Concentrated potassium solutions are for IV mixtures only and should never be used undiluted.

9. **Answer: a**

RATIONALE: When caring for an elderly patient who is being administered fluids, the nurse should carefully monitor the patient for signs and symptoms of fluid overload. The elderly are at an increased risk for fluid overload because the incidence of cardiac disease and decreased renal function may increase with age. The nurse observes the patient for difficulty in breathing, headache, flushing, nausea, vomiting, or signs of a hypersensitivity reaction when the patient is being administered lipid solutions. The nurse should monitor for signs of hypercalcemic syndrome and report the same to the primary health care provider when the patient is administered calcium. The nurse should test the patient's knee reflex before each dose of magnesium.

10. **Answer: d**

RATIONALE: The nurse should monitor the patient for systemic acidosis, which occurs because of the interaction of ammonium chloride and spironolactone. The interaction of ammonium chloride and spironolactone are not known to cause respiratory depression, heart block, and systemic alkalosis. Prolonged respiratory depression and apnea occur when magnesium is administered with the neuromuscular blocking agents. When magnesium is used with digoxin, heart block may occur. Prolonged use of oral sodium bicarbonate or excessive doses of IV sodium bicarbonate may result in systemic alkalosis.